Atlas of Critical Care Echocardiography

Alexis Salerno • Daniel J. Haase
Sarah B. Murthi
Editors

Atlas of Critical Care Echocardiography

Springer

Editors
Alexis Salerno
Department of Emergency Medicine
University of Maryland School of Medicine
Baltimore, MD
USA

Sarah B. Murthi
Department of Surgery, Program in Trauma
and Critical Care
R Adams Cowley Shock Trauma Center
Baltimore, MD
USA

Daniel J. Haase
Department of Surgery, Program in Trauma
and Critical Care
University of Maryland School of Medicine
Baltimore, MD
USA

ISBN 978-3-030-74685-8 ISBN 978-3-030-74687-2 (eBook)
https://doi.org/10.1007/978-3-030-74687-2

This Springer imprint is published by the registered company Springer Nature Switzerland AG
The registered company address is: Gewerbestrasse 11, 6330 Cham, Switzerland

I'd like to dedicate this book to a special mentor (who also happens to be creator of this book), Sarah B. Murthi. Your mentorship, friendship, and support have meant more than you could understand. Thank you for pushing me further than I could have anticipated.

This book is also dedicated to the fellows, faculty, and staff at the R Adams Cowley Shock Trauma Center, especially Dr. Thomas Scalea. Your excellence and dedication to the care of the critically ill and injured have motivated this book and so many other achievements. Thank you for supporting our vision of ultrasound and echocardiography.

Lastly, this book is dedicated to a close friend who has encouraged me, but also kept me grounded throughout everything – Ashley Aitken. You have supported me throughout my many personal and professional challenges. Thank you for telling me the perspective I always need to hear.

Daniel J. Haase

This book is dedicated to the residents and medical students who I have worked with over the last few years. The excitement of ultrasound learners when they see incredible pathology or learn new techniques keeps me energized in a field many describe as exhausting. This book is also dedicated to the University of Maryland Department of Emergency Medicine; our department chair Dr. Brian Browne, who has always supported ultrasound education; and our department ultrasound director Dr. Brian Euerle, who has mentored me since medical school.

I would also like to thank Dr. Sarah B. Murthi for the opportunity to collaborate with her on this project and for the wealth of knowledge I have learned from her through our numerous "nerdy talks" over the last 2 years.

Lastly, I would like to dedicate this book to my wonderful husband who helps me edit and even serves as an ultrasound model at times. And of course, our German Shephard puppy Kaiser!

Alexis Salerno

This book is dedicated to the Critical Care Fellows who I have worked with and learned from over the last 15 years. It is ultimately a collaboration between all of us. It came from years of picking through echocardiography and ultrasound to extract and develop new tools for taking care of critically ill patients. Two of them are my co-editors without whom this NEVER would have happened. The collaboration has been a true pleasure.

The book is also dedicated to The R Adams Cowley Shock Trauma Center and more specifically Thomas M. Scalea. He encourages all of us to blaze a trail while leaving a path to help others who have taken on the difficult task of acute care medicine.

Finally, the book is dedicated to my family: my husband Anand, our children Valon and Nina, and our two dogs Griffin and Ollie, whose warmth and support kept me sane. The dogs and I spent hours tucked in my office early in the morning and late at night bringing this project to completion.

Sarah B. Murthi

Preface

Point-of-care ultrasound is a growing discipline in acute care. As we were writing this book, the relevant metrics grew and grew, expanding outside of traditional echocardiography into vascular and body imaging. This new tool of hemodynamic ultrasound has the potential to improve how we manage shock and resuscitation along the continuum of care from pre-hospital management through recovery and on to hospital discharge. Also, the images you will obtain are beautiful and learning it will fundamentally change your understanding of the cardiovascular system. There is a steep learning curve, but we swear climbing it is rewarding – and it will make you a better doctor.

The book is designed to learn hemodynamic ultrasound and to refresh as needed. The first part describes how to obtain the windows and images. The second part outlines how to do measurements and analyze images. The final two parts are protocols which incorporate echocardiography into acute care medicine. The format is modular, and the parts are short, so you can tailor your experience to needs.

Enjoy! We loved writing it.

Baltimore, MD, USA — Alexis Salerno
Baltimore, MD, USA — Daniel J. Haase
Baltimore, MD, USA — Sarah B. Murthi

Acknowledgments

This is a collaboration between artists and physicians. Most of the illustrations were created by Vondel Mahon, Medical Illustrator. Misty Paccao also contributed figures and diagrams. Gary Wind, MD, FACS was deeply involved in the original conception of the project and created some of the images used.

The Department of Emergency Medicine granted us use of several images as did the Program in Trauma in the Department of Surgery at the University of Maryland.

Also, we would like to acknowledge the hard work and expertise of Syeda (Hina) Fatima, the cardiac sonographer who advised us throughout all aspects of manuscript conception and production.

Contents

Contributors

Ahmed Al Hazmi, MD, MBBS Jeddah, Saudi Arabia

Brooke Anderson, CRNP R. Adams Cowley Shock Trauma Center, University of Maryland, Baltimore, MD, USA

Sagar B. Dave, DO R. Adams Cowley Shock Trauma Center, University of Maryland, Baltimore, MD, USA

Michelle F. Dawson, CRNP University of Virginal Medical Center, Charlottesville, VA, USA

Syeda Fatima, RCS R. Adams Cowley Shock Trauma Center, University of Maryland, Baltimore, MD, USA

Kevin Flanagan, DO Department of Emergency Medicine, University of Maryland School of Medicine, Baltimore, MD, USA

Shannon Gaasch, CRNP R. Adams Cowley Shock Trauma Center, University of Maryland, Baltimore, MD, USA

David Gordon, MD Department of Medicine, University of Maryland School of Medicine, University of Maryland Medical Center, Baltimore, MD, USA

Daniel J. Haase, MD, RDMS, RCDS Department of Surgery, Program in Trauma and Critical Care, R Adams Cowley Shock Trauma Center, University of Maryland School of Medicine, University of Maryland Medical Center, Baltimore, MD, USA

Emily Hart, CRNP R. Adams Cowley Shock Trauma Center, University of Maryland, Baltimore, MD, USA

Allison Lankford, MD Department of Obstetrics and Gynecology and Reproductive Surgery, Division of Maternal Fetal Medicine, Anesthesia Critical Care, University of Maryland School of Medicine, R Adams Cowley Shock Trauma Center, Baltimore, MD, USA

Ann Matta, CRNP R. Adams Cowley Shock Trauma Center, Baltimore, MD, USA

Sarah B. Murthi, MD, RDCS, FACS Department of Surgery, Program in Trauma and Critical Care, R Adams Cowley Shock Trauma Center, University of Maryland School of Medicine, University of Maryland Medical Center, Baltimore, MD, USA

Erin Niles, PA-C R. Adams Cowley Shock Trauma Center, Baltimore, MD, USA

Brandon Masi Parker, DO Department of Surgery, University of Miami Miller School of Medicine, Miami, FL, USA

Alexis Salerno, MD Department of Emergency Medicine, University of Maryland School of Medicine, Baltimore, MD, USA

Rhea Votipka, CRNP Lahey Hospital and Medical Center, Pulmonary Critical Care Medicine, Burlington, MA, USA

Part I

Imaging

Obtaining, Interpreting, and Using Echo

Alexis Salerno and Sarah B. Murthi

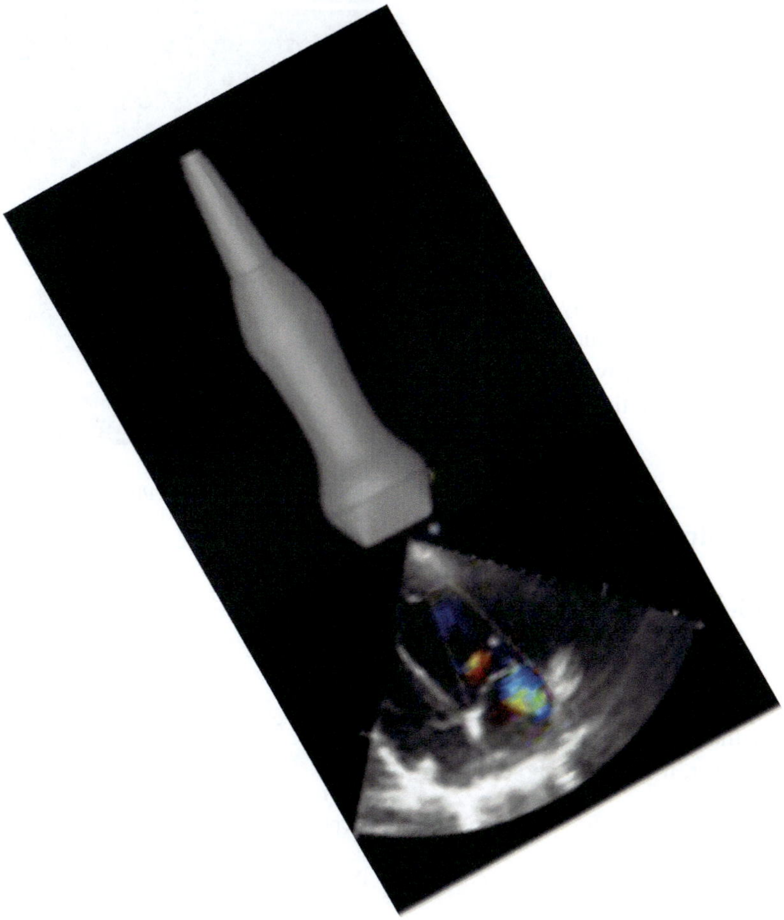

Supplementary Information The online version of this chapter (https://doi.org/10.1007/978-3-030-74687-2_1) contains supplementary material, which is available to authorized users.

A. Salerno
Department of Emergency Medicine, University of Maryland School of Medicine, Baltimore, MD, USA

S. B. Murthi (✉)
Department of Surgery, Program in Trauma and Critical Care, R Adams Cowley Shock Trauma Center, University of Maryland School of Medicine, University of Maryland Medical Center, Baltimore, MD, USA
e-mail: smurthi@som.umaryland.edu

A. Salerno et al. (eds.), *Atlas of Critical Care Echocardiography*, https://doi.org/10.1007/978-3-030-74687-2_1

Abbreviations

2D	Two-Dimensional
B Mode	Brightness Mode
CO	Cardiac Output
ECG	Electrocardiogram
EF	Ejection Fraction
LV	Left Ventricle
M Mode	Motion Mode
MHz	Megahertz
PLA	Parasternal Long Axis
POCUS	Point-of-Care Ultrasound
PSA	Parasternal Short Axis
SV	Stroke Volume
SX	Subxiphoid
VTI	Velocity Time Integral

1 Introduction

At first glance, the number of buttons on an ultrasound machine may be intimidating. But as with any skill, you just need to learn the language of ultrasound which is knobology. By using basic knobology, you can improve your ultrasound image. In this chapter we will review the basic ultrasound settings, modes and transducers.

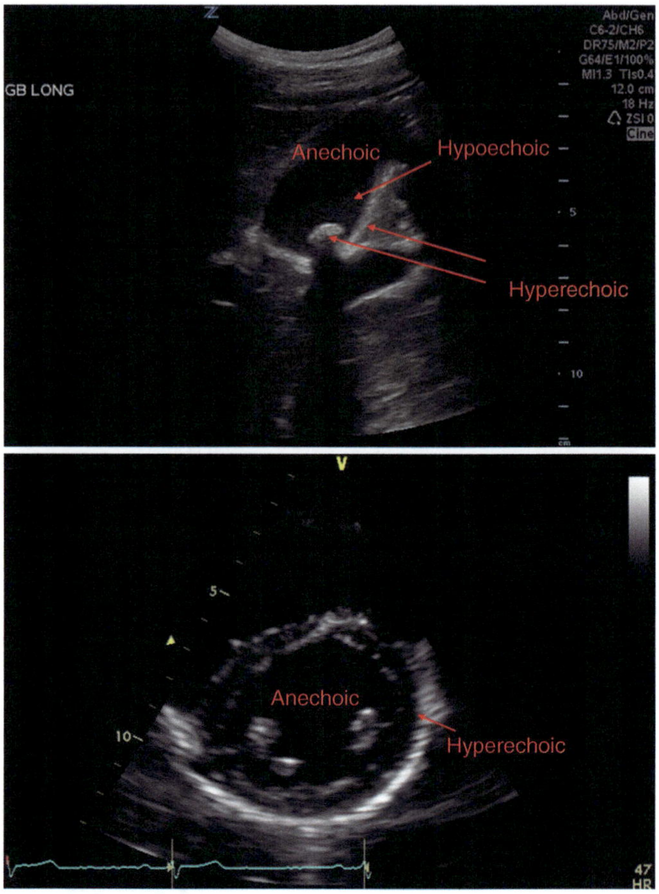

Fig. 1 Echogenicity. Upper panel: Abdominal ultrasound of the gallbladder with a stone. The gallstone is hyperechoic, the sludge around it is hypoechoic and the fluid in the gallbladder is anechoic. Lower panel: Echocardiogram of a parasternal short axis (PSA) view of the heart. The blood in the heart is anechoic and the pericardium around the heart is hyperechoic

2 Ultrasound Knobology

2.1 Echogenicity (Fig. 1)

- Echogenicity is the brightness of a structure. In POCUS it is described relative to a normal liver:
  - If a structure is darker than the liver, it is hypoechoic; if it is brighter than the liver, it is hyperechoic. If there is no color, it is called anechoic.

2.2 Knobs and Terms (Table 1)

Table 1 Knobs and actions

Knob	Action
Gain	Increases or decreases the white value of the image
Depth	Changes the imaging depth, there are 1 cm hash marks along the side of the monitor screen
iScan	Automatically optimizes gain and depth (name varies between systems)
Freeze	Freezes the ultrasound image
Caliper	Used to measure distances; remember to measure leading edge to leading edge
Still image	Often labeled save, stores a still photo of your image
Clips	Stores a video, can be adjusted either 5 heartbeats or 3–5 seconds
Zoom	Zooms in on a specific area of the image, can be done live or on a still image
Cine scroll	When the machine is on freeze, it will replay the last 5 seconds, good to review specific structures slowly for measurements

3 Ultrasound Scanning Modes

3.1 B Mode or Two-Dimensional (2D) (Fig. 2 Upper Panel, Video 1)

- B mode or brightness mode is the most used mode for ultrasound imaging. It is a 2D moving clip that is created by scan lines sequentially sent through a field at a specified frame rate.
- It is usually referred to as 2D imaging in echocardiography.
- Cardiac imaging requires higher frame rates for better temporal resolution of rapid valvular motion

3.2 M Mode (Fig. 2 Lower Panel)

- M mode or motion mode is used for precise measurements of change over time. A single crystal sends and receives the signal so there is no frame rate thus creating a continuous measurement.
- It can also be thought of as an ice pick view through a 2D image.

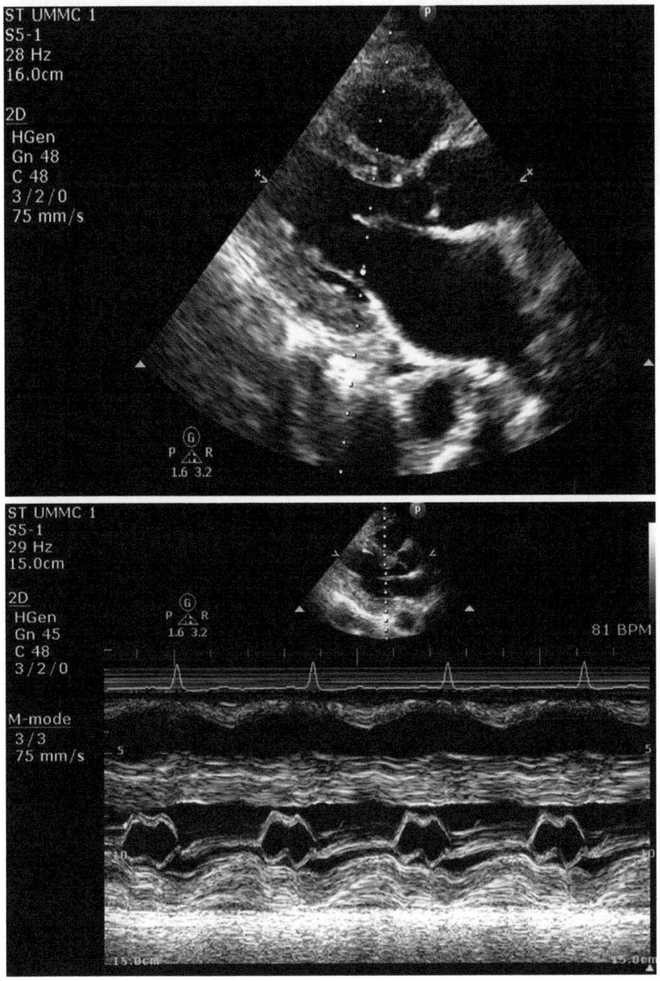

Fig. 2 2D and M mode imaging. Upper panel: A 2D image of the parasternal long axis (PLA) of the heart; the dotted line is the cursor. Lower panel: An M-mode image from the cursor in the upper panel

3.3 Doppler Modes (Fig. 3)

- Doppler is used to measure the velocity and direction of an object moving relative to the probe, most often blood.
- The ultrasound system calculates the Doppler change (shift) in the frequency between the sending and reflected signal.
  - Direction of the Doppler shift
    - Increase in the frequency: movement toward the transducer
    - Decrease in the frequency: movement away from the transducer
  - Amount of the shift
    - Velocity of movement; more shift, higher velocity flow

3.3.1 Types of Doppler

- Pulsed wave Doppler
  - A single crystal is used to send a pulsed signal:
    - Pause period allows the return signal to be heard.
  - Movement is displayed around a baseline:
    - Flow toward the probe, above
    - Flow away from the probe, below
  - Allows listening at a specific point on the cursor.
  - At high flows the Nyquist limit is reached, unable to measure and aliasing will occur.
  - Uses: Stroke volume measurement, assessing portal and hepatic venous flow
- Continuous wave Doppler
  - Two crystals are used. One continuously sends, while the other receives the return signal.
  - Movement is displayed around a baseline.
  - Listens along the entire cursor.
  - Cannot measure flow at a specific point.
  - Aliasing does not occur so there is no limit, able to measure high flow.
  - Uses: Tricuspid jet to assess for elevated pulmonary artery pressure and grade of aortic stenosis
- Color flow Doppler
  - Color is a type of pulsed wave Doppler.
  - A color value is assigned to a positive and negative Doppler shift:
    - Red is classically movement toward the transducer.
    - Blue is classically movement away from the transducer.
    - Brightness is velocity of flow.
  - Uses: Locate blood flow and identify pathologic flow (i.e., a ventricular septal defect (VSD)).
- Tissue Doppler imaging
  - Pulsed wave Doppler.
  - Setting detects the low-frequency change of tissue movement.
  - Measures tissue movement not blood flow.
  - Uses: Assessment of diastolic function.

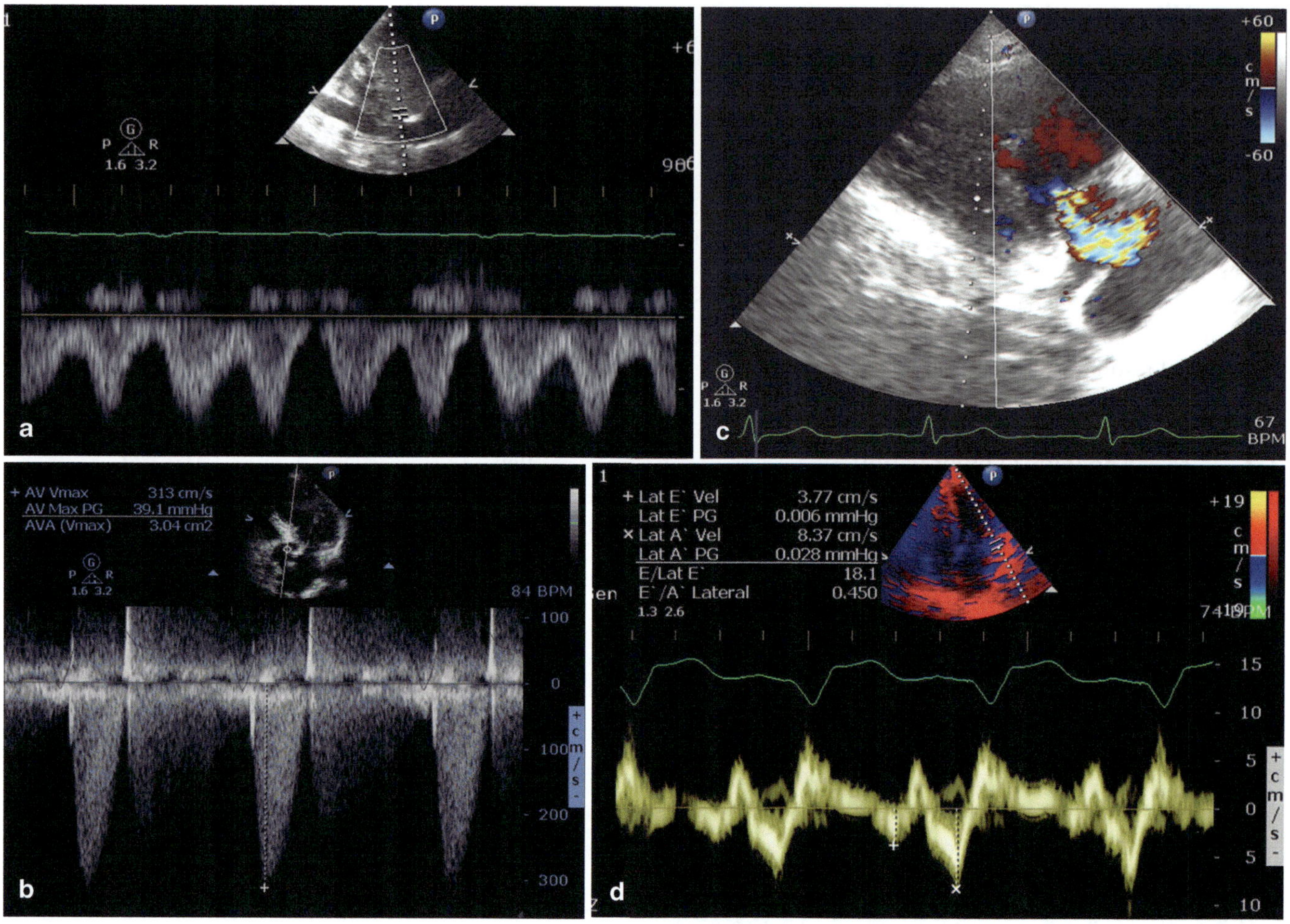

Fig. 3 Doppler modes. (**a**) Pulsed wave Doppler (PWD). (**b**) Continuous wave Doppler (CWD). (**c**) Color flow Doppler (CFD). (**d**) Tissue Doppler imaging (TDI)

4 Ultrasound Transducers (Fig. 4)

4.1 Curvilinear

- Low frequency
  - 2–5 MHz
- Image output shaped like a pyramid without the top
- Uses: Imaging deeper structures such as abdominal structures

4.2 Linear

- High frequency
  - 5–12 MHz
- Image output shaped like a vertical rectangle
- Uses: Superficial imaging, vascular studies, and procedure guidance

4.3 Phased Array

- Low frequency
  - 2–5 MHz
- A smaller footprint than the curvilinear probe
  - Ideal for fitting between rib spaces
- Image output shaped like a triangle
- Uses: Cardiac, thoracic, and superficial abdominal structures

5 Transducer Movements (Fig. 5)

There are common movements in ultrasound, all of which are used during echocardiography (Table 2). In the parasternal short axis (PSA), you *fan* through the heart. To obtain the parasternal long axis (PLA), you *rock* under the sternum. To get the subxiphoid (SX) window, you *compress* under the

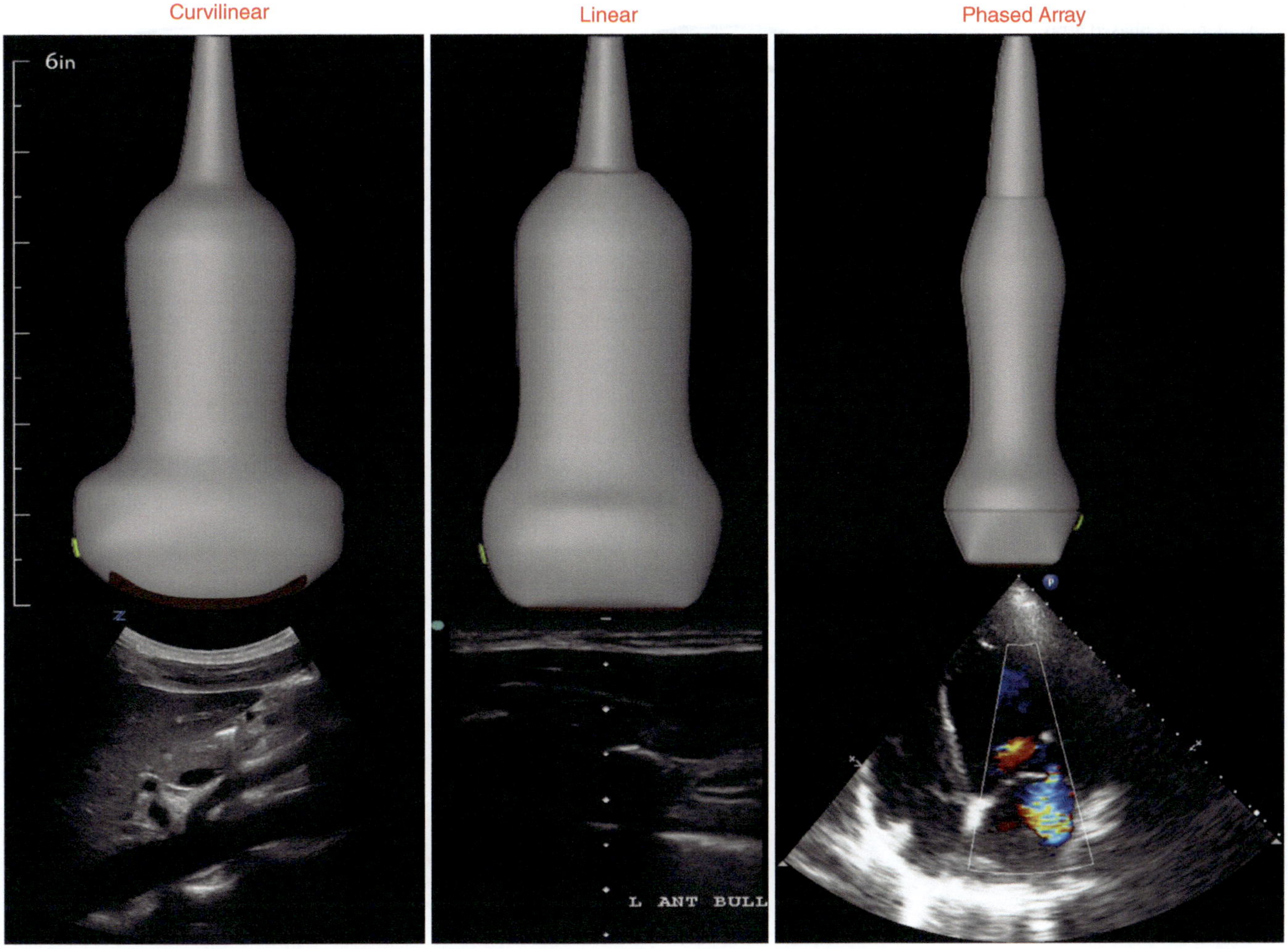

Fig. 4 Transducers. Transducers are shown above images that are generated on an ultrasound display screen

xiphoid. To move from the PSA to the apical window, you *slide* across the chest, and to transition from the PLA to the PSA, you *rotate* the transducer.

6 Exam Types and Presets (Fig. 6)

Ultrasound systems come with imaging software packages called presets or exam type depending on the manufacturer. It is important to select the best presets for the type of imaging.

- Cardiac imaging (Fig. 6 upper panel; Video 1)
  - Indicator/grove is displayed on the right of the screen:
    - By convention, possibly to align better with cardiac catheterization imaging
  - ECG leads are active and displayed at the bottom of the screen.
  - Higher frame rate/less scan lines:
    - Better for assessing for rapid valvular movement
    - Better for assessing cardiac function
    - Grainy still image
  - Less black white compression:
    - Better for differentiating the endocardium and epicardium
- Abdominal and lung imaging (Fig. 6 lower panel; Video 2)
  - Indicator/grove is displayed on the left of the screen:
    - Appears like a mirror image of a cardiac still
  - No ECG leads.
  - Lower frame rate/more scan lines:
    - More resolution of still structures (i.e., liver or kidney)
    - Worse for assessing rapid movement
      - The heart may falsely appear dysfunctional.
  - More compression:
    - Smoother image

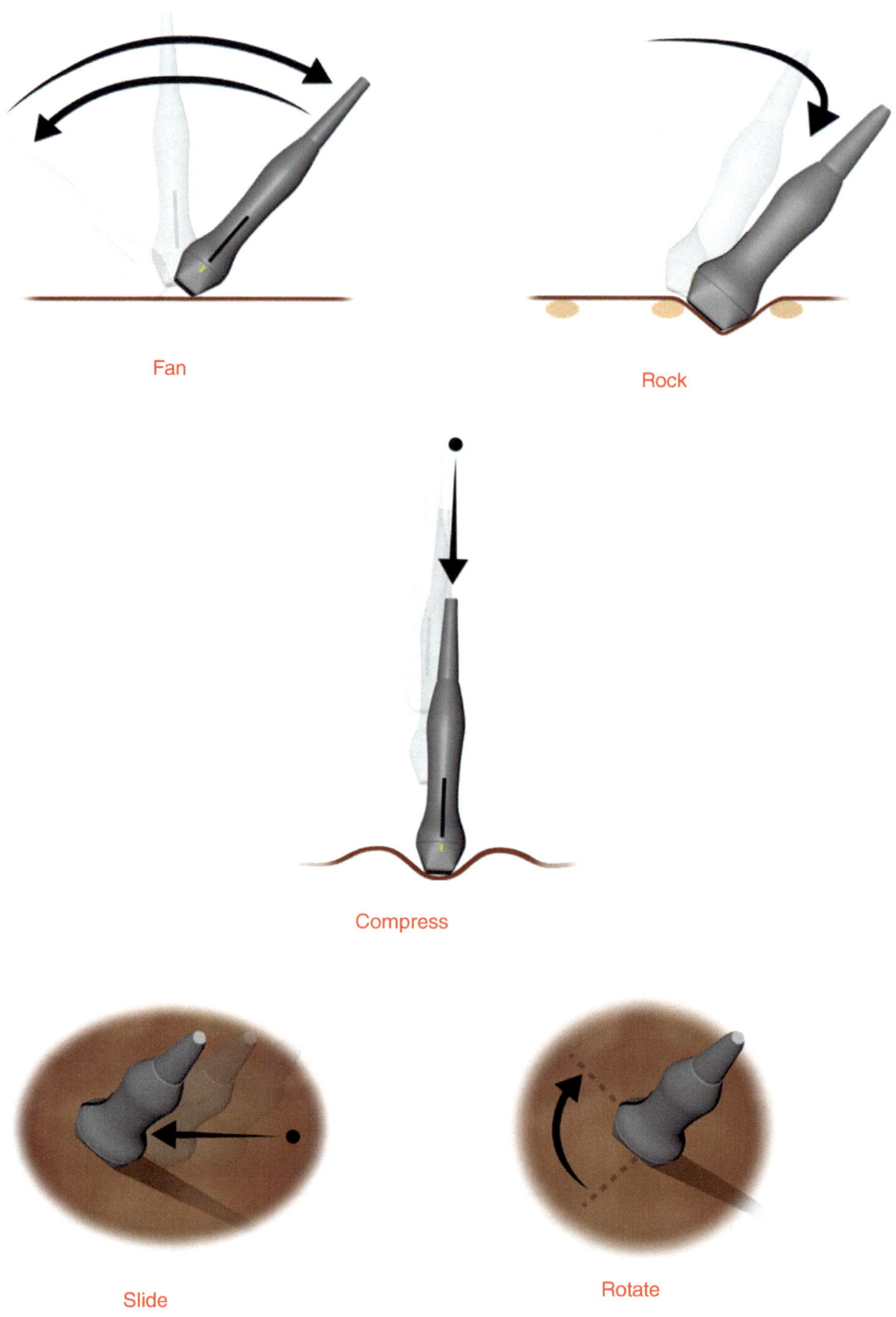

Fig. 5 Transducer movements. A phased array probe is demonstrating the most common transducer movements

Table 2 Common movements in ultrasound

Motion	Action	Example
Fan	Scans through an image	Fanning through the heart in the PSA
Rock	Centers on a structure by tilting	Under the sternum to get the PLA
Compress	Pressing down with probe	Under the xiphoid to get SX
Slide	Moving the probe on the surface	From the PLA to the apical
Rotate	Changes the image axis	From PLA to PSA

7 Measurements in Point-of-Care Ultrasound

Objective quantitative measurements are relatively new to POCUS, especially compared to radiology and cardiology. Cardiology has been evaluating function for decades; therefore, there are established assessments like left ventricular ejection fraction (LVEF) and the LV velocity time interval (VTI). Conversely measurements of volume status are new and in flux.

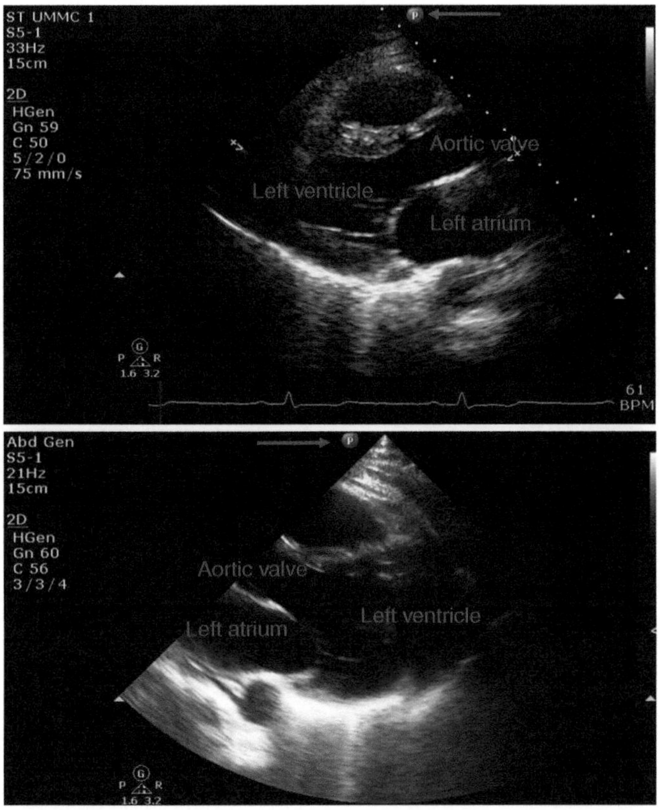

Fig. 6 Cardiac vs. abdominal presets. Upper panel: The heart imaged in cardiac presets. Lower panel: The heart imaged in abdominal presets. The arrow points to the dot on the screen that shows the direction of the indicator on the probe

- *Helpful*
  - Measurements need to be used carefully, but they can be very helpful.
  - Trend changes over time in the same patient.
  - Example: Doppler measurement through the left ventricular outflow tract can be used to calculate stroke volume (SV). From this the cardiac output (CO) can be measured, and if the mean arterial blood pressure is known, then the systemic vascular resistance can be calculated.
- *Categories and large ranges are better*
  - It is far better to use ultrasound in grades and categories rather than a continuous variable:
    - More accurate interpretation of the data
    - Not able to tell a cardiac index of 2.7 from one of 2.9, but can assess likely low, normal, or high
  - Example: The LVEF is a great measurement; the large ranges and rounded cutoffs make it intuitive and reproducible.
- *POCUS research pitfall; specific cutoff values*
  - Specific, non-reproducible, cutoff values based on a receiver operating curve (ROC) to detect a finding are frequent in POCUS literature:
    - Because ultrasound systems are common in the emergency department and ICU, it is easy to start using the value before it has been fully assessed.
    - Pattern of initial paper published defining a value, and then a series of follow-up papers discrediting that value and reporting a new specific number.
    - Example: IVC diameter change and specific values of 18%.
  - Means accepting that US will not always provide an answer.
  - Even if a discrete number is generated with ultrasound, it is only a semiquantitative tool.
- *Be smart*
  - Different measurements have different sources of error:
    - Know where the error is in the measurements you commonly use.
  - Assess the same property in several ways:
    - Allows you to check one value against the other
    - Allows a better understanding of cardiac physiology
  - Example: Assess the LVEF and measure the SV and CO. Not only can you check the SV measurement against your global assessment of LVEF, you learn how well the LV is working *and* how much it is putting out.
- *Practice, play, and check*
  - Before using a measurement, become comfortable with it.
- *Better software for POCUS is needed*
  - Currently measurements require expertise and are cumbersome to perform.
  - Manufactures will develop new tools to make measurements easier, faster, and more reproducible.

Suggested Reading

Chan V, Perlas A. Basics of ultrasound imaging. In: Atlas of ultrasound guided procedures in interventional pain management. New York: Springer; 2011. p. 13–9.

Parasternal Long Axis

Sarah B. Murthi and Syeda Fatima

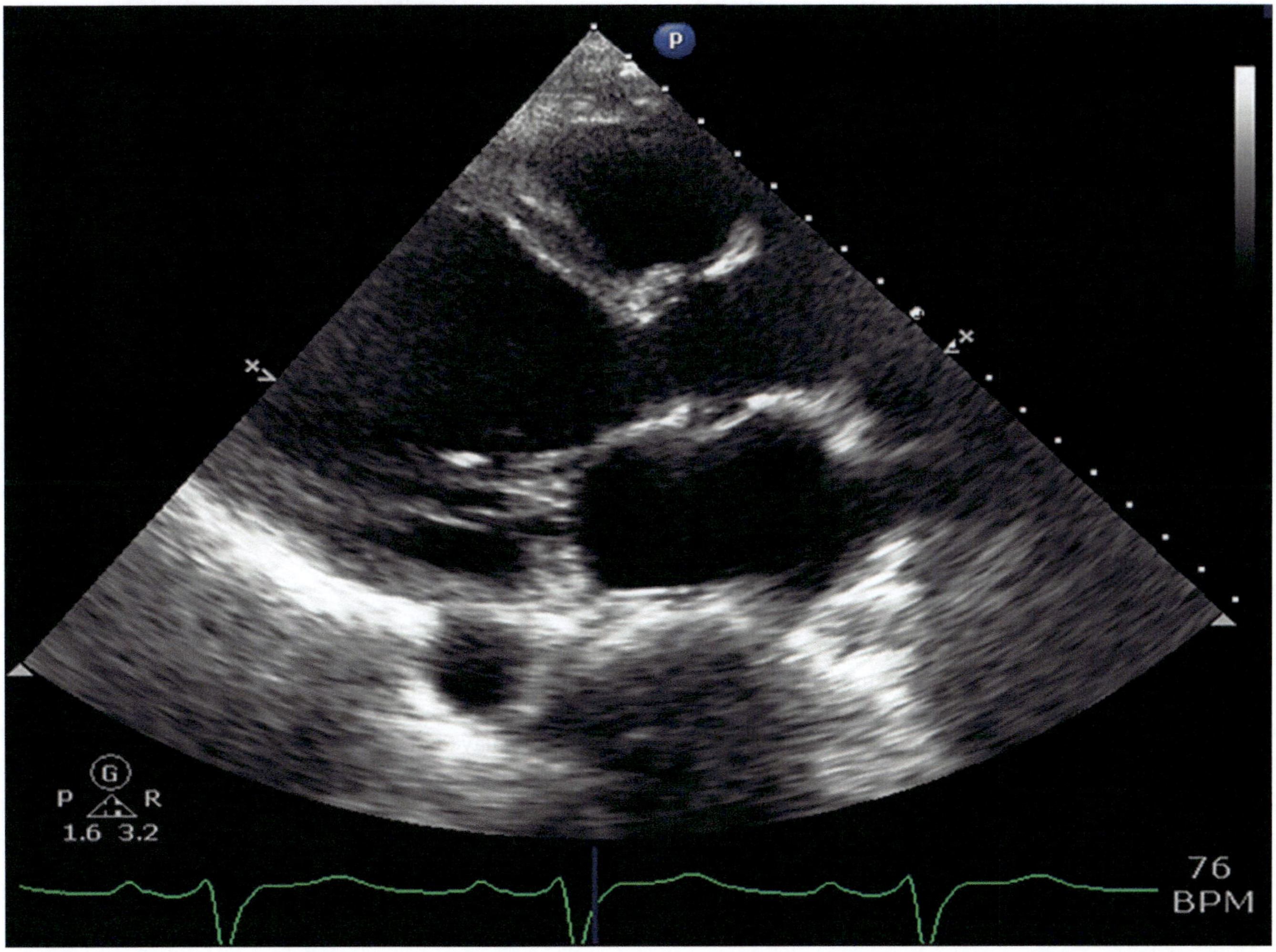

S. B. Murthi (✉)
Department of Surgery, Program in Trauma and Critical Care, R Adams Cowley Shock Trauma Center, University of Maryland School of Medicine, University of Maryland Medical Center, Baltimore, MD, USA
e-mail: smurthi@som.umaryland.edu

S. Fatima
R. Adams Cowley Shock Trauma Center, University of Maryland, Baltimore, MD, USA

A. Salerno et al. (eds.), *Atlas of Critical Care Echocardiography*, https://doi.org/10.1007/978-3-030-74687-2_2

Abbreviations

EF	Ejection fraction
ICU	Intensive care unit
LV	Left ventricle
LVOTD	Left ventricular outflow tract diameter
PLA	Parasternal long axis
RV	Right ventricle
TTE	Transthoracic echocardiogram

1 Introduction

The parasternal long axis (PLA) is the first image in a transthoracic echocardiogram (TTE). It is an important window because it allows assessment of the left ventricular ejection fraction (LVEF) and measurement of the LV outflow tract diameter (LVOTD).

The PLA can be hard to obtain in ICU patients. Positive airway pressure from mechanical ventilation expands the lungs and pushes the heart more medially and inferiorly under the sternum. Even so assessments of LVEF can usually be made in the PLA.

The orientation of the heart on the display screen is hard to understand at first. In TTE the transducer indicator is displayed on the right of the screen. In most other ultrasound imaging, it is on the left. This can be confusing. Stick with it, the PLA is an important window, and you will find it invaluable once conquered.

2 Obtaining the PLA

The ideal PLA view includes the midportion and base of the left ventricle, both leaflets of the mitral valve, the aortic valve and the aortic root, the left atrium, and the right ventricle (Fig. 1). The PLA is obtained with the transducer placed in the third or fourth intercostal space with the marker pointed to patient's right shoulder. This will place the heart's longest axis in view in most patients, but slight clockwise or counterclockwise rotation may be required for variable lie of the heart. Slight medial and lateral angulation may be required to achieve optimal view of LV largest diameter and mitral valve maximal excursion.

Placing the patient in left lateral decubitus may improve images.

- Place the transducer to the left of the sternum:
  - 2–6th rib space
  - May be lower and more medial in patients on a ventilator

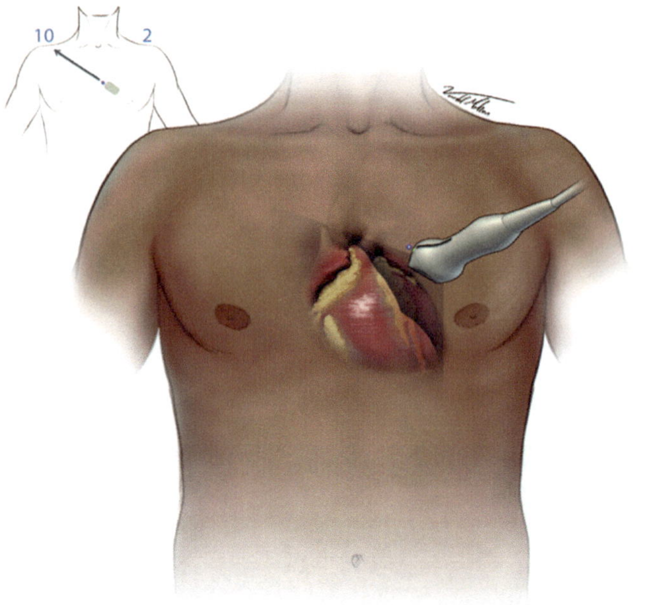

Fig. 1 Transducer placement in the PLA: The transducer is placed just to the left of the sternum between the second and sixth rib spaces. The indicator is aimed at the patient's shoulder bisecting the right clavicle, at the 10 o'clock position

- The indicator bisects the patient's right clavicle:
  - 10 o'clock position
- Slightly rock the transducer under the sternum:
  - Once under the sternum, tilt the face up to open the left ventricle.

2.1 Image Orientation (Fig. 2)

- In transthoracic cardiac exams by convention, the indicator is displayed on the right of the screen:
  - In abdominal and all other ultrasound imaging, it is displayed on the left.
- In the PLA the indicator is on the imager's left but displayed on the right of the screen:
  - Making the PLA orientation on the screen is difficult to understand.
  - Imagine rotating the image under the transducer 180° and floating on the screen.
- In the other cardiac windows, the transducer is on the imager's right, so the right display is more intuitive:
  - Easier to understand.
  - Imagine the image under the transducer floating on to the screen.

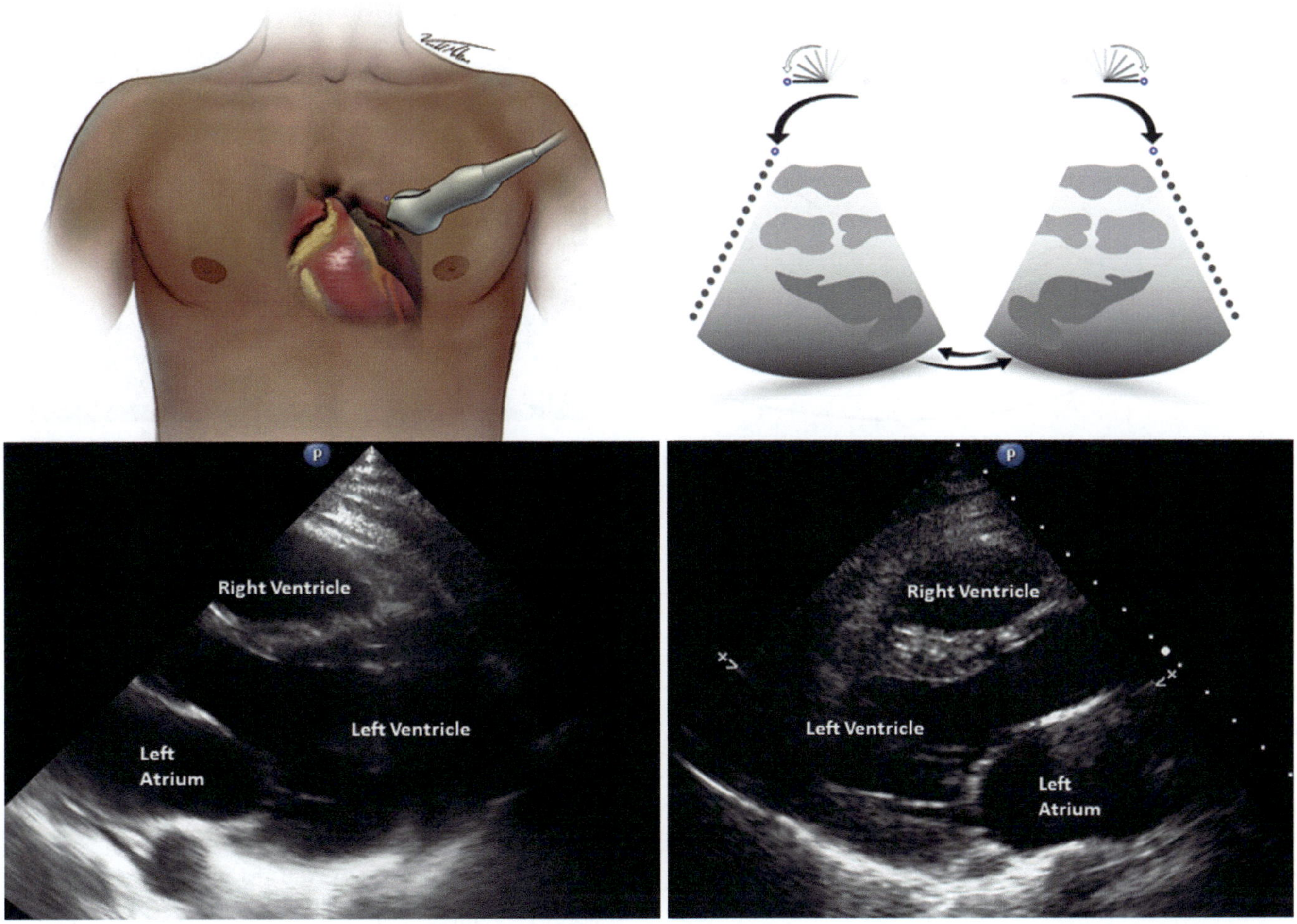

Fig. 2 Transducer orientation in the PLA: The orientation of the heart on the display screen depends on the exam type, or presets selected. In abdominal presets (lower left panel), the transducer indicator (purple ball; all panels) is displayed on the left of the screen. In cardiac imaging presets (lower right panel), the indicator is displayed on the right of the screen

3 Assessments and Measurements

- LV ejection fraction
  - Visual assessment.
  - E-point septal separation.
  - See chapter "Left Ventricular Ejection Fraction and E-point Septal Separation".
- Aortic valve
  - Aortic stenosis
  - Aortic insufficiency
- Left ventricular outflow tract diameter
  - Needed for stroke volume and cardiac output measurements.
  - See chapter "Stroke Volume, Cardiac Output, and Systemic Vascular Resistance".
- Left atrial size
- Mitral valve function
  - Regurgitation
- RV function
  - May provide the first indication of dysfunction.
  - See chapter "Right Ventricular Systolic Function".
- Posterior pericardial effusion

4 Ideal Image (Fig. 3)

- The LV appears oval, often football shaped.
- The RV is small and seen above the LV.
- The left atria, mitral valve, aortic valve, papillary muscles, aortic root, and descending aorta can be visualized.

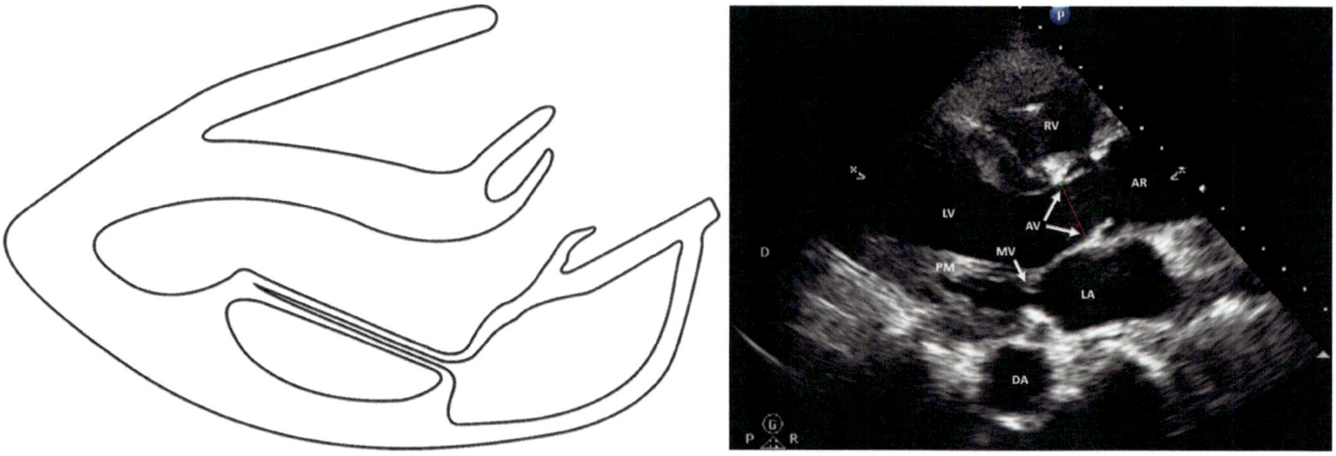

Fig. 3 Ideal PLA window: RV right ventricle, LV left ventricle, PM papillary muscle, MV mitral valve, AV aortic valve, LA left atria, DA descending aorta

5 Tips and Pointers

- If the LV is round rather than oval, image is foreshortened:
  - Come slightly off the sternum.
  - Tilt the transducer face up to open the left ventricle and the left ventricular outflow tract.
- If the RV is large, the transducer may be too high:
  - Come down a rib space.

6 Special Considerations

- Often the ideal image cannot be obtained:
  - But assessments of overall LV function can usually be made.
- On a ventilator the heart is lower and more medial
  - May be helpful to prop, or turn the patient right side-up.
  - Usually the PLA can be performed with the patient supine.

Suggested Reading

Lichtenstein D, van Hooland S, Elbers P, Malbrain ML. Ten good reasons to practice ultrasound in critical care. Anaesthesiol Intensive Ther. 2014;46(5):323–35. https://doi.org/10.5603/AIT.2014.0056. PMID: 25432552.

Moreno O, Ochagavía A, Artigas A, Barbadillo S, Tomás R, Bosque MD, et al. Impact of goal directed basic echocardiography on diagnostic and therapeutic management in an ICU of cardiac surgery. Med Intensiva. 2020;44(9):534–41. https://doi.org/10.1016/j.medin.2019.06.009. English, Spanish. Epub 2019 Aug 29. PMID: 31474457.

Vieillard-Baron A, Millington SJ, Sanfilippo F, Chew M, Diaz-Gomez J, McLean A, et al. A decade of progress in critical care echocardiography: a narrative review. Intensive Care Med. 2019;45(6):770–88. https://doi.org/10.1007/s00134-019-05604-2. Epub 2019 Mar 25. Erratum in: Intensive Care Med. 2019 Apr 15; PMID: 30911808.

Parasternal Short Axis

Allison Lankford

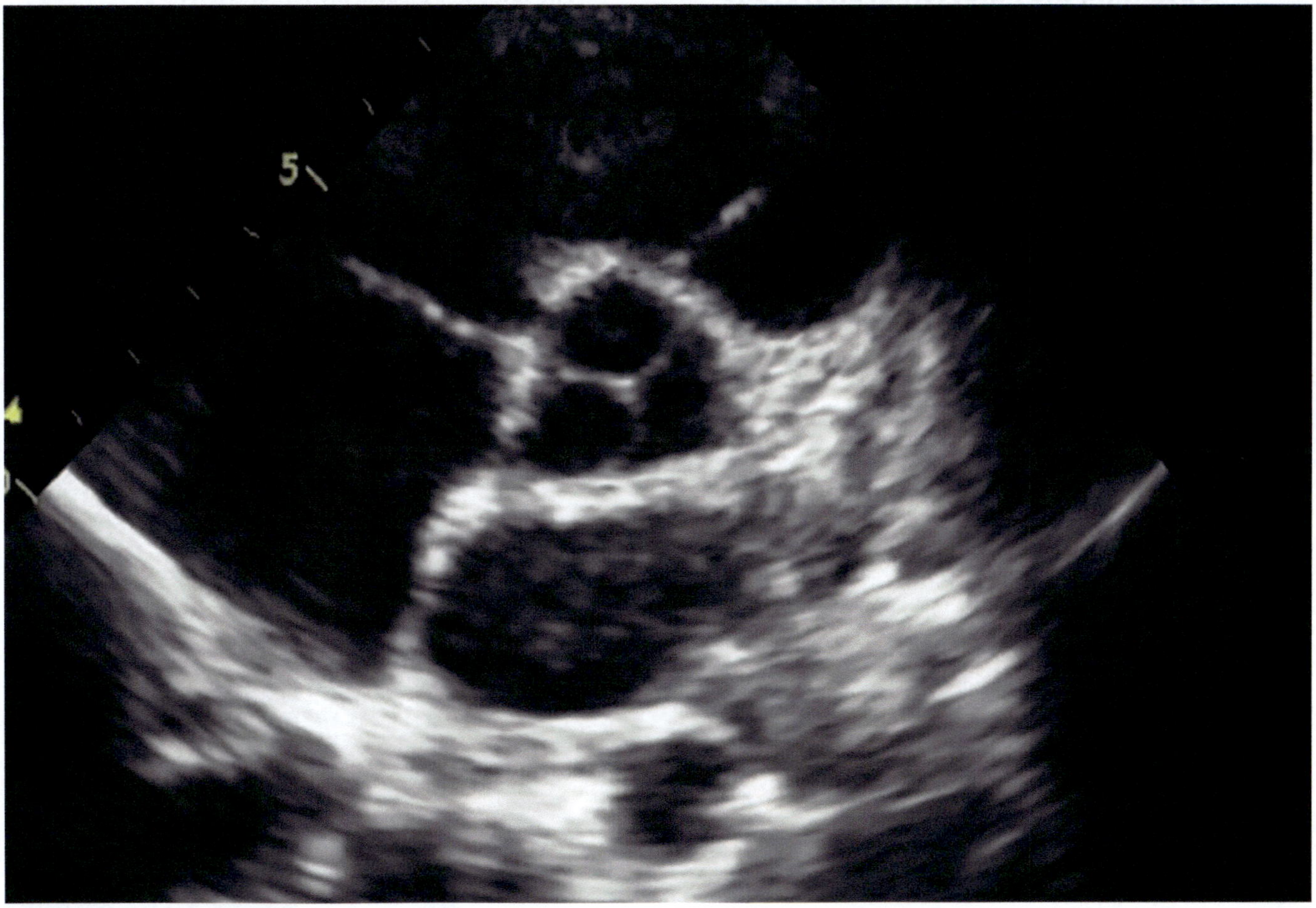

A. Lankford (✉)
Department of Obstetrics and Gynecology and Reproductive Surgery, Division of Maternal Fetal Medicine, Anesthesia Critical Care, University of Maryland School of Medicine, R Adams Cowley Shock Trauma Center, Baltimore, MD, USA
e-mail: allison.lankford@som.umaryland.edu

A. Salerno et al. (eds.), *Atlas of Critical Care Echocardiography*, https://doi.org/10.1007/978-3-030-74687-2_3

1 Introduction

The parasternal short axis (PSA) is the second window in a transthoracic echocardiogram (TTE). It is one of the most overlooked images in the TTE. The PSA allows for qualitative assessment of left ventricular (LV) function, and LV hypertrophy. It is also important in assessing right ventricular (RV) function, and assessing for RV pressure volume overload evidenced by a D-shaped LV, or flat interventricular septum. The measurement of tricuspid regurgitant velocity in the aortic valve window is a predictor for pulmonary hypertension.

2 Obtaining the Parasternal Short Axis

There are four slices within the PSA, defined by the level at which the transducer is transecting the heart from the base of the LV to its apex (Fig. 1). The aortic valve (AV) is at the base of the heart. The AV, left atrium (LA), right atrium (RA), tricuspid valve (TV), right ventricle (RV), and pulmonic valve (PV) can be seen. At the level of the mitral valve (MV), both leaflets of the mitral valve, the LV, and RV are visualized. At the level of the papillary muscles, a short axis view of the middle of both the RV and LV is apparent. At the apex a short axis view of the tip of the LV is seen. Some centers image down to up (apex, papillary, mitral, AV); either is fine provided the approach is systematic and complete.

Transducer Position

- From the parasternal long axis (PLA), rotate the transducer clockwise approximately 90°:
  - From the 10 o'clock to 2 o'clock position.
  - The indicator bisects the left clavicle.
    - Do not go past the left shoulder.
  - Focus on the aortic valve.
  - Other than rotating it, try not to move the transducer.
- By tilting the transducer base to the apex, obtain different short axis images.

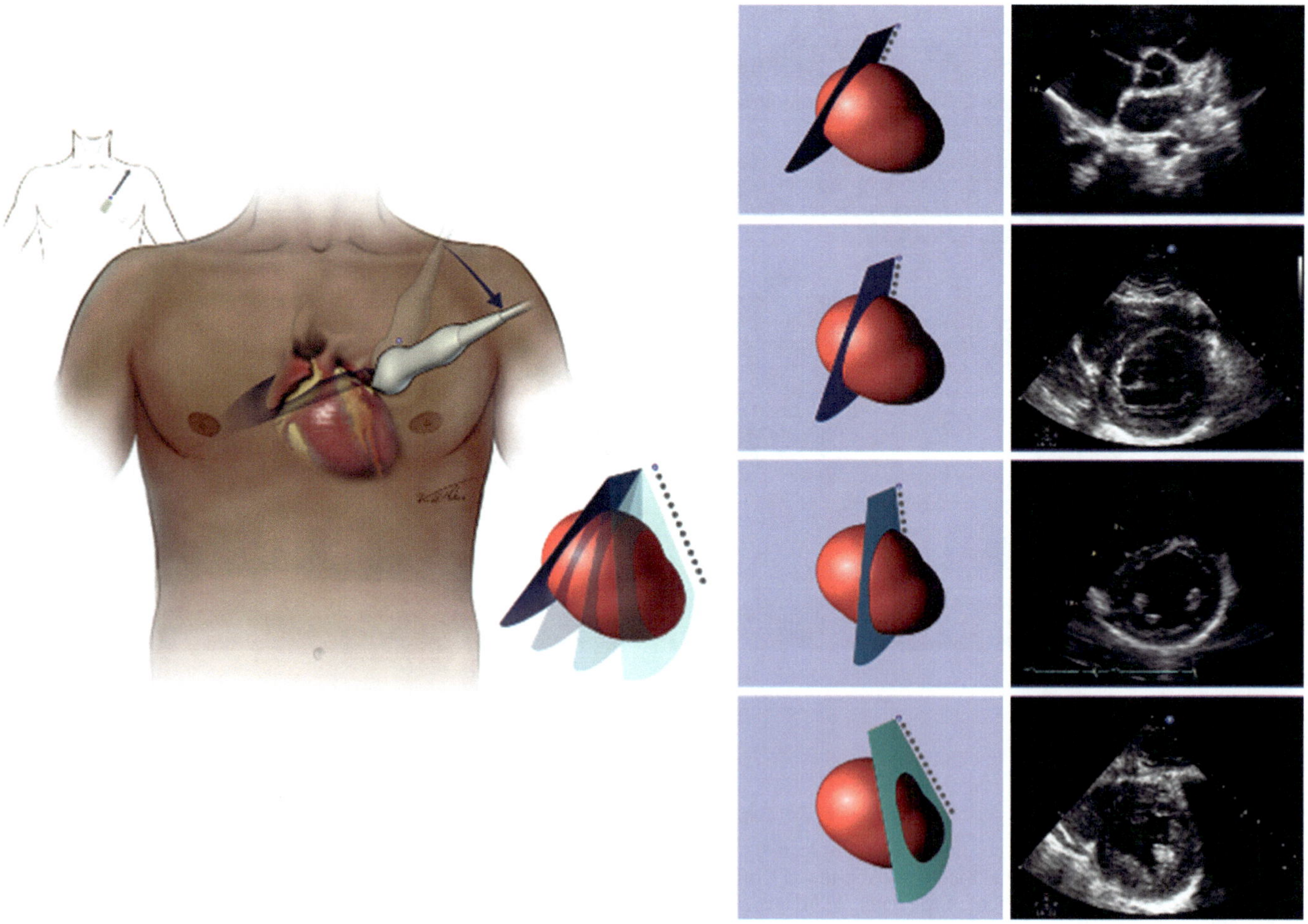

Fig. 1 Transducer placement for the parasternal short axis view. The left panel shows correct transducer placement. The right panel displays the aortic valve, mitral valve, papillary, and apical levels

Aortic Valve

- Tilt/fan the transducer up toward the patient's head to see the centrally located AV which comes into view:
  - Adjust until the AV appears a perfect quarter-sized circle in the middle of the screen.

Mitral Valve

- If the MV is seen first, tilt the transducer face slightly up to get the AV window:
- From the AV view tilt the transducer face down to open the mitral valve.

Papillary Muscle

- From the MV view continue to tilt the face down until the round papillary muscles are seen.
- Adjust the depth so that the LV fills about three quarters of the screen.

Apex

- Continue to tilt the transducer down toward the patient's feet to obtain an image of the tip of the LV.

2.1 Image Orientation (Fig. 2)

Aortic Valve Level

- The aortic valve is in the center of the screen. It is enclosed by the LA, RA, RV, and main pulmonary artery.
- A normal AV resembles a Mercedes-Benz symbol.
- The RV is on the left and upper side of the screen.

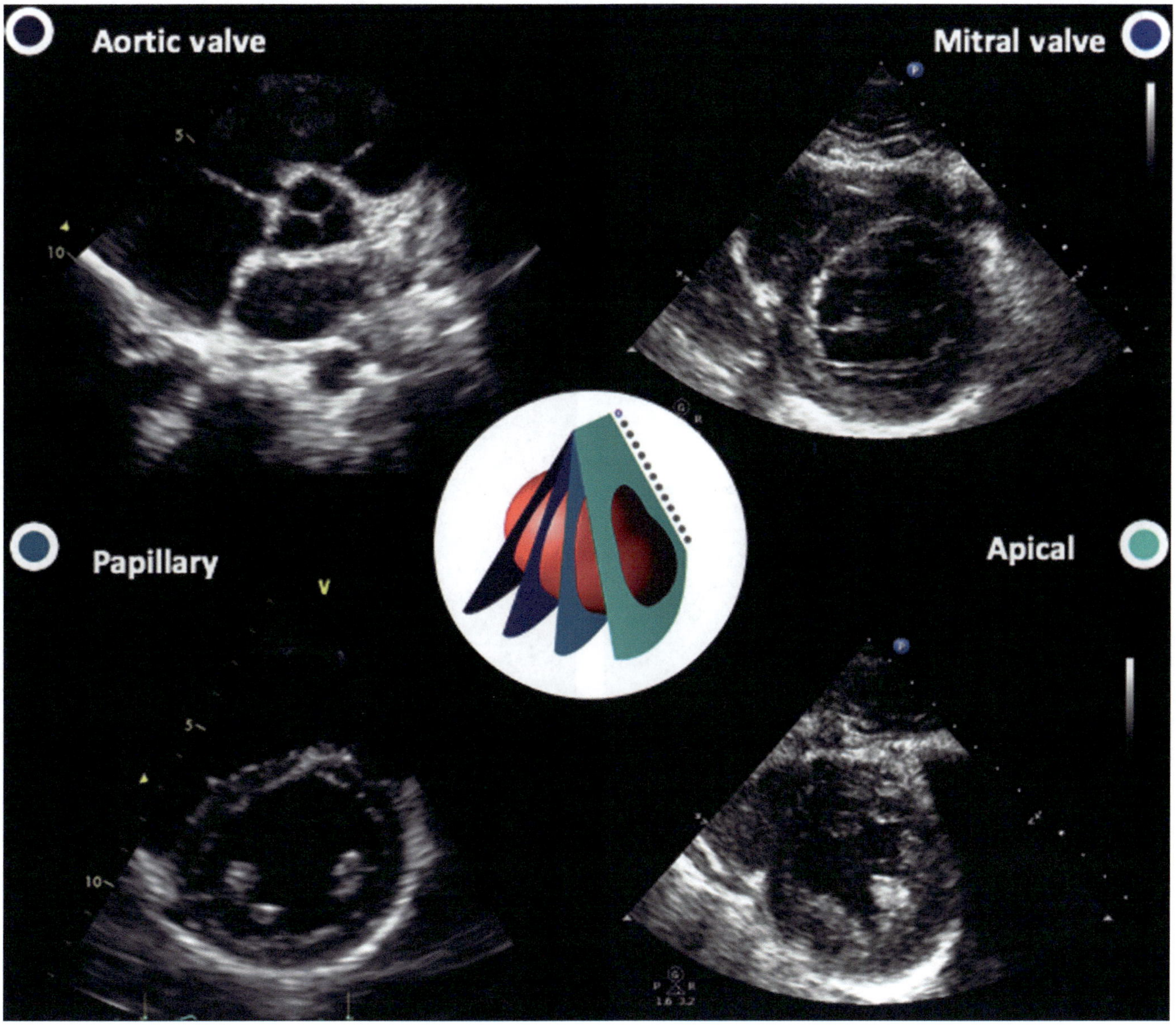

Fig. 2 Standard views for the parasternal short axis window

Mitral Valve Level

- The anterior leaflet is superior; the posterior is inferior.

Papillary Level

- The LV is in the center of the screen.
- The RV is superior and to the left.
  - Best image for assessing RV function and pressure volume overload

Apex Level

- The LV apex is seen in the center of the screen.
  - Best view for assessing apical

2.2 Ideal Images

Aortic Valve Level (Fig. 3)

- The aortic valve is in the center of the screen; ideally it will appear as a quarter-shaped circle:
  - Evaluate the opening and closing of the AV.
  - Look for a bicuspid valve.
- The tricuspid valve should be well visualized to the left, the RA is below the TV, and the RV is above it:
  - Apply color flow Doppler to find the tricuspid jet.
  - Apply continuous wave Doppler to measure the peak flow, which can be used to estimate the systolic pulmonary artery pressure.
  - A generalized assessment of RV function can be made.
- Often the pulmonic valve is in the upper right, above the AV.
- Sometimes the descending aorta can be seen in the lower right corner.

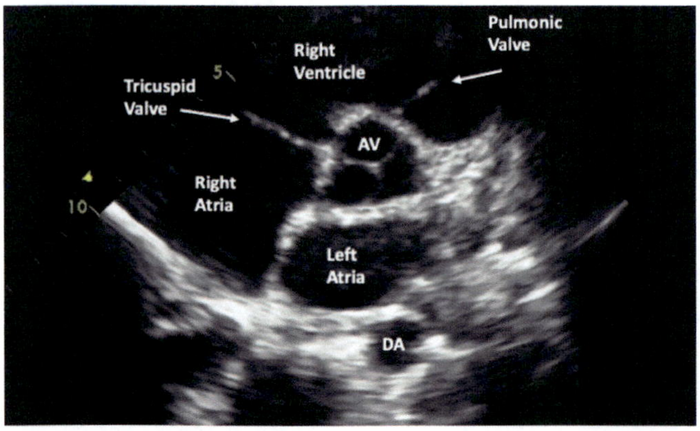

Fig. 3 Ideal image of the parasternal short axis; aortic valve level. AV aortic valve, DA descending aorta

Mitral Valve Level (Fig. 4)

- Both the anterior and posterior leaflets are well visualized.
- Evaluate the opening and closing of the valve.
- It has a heart-shaped opening at times in the cycle!

Papillary Level

- The LV is in the center of the screen.
- The center of the papillary muscles is well seen:
  - Position and size will vary between patients.
- The RV is superior and to the left, which surrounds the LV:
  - 9–12 o'clock positions.
  - It looks like a crescent moon with normal RV function:
    - With RV dysfunction it will appear fuller and more circular.
  - Interventricular septum should appear curved like the letter C:
    - With RV overload it will appear flat like the straight part of the letter D.
  - Best level for assessing RV function.
  - Best level for assessing RV pressure and volume overload.

Apex Level

- The LV apex is seen in the center of the screen:
  - Look for apical akinesis.

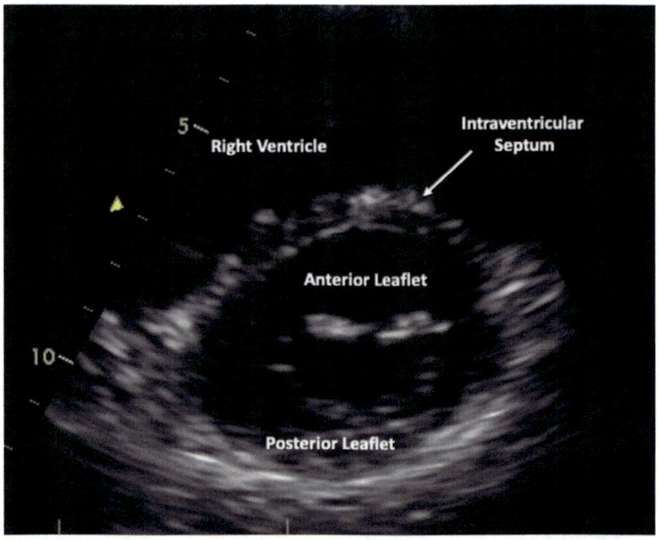

Fig. 4 Ideal image of the parasternal short axis; mitral valve level. Not the heart-shaped opening of the mitral valve

3 Assessment and Measurements

- LV ejection fraction
  - Visual assessment
- LV hypertrophy
  - Visual assessment
- RV size
  - Visual assessment
  - May confirm findings from PLA
    - RV may appear large and dilated due to an underlying pathology.
    - Diastolic collapse of RV.
- Interventricular septum
  - Flat versus curved
    - Flattening of the interventricular septum may be another indication of an underlying pathology such as a pulmonary embolism.
- Tricuspid regurgitation
  - At the level of the aortic valve.
  - Helpful for assessing for pulmonary hypertension (PTHN).
  - Estimation of the pulmonary artery systolic pressure (PASP) can be accomplished by measuring the peak tricuspid regurgitant jet velocity (TRV) and adding it to the right atrial pressure.
  - Peak TRV alone can estimate the probability of PTHN.

4 Tips and Pointers

- Acquisition of the papillary muscle, mitral valve, and aortic valve may not take place in that exact sequence.
- ICU patients are challenging, and as you turn the transducer from the parasternal long to the parasternal short axis, one of these three structures may pop into view. From there you can obtain the remaining two structures by simply fanning the transducer to the patient's head or feet.
- If the LV appears oval, instead of round, move up or down one or two rib spaces to maintain a round appearance of the LV.

Suggested Reading

Augustine DX, Coates-Bradshaw LD, Willis J, Harkness A, Ring L, Coghlan G, et al. Echocardiographic assessment of pulmonary hypertension: a guideline protocol from the British Society of Echocardiography. Echo Res Pract. 2018;5(3):G11–24. https://doi.org/10.1530/ERP-17-0071.

Labovitz AJ, Noble VE, Bierig M, Goldstein SA, Jones R, Kort S, Porter TR, et al. Focused cardiac ultrasound in the emergent setting: a consensus statement of the American Society of Echocardiography and American College of Emergency Physicians. J Am Soc Echocardiogr. 2010;23(12):1225–30.

Oren-Grinberg A, Talmor D, Brown SM. Focused critical care echocardiography. Crit Care Med. 2013;41(11):2618–26. https://doi.org/10.1097/CCM.0b013e31829e4dc5.

Apical 4 Chamber and Apical 5 Chamber

Erin Niles, Ann Matta, and Sarah B. Murthi

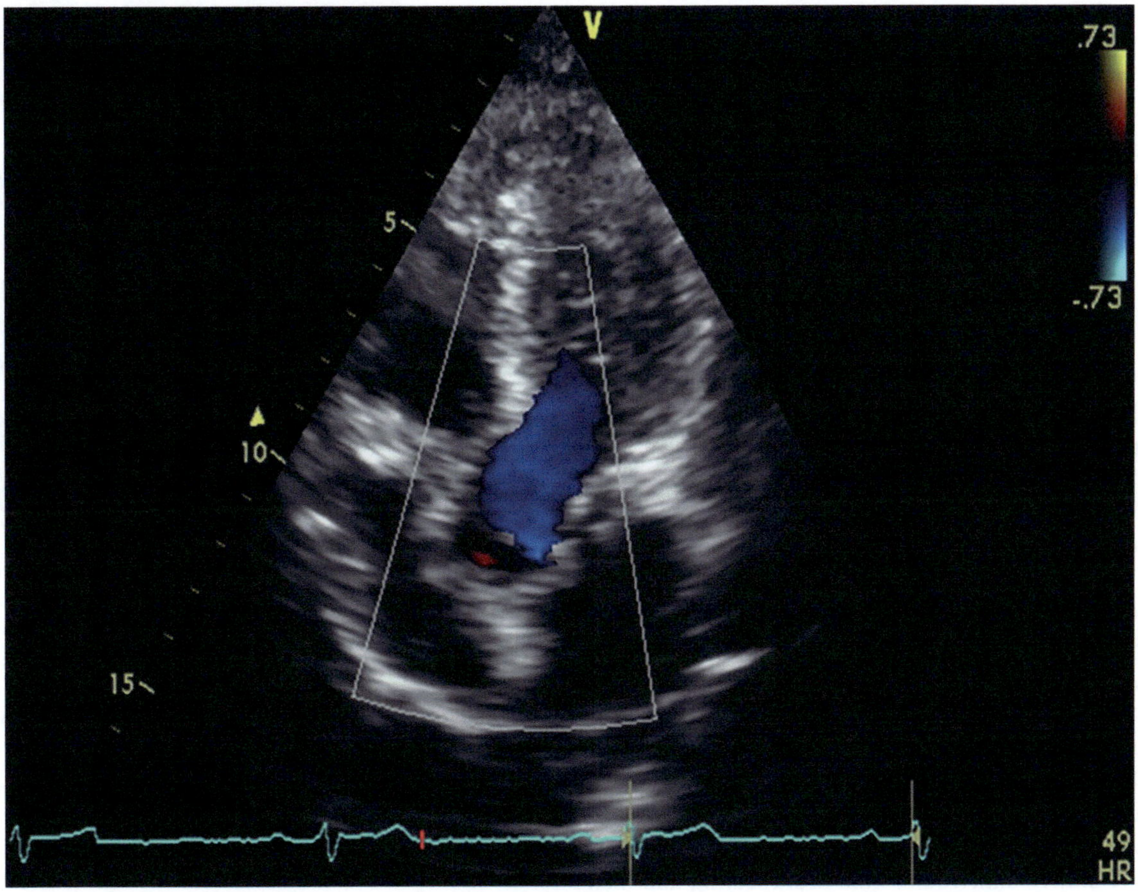

Supplementary Information The online version of this chapter (https://doi.org/10.1007/978-3-030-74687-2_4) contains supplementary material, which is available to authorized users.

E. Niles · A. Matta
R. Adams Cowley Shock Trauma Center, Baltimore, MD, USA

S. B. Murthi (✉)
Department of Surgery, Program in Trauma and Critical Care, R Adams Cowley Shock Trauma Center, University of Maryland School of Medicine, University of Maryland Medical Center, Baltimore, MD, USA
e-mail: smurthi@som.umaryland.edu

A. Salerno et al. (eds.), *Atlas of Critical Care Echocardiography*, https://doi.org/10.1007/978-3-030-74687-2_4

Abbreviations

2D	Two dimensional
AP 4C	Apical four chamber
AP 5C	Apical five chamber
CO	Cardiac output
LV	Left ventricle
LVOT	Left ventricular outflow tract
RV	Right ventricle
SV	Stroke volume
TAPSE	Tricuspid annular plane systolic excursion
VTI	Velocity time integral

1 Introduction

The apical four- (AP 4) and apical five- (AP 5) chamber views are high-yield windows in transthoracic echocardiography. Once obtained, they provide valuable information about right ventricular (RV) and left ventricular (LV) function, atrial size, and the visualization of pathology including atrial septal defects and ventricular septal defects. Mitral and tricuspid valve function and structure are assessed in the AP 4, as is diastolic function with Tissue Doppler imaging. Pulsed Wave Doppler measurement of the velocity time integral (VTI) through ventricular outflow tract (LVOT) is measured in the AP 5.

1.1 Obtaining the AP 4

Usually, the AP 4 is obtained first and then the AP 5 (Figs. 1 and 2). From the short axis view, the transducer is moved inferiorly and laterally.

- Place the transducer at the patient's point of maximal impulse:
  - This may be difficult to estimate; start lateral to the midclavicular line at the 4th–5th intercostal space and move medially.
  - Move slowly until you see the heart beating and then optimize your view.
  - May be more lateral and caudal in patients with left ventricular hypertrophy.
  - May be more medial in thin patients.
  - May be more medial and inferior in patients on positive pressure ventilation.
  - Might need to increase depth from the short axis view.
  - In patients with pendulous breast tissue, elevate the tissue and place the transducer under the breast fold.
- The indicator points to the patient's left midaxillary line:
  - 3 o'clock position, aimed down toward the bed
- To obtain the RV-focused view:
  - Slightly fan counterclockwise while maintaining the level.

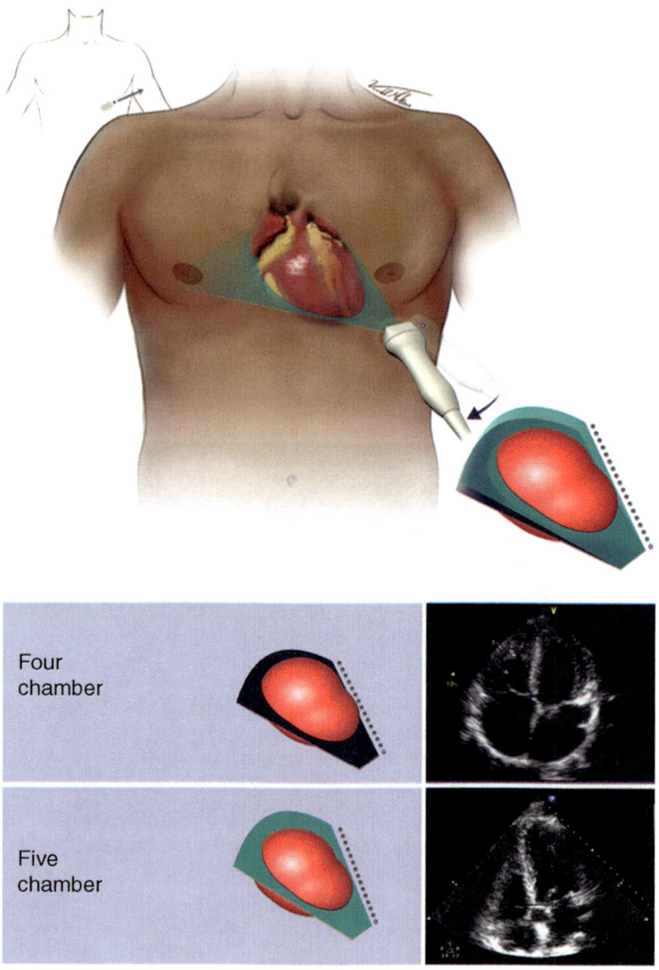

Fig. 1 Transducer placement for apical four- and five-chamber views. The AP 4 (dark blue, upper panel) window is obtained, and then the transducer face is angled up to open the AP 5 (teal, lower panel)

- Tilt the transducer cranially to fully open the ventricles and avoid foreshortening:
  - A coronal view of the heart will come into focus.
  - Continue to adjust the image until the septum is vertically midline near the center of the ultrasound screen image.

1.2 Obtaining the AP 5

After obtaining the AP 4 and completing the measurements, tilt the face of the transducer up to obtain the AP 5 (Figs. 1 and 2). It's a small movement (Video 1):

- Obtain the AP four-chamber view.
- Tilt the transducer head up (ventrally) to visualize the LVOT, aortic valve, and proximal aorta (Fig. 2).
- To obtain a good five-chamber view, you may need to move the transducer more laterally so that the septum is parallel to the transducer.
  - Important in obtaining the LVOT VTI used to the stroke volume (SV) and cardiac output (CO)

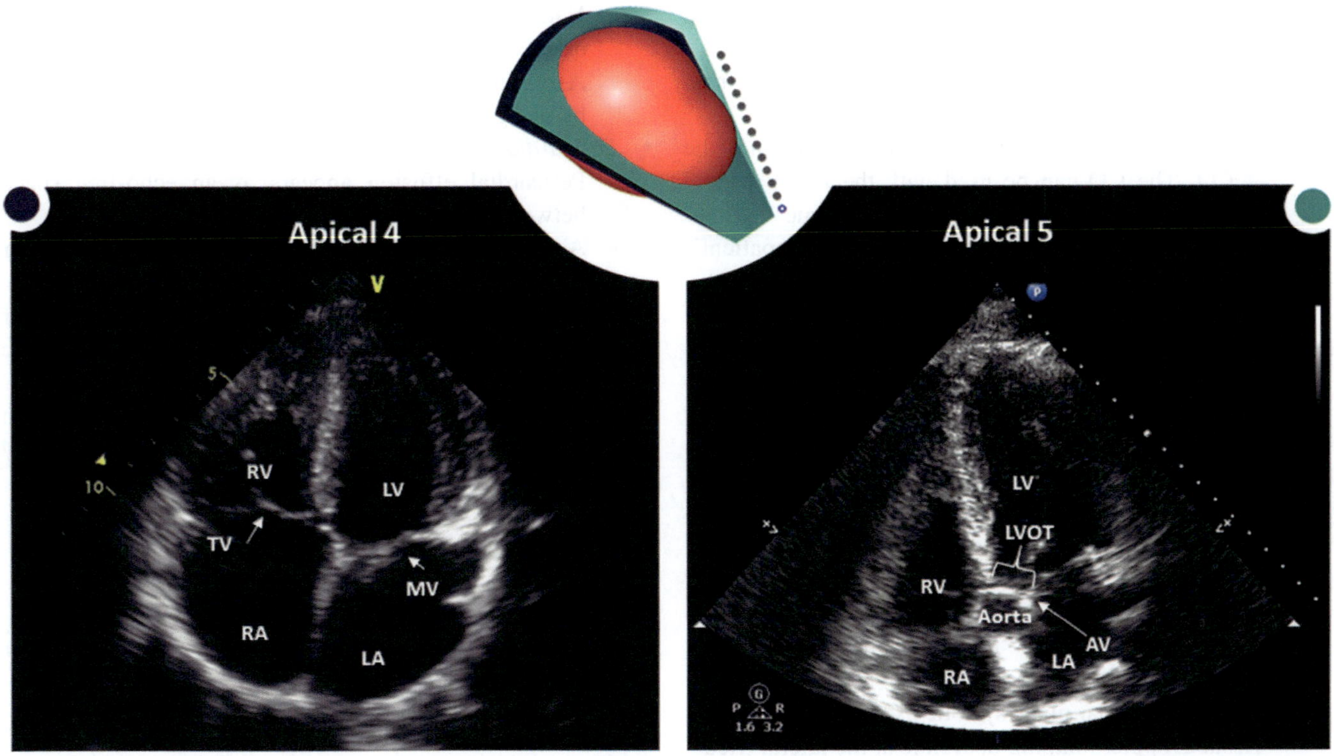

Fig. 2 Anatomy for apical four- and five-chamber windows. Left panel: AP 4, RV right ventricle, TV tricuspid valve, RA right atrium, LV left ventricle, MV mitral valve, LA left atrium. Right panel: AP 5 LVOT left ventricular outflow tract

1.3 Image Orientation

- The image is displayed as a coronal cut of the heart:
  - The atria are at the bottom of the screen and the ventricles which are closest to the transducer at the top.
  - The left side of the heart is on the viewer's right, and the right side of the heart is on the viewer's left.
  - In the AP 5 the aortic valve is considered the "fifth" chamber.

1.4 Ideal Image (Fig. 2)

- *Apical four chamber*
  - LV apex is visualized.
  - RV free wall is visualized.
  - The intraventricular septum is in the center of the screen.
  - The heart appears long like a football, not foreshortened, and round like a softball.
  - To obtain the RV-focused view, the transducer should be slightly rotated counterclockwise while maintaining at the level of the apex.
- *Apical five chamber*
  - Aortic valve is now visible allowing for VTI measurements.
  - Ideally the septum and blood flow through the aortic valve should be parallel to a cursor dropped from the center of the screen.
  - The left atrium is harder to see and may be obscured by the LVOT.

1.5 Assessments and Measurements

- *LV structure and focal wall motion*
  - Regional myocardial function is assessed by observing LV wall thickness and regional myocardial wall motion:
    - The inferoseptal, lateral wall, and apex can be visualized.
  - Each segment can be analyzed individually for evidence of normality, hyperkinetic, hypokinetic, akinetic, or dyskinetic function.
- *LV function*

  Systolic (see chapter "Left Ventricular Ejection Fraction and EPSS")
  - Visual assessment of ejection fraction

  Diastolic (see chapter "Diastolic Function"*)*
  - Pulsed wave Doppler through the mitral valve
  - Tissue Doppler imaging at the lateral mitral annulus
- *Stroke volume, cardiac output, and systemic vascular resistance* (*see* chapter "Stroke Volume, Cardiac Output, and Systemic Vascular Resistance")

  - Pulsed wave Doppler at the outflow tract to obtain the LVOT VTI
    - Used with the LVOT diameter measurement from the parasternal long axis to measure the SV.
    - The SV multiplied by the heart rate estimates the CO. The CO can be used with the mean arterial blood pressure to calculate the systemic vascular resistance. Also, it can be divided by the patient's body surface area to obtain the cardiac index.
- *Grade aortic valve stenosis (see* chapter "Potpourri of Pathology"*)*
  - Continuous wave Doppler through the AV to obtain the AV VTI
    - Used in conjunction with the LV VTI to grade aortic valve stenosis
- *LV to RV size*
  - Visual comparison of LV to RV size
    - Normal RV should be two-thirds the size of LV.
- *RV function*

  Systolic (see chapter "Right Ventricular Systolic Function"*)*
  - Tricuspid annular plane systolic excursion (TAPSE)
  - Tissue Doppler imaging in systole at the lateral tricuspid annulus
  - Visual assessment

  Diastolic (see chapter "Diastolic Function"*)*
  - Pulsed wave Doppler through the tricuspid valve
  - Tissue Doppler imaging at the lateral tricuspid annulus in diastole
- *Aortic valve, mitral valve, and tricuspid valve function and structure*
  - Narrow 2D sector and/or zoom to improve image quality.
  - Stenosis and regurgitation:
    - Use color Doppler flow to visually assess flow/jet velocities through valves.
  - Look for leaflet abnormalities.
- *Intraventricular septum*
  - Narrow 2D sector and/or zoom to improve image quality.
  - Assess for ventricular septal defects by using Doppler color.
- *Left and right atrial size and defects*
  - Narrow 2D sector and/or zoom to improve image quality.
  - Assess for atrial septal defects or patent foramen ovale by using Doppler color.
- *Pericardial effusion*
  - Pericardial effusion appears as an echo-free space between the two layers of the pericardium.
  - Assess if the pericardial effusion is global or localized.
  - If there is presence of a pericardial effusion, assess for evidence of echocardiographic evidence of cardiac tamponade physiology:
    - Duration of atrial collapse (collapse longer than one-third of the cardiac cycle) has a high sensitivity and specificity for cardiac tamponade.
- *Descending aorta*
  - Visualized in cross section near the left atrium.
  - Evaluate for dilation or dissection.
- *Thrombi/masses*
  - Evaluate all four chambers for presence of thrombi or masses.

1.6 Troubleshooting/Pointers

- *Difficulty obtaining a good view*
  - Usually, the window is more inferior and medial in an intubated patient.
  - Occasionally the AP 4 and 5 can be seen from the subxiphoid window.
  - Have the patient lie in a left lateral position to bring the heart more anterior and toward the chest wall.

Suggested Reading

https://www.asecho.org/wp-content/uploads/2018/10/Guidelines-for-Performing-a-Comprehensive-Transthoracic-Echocardiographic-Examination-in-Adults.pdf

https://fpnotebook.com/cv/rad/ApclFrChmbrEchcrdgrmVw.htm

https://intensivecarenetwork.com/lesson/4-basic-cardiac-echo-how-to-pre-reading-for-fcus-course/

https://www.asecho.org/wp-content/uploads/2016/02/2015_ChamberQuantificationREV.pdf

Subxiphoid Cardiac and Inferior Vena Cava Views

Rhea Votipka and Shannon Gaasch

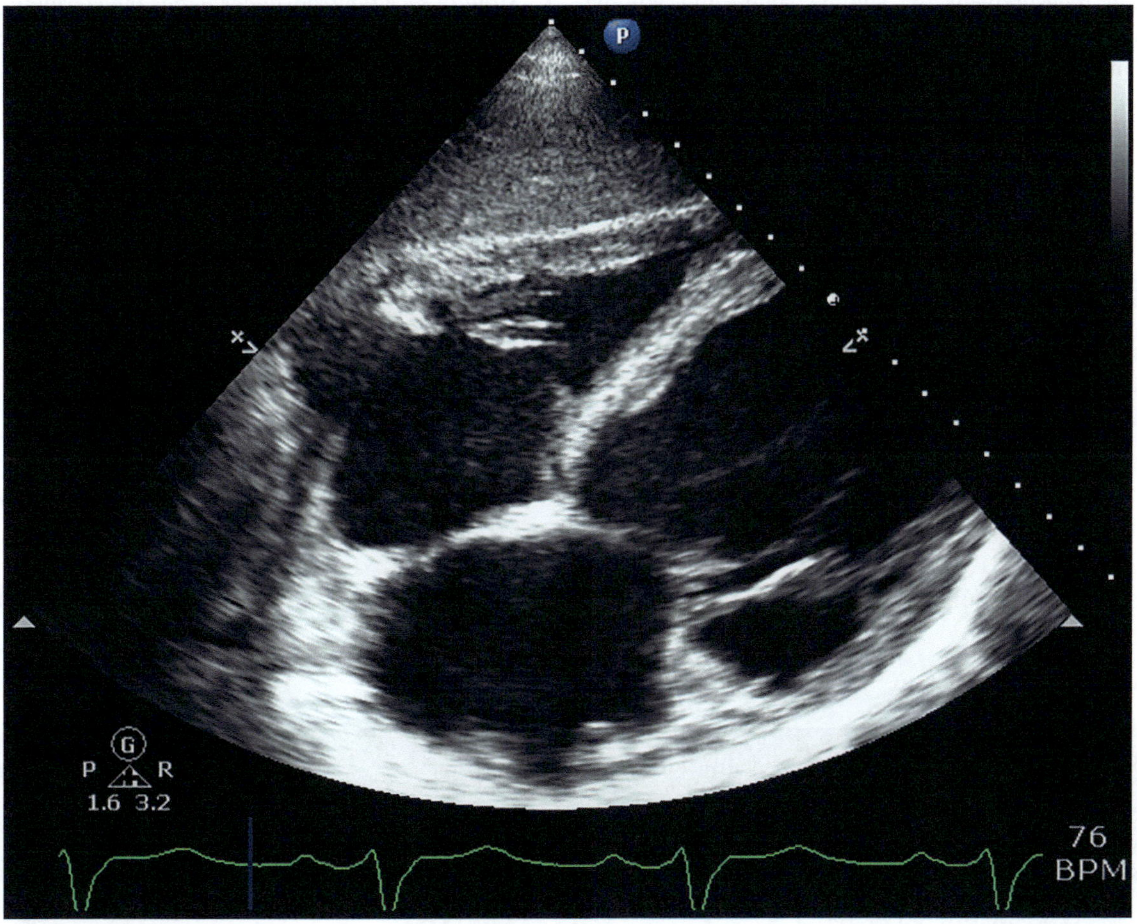

Supplementary Information The online version of this chapter (https://doi.org/10.1007/978-3-030-74687-2_5) contains supplementary material, which is available to authorized users.

R. Votipka
Lahey Hospital and Medical Center, Pulmonary Critical Care Medicine, Burlington, MA, USA

S. Gaasch (✉)
R. Adams Cowley Shock Trauma Center, University of Maryland, Baltimore, MD, USA
e-mail: shannon.gaasch@umm.edu

A. Salerno et al. (eds.), *Atlas of Critical Care Echocardiography*, https://doi.org/10.1007/978-3-030-74687-2_5

1 Introduction

The subxiphoid (SX) view, also referred to as the subcostal, can be helpful in a patient with difficult parasternal or apical windows due to air trapping, high positive end expiratory pressure, or patient anatomy. The SX is the easiest view during cardiac arrest and for rapid assessment of the heart. It is the primary cardiac window in both the Focused Assessment Sonogram for Trauma (FAST) and Rapid Ultrasound in SHock (RUSH) examinations. Using the SX, providers can examine for pericardial effusions, RV dilation, and overall cardiac function. In the same window, with minor adjustments, is the inferior vena cava (IVC). The IVC is responsible for returning blood to the heart and has been considered a surrogate measurement for volume status and volume responsiveness (VR), or the likelihood that the stroke volume will increase with a fluid bolus.

2 Obtaining the Subxiphoid View

The ideal subxiphoid view includes all four chambers of the heart as well as a view of the inferior portion of the pericardium (Fig. 1, left panel). In general, the SX should be performed in cardiac presets, but for the RUSH and FAST, it is done in abdominal presets to allow rapid imaging of both the abdomen and heart in an unstable patient.

- *Overhand grip.*
- *Place the transducer 1–2 cm below the xiphoid process.*
- *Directed underneath the ribcage, toward the patient's left shoulder:*
  - 2-o'clock position, angle typically less the 20°
- *May need to increase depth to 20 cm.*
- *Slightly rock the transducer under the sternum:*
  - Once under the sternum, tilt the face up to open the left ventricle.

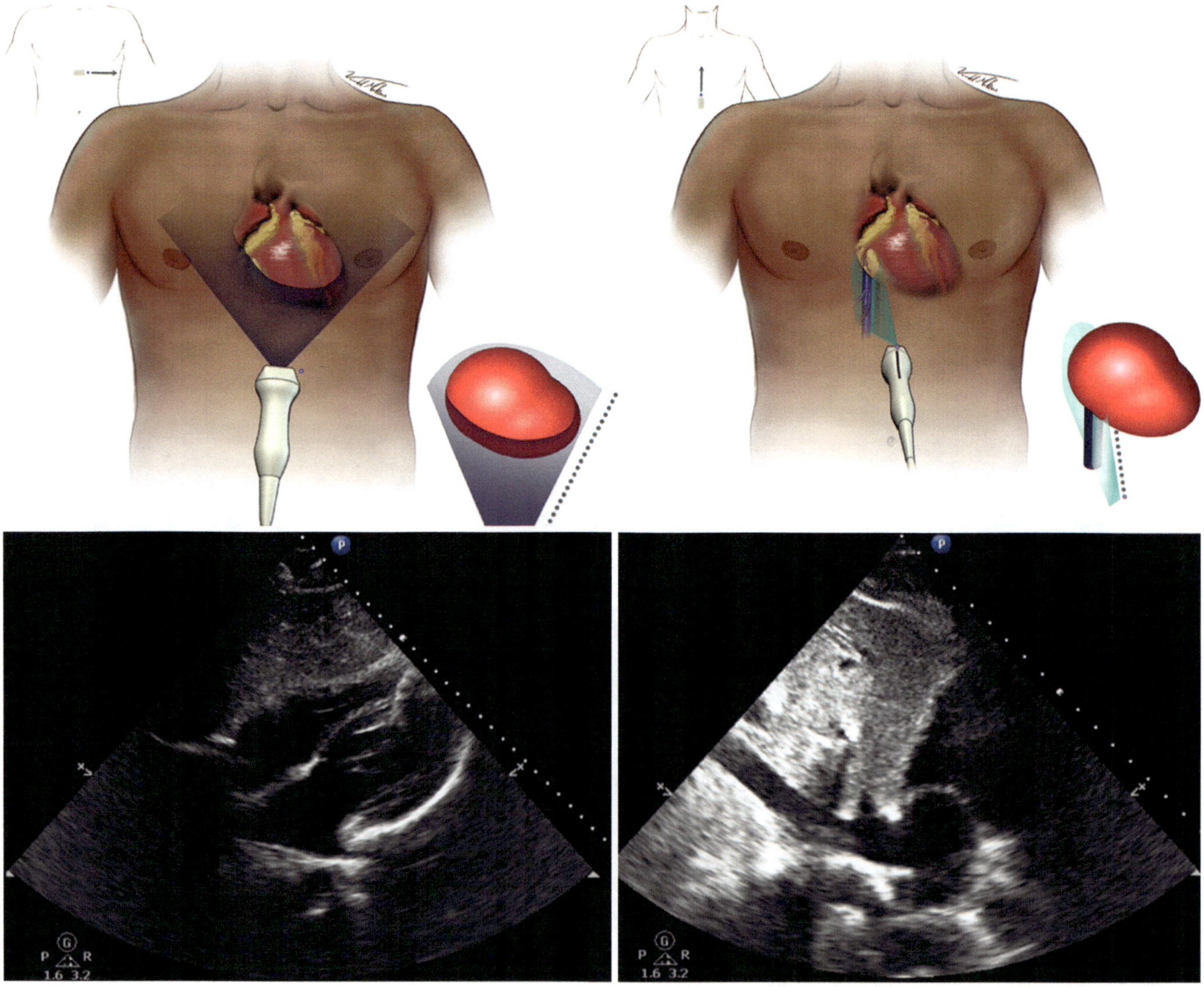

Fig. 1 Obtaining the subxiphoid and inferior vena cava windows. Left panel is the SX. Right panel is the IVC

3 Obtaining the IVC Window

The ideal IVC view is found using a longitudinal approach. It allows visualization of the IVC coursing through the liver, entering the right atrium (Fig. 1, right panel).

- *Place the transducer in the subxiphoid position*
  - Once the right ventricle and atrium are identified, rotate the probe counterclockwise 90°.
  - Longitudinal images are best obtained for IVC measurements (Video 1).
- *The indicator in the cranial or caudal position*
  - 12-o'clock position, transducer aimed up (Fig. 1, left panel).
  - Some centers use the caudal position (indicator aimed down at 6 o'clock); either will open the IVC in long axis.
- *Slightly rock the transducer laterally to the patient's right*
  - Follow the IVC inferiorly as it passes through the liver.
  - Look for the confluence of the hepatic vein with the IVC.
  - The IVC can be differentiated from the aorta by its thinner walls and collapse during respirations.

4 Image Orientation Cardiac Presets

For the subxiphoid view, the indicator is toward the patient's left:

- The left hepatic lobe will be viewed in the near field of the image.
- The subxiphoid four-chamber view of the heart can be found deep to the liver.
  - Indicator on the right of the screen
- For the IVC longitudinal view, the indicator is toward the patient's head (or feet).
  - Indicator on the right of the screen

5 Image Orientation Abdominal Presets for the FAST and RUSH

Abdominal presets are ideal for visceral imaging, not the rapidly moving heart (Fig. 2, Video 2). A slower sweep speed which allows for more scan lines and more compression makes the liver appear smoother and more resolved than it does in cardiac presets. But the moving heart will appear less clear. The FAST and RUSH use abdominal presets to allow rapid imaging of both the heart and abdomen. If a more complete cardiac assessment is needed, then cardiac presets should be used.

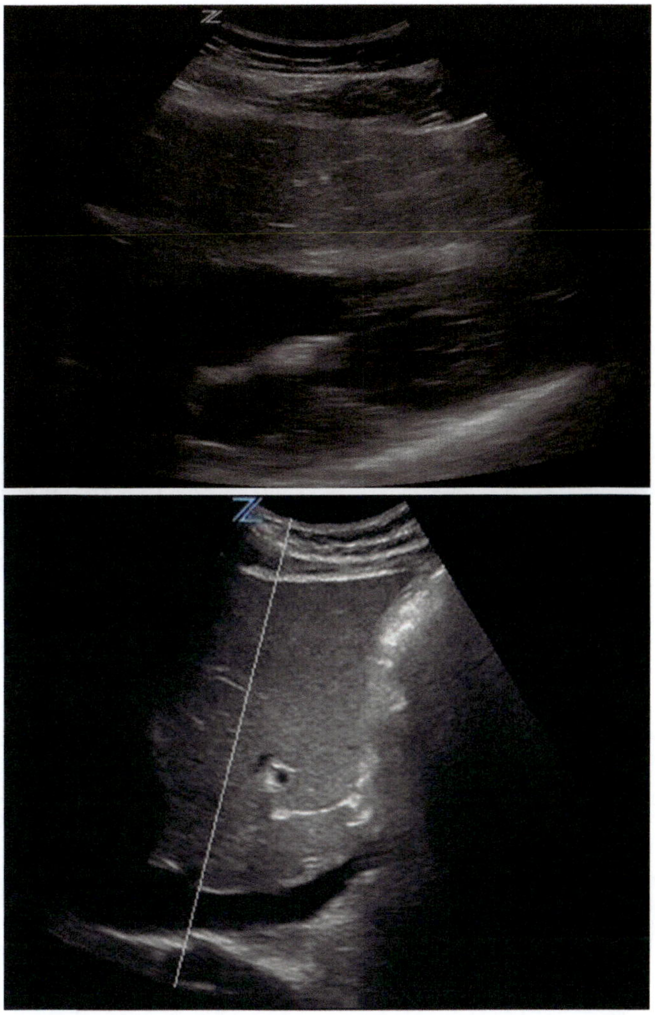

Fig. 2 Subxiphoid (SX) and inferior vena cava (IVC) in abdominal presets. Abdominal presets are used in the FAST and RUSH; note the Z indicator on the left of the image. The upper panel is the SX; the lower panel is the IVC

- SX: the transducer grove is toward the patient's right:
  - Indicator on the left side of the screen
- IVC: the indicator is toward the patient's head:
  - Indicator on the left of the screen

6 Ideal Image

- Subxiphoid view (Fig. 3)
  - Similar to the apical four-chamber view, but the apex is oriented toward the upper right.
  - The RV and LV are triangular in shape with the RV roughly two thirds the size of the LV.
- IVC view (Fig. 4)
  - Visualization of the IVC entering the right atrium
  - Visualization of the hepatic vein entering the IVC

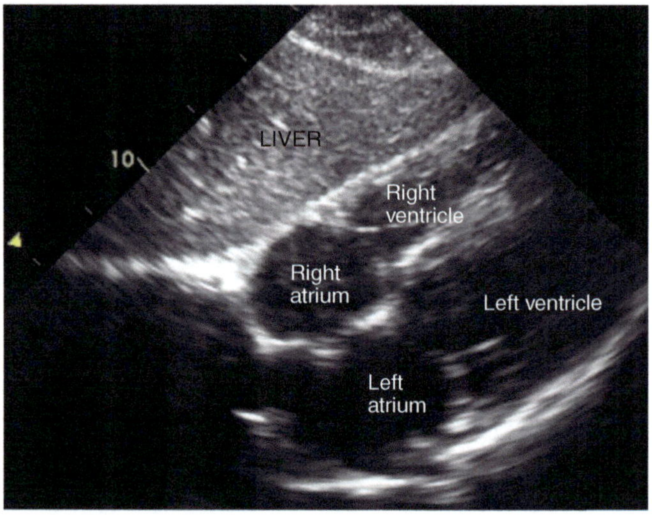

Fig. 3 Ideal subxiphoid (SX) image. In the ideal SX image, the liver, right atrium, right ventricle, left atrium, and left ventricle can be seen

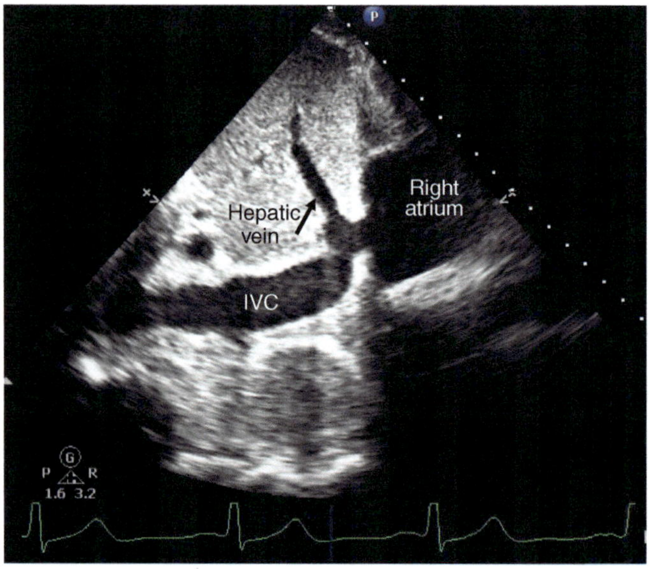

Fig. 4 Ideal inferior vena cava (IVC) image. In the ideal IVC image, the IVC can be seen entering the right atrium and the hepatic vein can be seen entering the IVC

7 Assessments and Measurements

For the subxiphoid view
- RV and LV function
  - Visual assessment
- Biatrial size
- Tricuspid valve
  - Visual assessment
  - Color Doppler
- Mitral valve
- Pericardial effusion

For the IVC view
- IVC diameter
- IVC diameter change with respiration

8 Tips and Pointers

- Subxiphoid view
  - Best obtained in the supine position with relaxed abdominal wall.
  - To improve the view, have the patient take a deep breath in and hold.
  - To relax the abdominal muscles, bend the patient's knees if possible.
  - Recent abdominal surgery, bowel gas, abdominal discomfort, or large abdominal girth may limit the ability to acquire this image.
- IVC view
  - Bowel gas may obstruct view of IVC:
    - Apply slight pressure on the abdomen with the probe to displace the bowel.
  - A plethoric IVC could be indicative of other pathology not just fluid tolerance:
    - RV failure, tricuspid regurgitation, and cardiac tamponade
    - High PEEP and COPD/asthma exacerbation
  - Intra-abdominal hypertension can cause the IVC to be smaller than expected.

Suggested Reading

Denault AY, Langevin S, Lessard MR, Courval JF, Desjardins G. Transthoracic echocardiographic evaluation of the heart and great vessels. Can J Anesth/Journal canadien danesthésie. 2018;65(4):449–72. https://doi.org/10.1007/s12630-018-1068-4.

Millington SJ. Ultrasound assessment of the inferior vena cava for fluid responsiveness: easy, fun, but unlikely to be helpful. Can J Anesth/Journal canadien danesthésie. 2019;66(6):633–8. https://doi.org/10.1007/s12630-019-01357-0.

Mitchell C, Rahko PS, Blauwet LA, Canaday B, Finstuen JA, Foster MC, et al. Guidelines for performing a comprehensive transthoracic echocardiographic examination in adults: recommendations from the American Society of Echocardiography. J Am Soc Echocardiogr. 2019;32(1):1–64.

Via G, Tavazzi G, Price S. Ten situations where inferior vena cava ultrasound may fail to accurately predict fluid responsiveness: a physiologically based point of view. Intensive Care Med. 2016;42(7):1164–7. https://doi.org/10.1007/s00134-016-4357-9.

Liver Doppler

David Gordon and Sarah B. Murthi

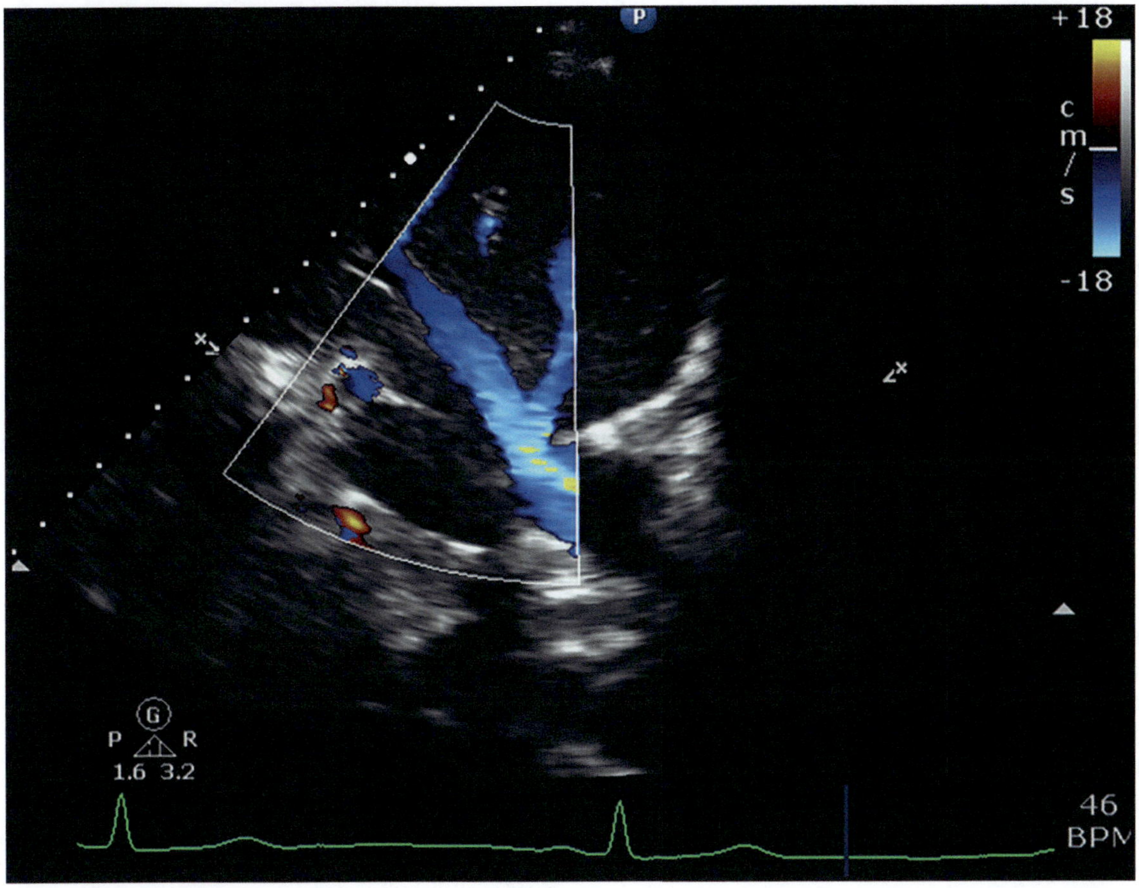

Supplementary Information The online version of this chapter (https://doi.org/10.1007/978-3-030-74687-2_6) contains supplementary material, which is available to authorized users.

D. Gordon
Department of Medicine, University of Maryland School of Medicine, University of Maryland Medical Center, Baltimore, MD, USA

S. B. Murthi (✉)
Department of Surgery, Program in Trauma and Critical Care, R Adams Cowley Shock Trauma Center, University of Maryland School of Medicine, University of Maryland Medical Center, Baltimore, MD, USA
e-mail: smurthi@som.umaryland.edu

A. Salerno et al. (eds.), *Atlas of Critical Care Echocardiography*, https://doi.org/10.1007/978-3-030-74687-2_6

Abbreviations

a	Atrial wave
CFD	Color flow Doppler
D	Diastolic wave
ECG	ElectroCardioGram
IVC	Inferior vena cava
PWD	Pulsed wave Doppler
S	Systolic wave
SX	Subxiphoid

1 Introduction

Assessing for evidence of venous congestion is an important element in fluid management. Elevations in atrial pressure resulting from excessive fluid boluses can cause venous congestion which results in decreased resorption of plasma in the capillary beds causing tissue edema and organ dysfunction. Venous congestion on the left side presents as pulmonary edema and respiratory dysfunction. Often diffuse B lines are present and can be seen with ultrasound. Elevated right atrial pressure is harder to detect clinically. Interestingly changes in the portal and hepatic venous pulsed wave Doppler (PWD) waveforms reflect elevations in right atrial pressure causing venous congestion. The Chapter Right Atrial Pressure describes how to interpret the findings.

2 Obtaining the Hepatic PWD

The hepatic and portal veins can be seen from the subxiphoid (SX) window. If the patient has had abdominal surgery or has an open abdomen, then the transducer may be placed somewhere between the midclavicular line and anterior axillary line below the rib cage on the patient's right. Color flow Doppler (CFD) is useful in identifying measurable flow.

- Phased array probe
  - Cardiac presets/exam type
  - ECG leads in place
- From the subxiphoid (SX) window fan to the patient's right (Fig. 1)
- Surgical incision, open abdomen, or disrupted SX window
  - Find space between the midclavicular line and anterior axillary line.
  - Identify the hepatic veins entering the inferior vena cava (IVC).
- Indicator toward the patient's head
- Rock and fan until the ideal image is obtained (Fig. 2)

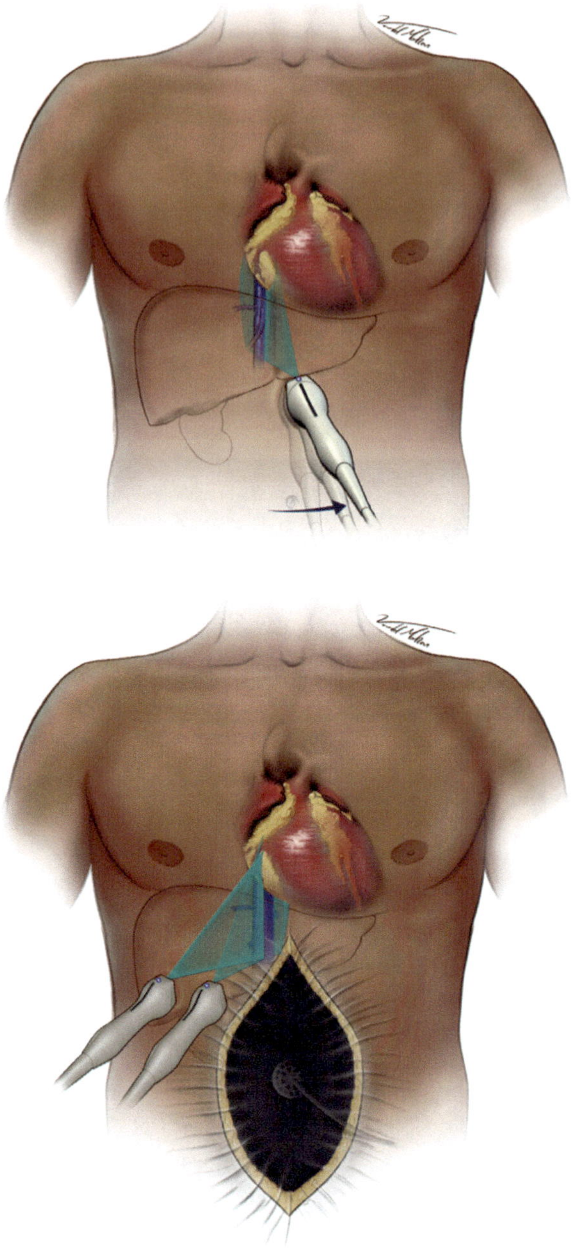

Fig. 1 Hepatic and portal vein transducer placement. *Upper panel*, most common probe location. *Lower panel*, placement if the subxiphoid window is disrupted

- Identify the hepatic veins draining into the IVC
  - The hepatic vein is a large hypoechoic thin-walled vessel.
- Apply color flow Doppler to identify the area of measurable blood flow (Video 1)
- Select PWD to activate cursor
  - Set cursor location.
  - Optimize the gate.
- Select PWD again to activate tracing

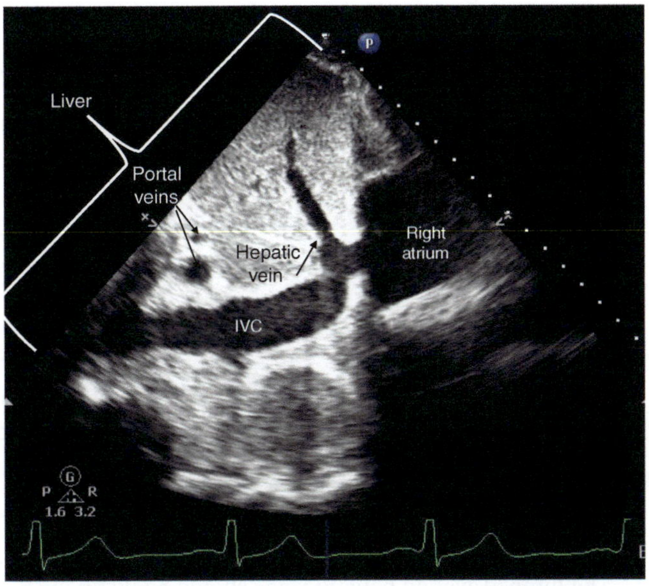

Fig. 2 Ideal image of the hepatic and portal veins. IVC inferior vena cava

- Record tracing
- *Normal hepatic venous waveform* (Fig. 3)
  - Atrial contraction (a) waveform
    - Above the baseline.
    - Blood flows retrograde toward the transducer.
    - Occurs just before the QRS wave on the ECG tracing.
  - Systolic (S) filling waveform
    - Below the baseline.
    - Blood flows rapidly into the right atrium away from the transducer. With normal flow systolic velocity is higher then diastolic velocity.
    - Occurs in the middle of the QRS.
    - The first waveform on or after the QRS.
  - Diastolic (D) filling waveform
    - Below the baseline.
    - Blood flows into the right atrium away from the transducer.
    - The second waveform after the S.
      - On the T-wave of the ECG

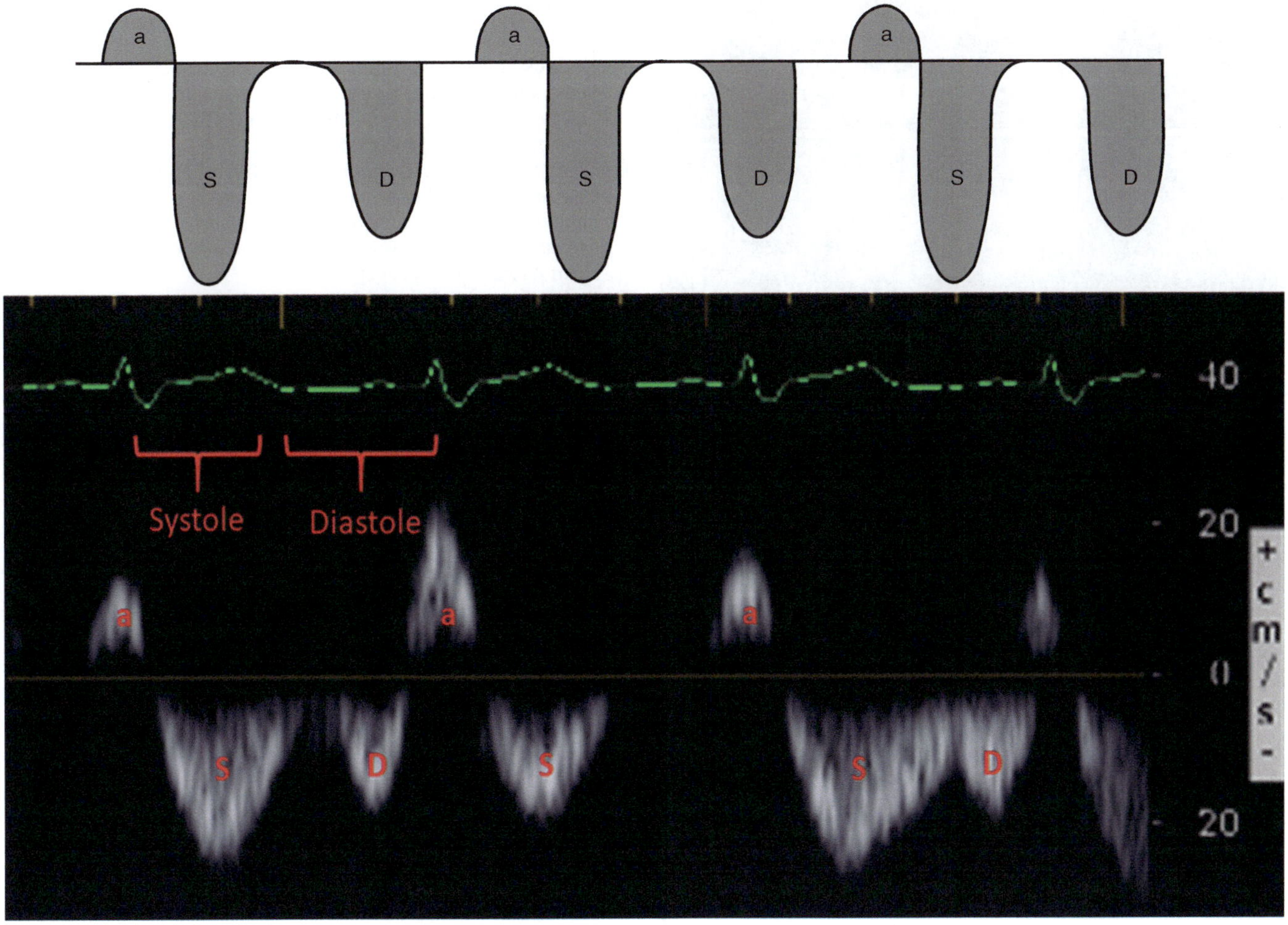

Fig. 3 Identifying the atrial contraction (a), systole (S), and diastole (D) waves of the hepatic vein

3 Obtaining the Portal Pulsed Wave Doppler

- Initial setup is identical to hepatic assessment
- Identify a portal vein (see Fig. 2)
  - Smaller, thicker-walled, hyperechoic vessels
  - Usually seen in cross section so they appear round
- Apply color flow Doppler to identify the area of measurable blood flow
- Select PWD to activate cursor
  - Set cursor location.
  - Optimize the gate.
- Select PWD again to activate tracing
- Record tracing
- *Normal portal waveform* (Fig. 4)
  - Continuous flow above the baseline
  - May sometimes see the hepatic arterial flow superimposed over the portal:
    - This is not portal vein pulsatility.
    - Try to adjust the sample window to only have portal flow.

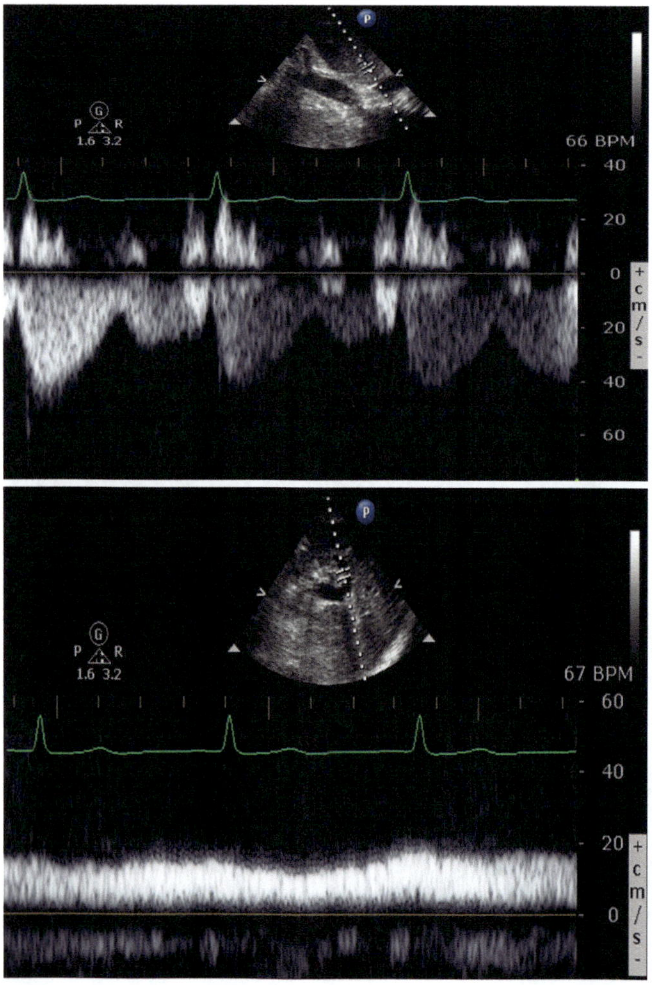

Fig. 4 Normal hepatic and portal vein pulsed wave Doppler. *Upper panel*, normal hepatic venous flow. *Lower panel*, normal portal venous flow

4 Tips and Pointers

- Portal flow is easier to interpret, but hepatic flow is easier to obtain.
- It is possible to assess hepatic flow without an ECG, but it is less reliable especially in atrial fibrillation. Also there is often noise above the baseline, and it can be difficult to identify the a-wave.
  - Find the a-wave above the baseline.
  - The next wave is the S-wave followed by the D-wave.
- The thinned-walled hepatic veins should be distinguished from the thick hyperechoic walled portal vein, and can be seen entering the IVC.

Suggested Reading

Spiegel RS, Teeter W, Sullivan S, Tupchong K, Mohammed N, Sutherland M, et al. The use of venous Doppler to predict adverse kidney events in a general ICU cohort. Crit Care. 2020;24:615. https://doi.org/10.1186/s13054-020-03330-6.

Beaubien-Souligny W, Benkreira A, Robillard P, Bouabdallaoui N, Chasse M, Desjardins G, et al. Alterations in portal vein flow and intrarenal venous flow are associated with acute kidney injury after cardiac surgery: a prospective observational cohort study. J Am Heart Assoc. 2018;7(19):e009961.

Gallix BP, Taourel P, Dauzat M, Bruel JM, Lafortune M. Flow pulsatility in the portal venous system: a study of Doppler sonography in healthy adults. AJR Am J Roentgenol. 1997;169(1):141–4.

Renal Doppler

Sarah B. Murthi

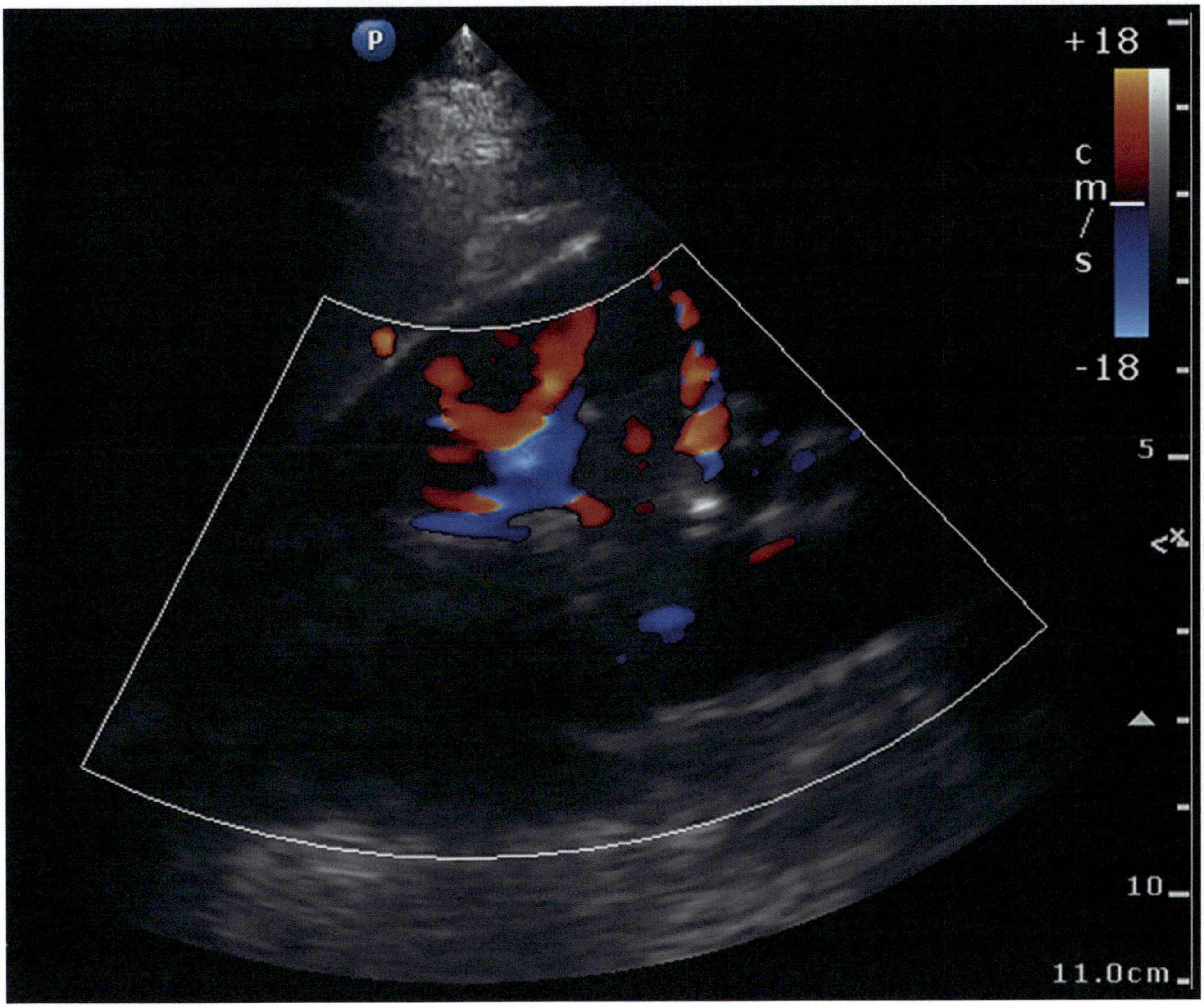

S. B. Murthi (✉)
Department of Surgery, Program in Trauma and Critical Care,
R Adams Cowley Shock Trauma Center, University of Maryland
School of Medicine, University of Maryland Medical Center,
Baltimore, MD, USA
e-mail: smurthi@som.umaryland.edu

A. Salerno et al. (eds.), *Atlas of Critical Care Echocardiography*, https://doi.org/10.1007/978-3-030-74687-2_7

Abbreviations

CFD	Color flow Doppler
EDV	End-diastolic velocity
PSV	Peak systolic velocity
PWD	Pulsed wave Doppler
RAP	Right atrial pressure
RRI	Renal resistive index

1 Introduction

Acute renal failure is associated with increased mortality in critically ill patients. Doppler ultrasound of the kidney holds promise as a novel form of monitoring renal perfusion. Measures of venous congestion may indicate when fluid is becoming harmful, while the assessment of renal arterial flow may help detect early acute renal injury.

2 Obtaining the Renal Doppler Image

- Phased array transducer or curvilinear transducer.
  - Abdominal exam type
- From the liver window, move inferiorly 1–2 cm and laterally 1–2 cm:
  - Between the anterior axillary and midclavicular lines
  - Around the 11–12th rib space (Fig. 1, upper panel)
- Transducer indicator toward the patient's head.
- Adjust the depth to the center on the kidney; fan and rock to obtain the ideal image (Fig. 1, lower panel):
  - The liver will be on top of the kidney.
- Apply color flow Doppler (CFD) (Fig. 2).
  - Optimize the scale:
    - If in cardiac presets, you will need to decrease the scale.
    - If in abdominal presets, the scale is usually correct.
    - Most patients fall between 15 and 18 cm/sec.
    - If unable to see color flow at 10 cm/sec, it likely will not be able to measure with PWD.
- Select pulsed wave Doppler (PWD); place the sample area in a region of high flow.

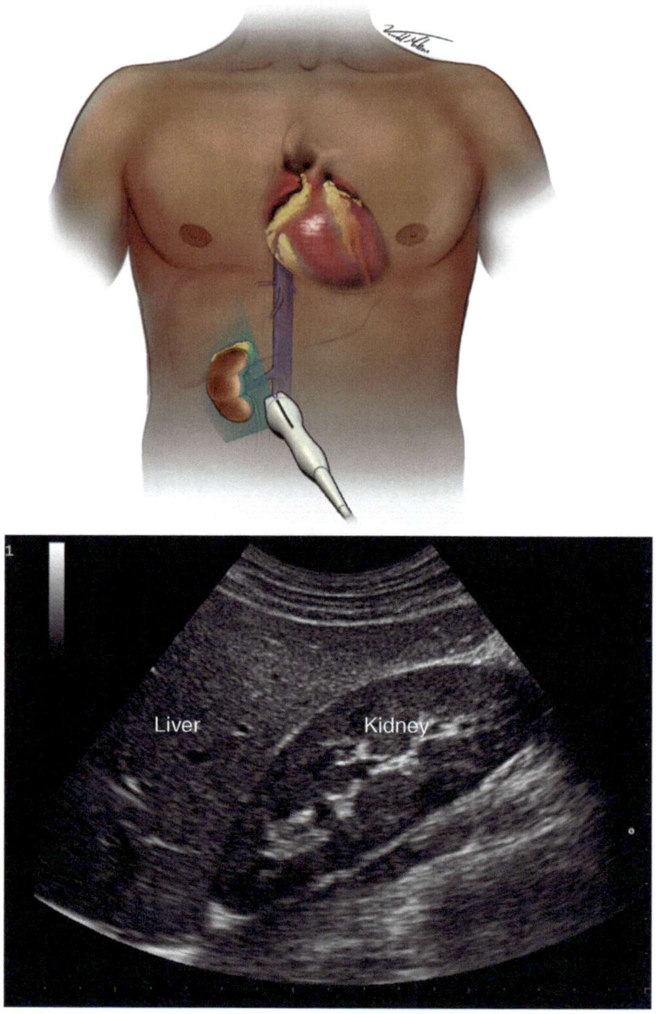

Fig. 1 Transducer placement for renal assessment. Upper panel: Correct transducer placement. The probe is placed with the indicator cephalad between the anterior axillary and midclavicular lines. Lower panel: Ideal image of the kidney

- Select PWD again to obtain waveform.
- Adjust scale and baseline to optimize PWD waveform.
- Try to obtain a tracing in which both arterial and venous flow can be seen:
  - The artery is above the baseline and the vein is below it.
  - Sometimes only one flow pattern can be optimized.
  - Save the image.

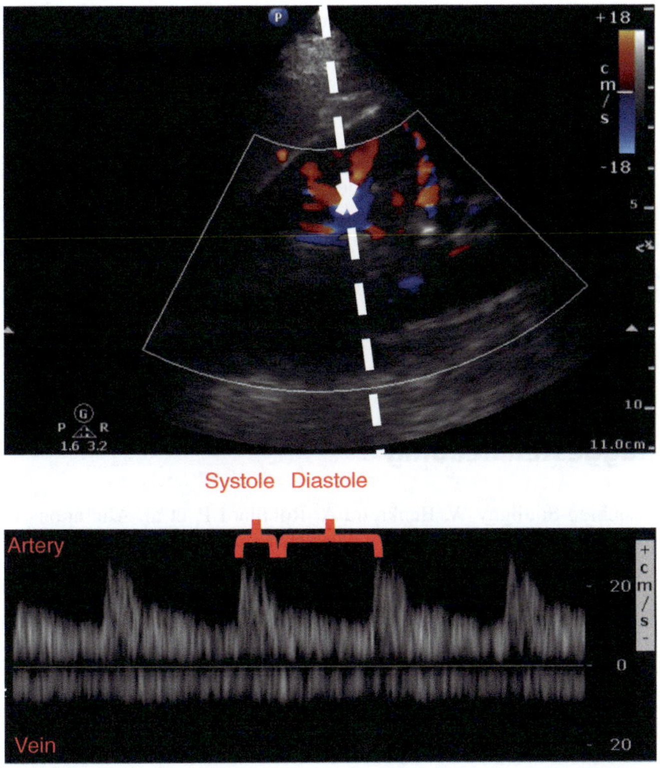

Fig. 2 Renal pulsed wave Doppler. Upper panel: color flow Doppler. The PWD cursor is placed in an area of high flow; ideal sample volume placement is marked with a white X. Lower panel: Pulsed wave Doppler tracing. Arterial flow is above the baseline. Venous flow is below the baseline

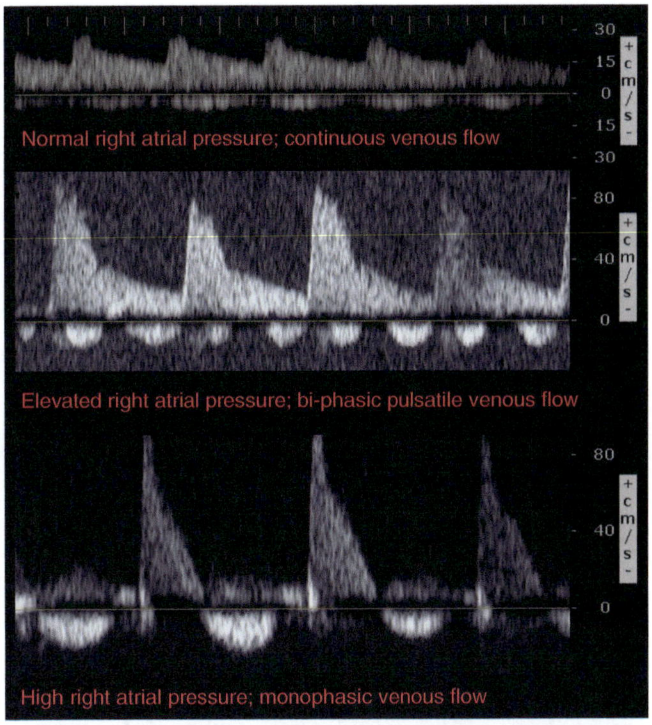

Fig. 3 Changes in renal venous flow with increases in right atrial pressure. Upper panel: Normal venous flow. Flow is continuous throughout the cycle. Middle panel: elevated right atrial pressure causes venous congestion creating a biphasic pulse in the vein, so there is no drainage during parts of systole and diastole. Lower panel: High right atrial pressure results in monophasic diastolic flow. There is no venous drainage during systole

3 Renal Venous Assessments

Elevations in right atrial pressure (RAP) from fluid boluses and right ventricular dysfunction can cause venous congestion (Fig. 3). There is more data in heart failure, but recently there is interest in using venous flow changes as an indication that ongoing fluid boluses are becoming harmful, and perhaps diuresis is indicated in shock with normal cardiac function. How to use renal, portal, and hepatic flow to assess RAP is discussed in "Right Atrial Pressure Assessment".

- Normal renal venous flow is continuous, minor pulsations may be present, but there is flow throughout the cardiac cycle.
- As RAP becomes elevated, flow becomes clearly biphasic and pulsatile, with no flow in between systole and diastole.
- With high RAP renal venous flow transitions to monophasic with no systolic venous flow.

4 Renal Arterial Assessments

How to use the renal arterial Doppler flow pattern in shock is not yet established, but it is intriguing that the arterial and venous flow patterns can be seen at the same time. It is possible that in the future, this could lead to renal-protective resuscitation in shock.

- The renal resistive index (RRI) (Fig. 4):
  - (PSV-EDV)/PSV
    - PSV: peak systolic velocity
    - EDV: end-diastolic velocity (lowest diastolic velocity)
- With normal renal artery flow, there is inflow throughout the cardiac cycle; with renal injury there is more resistance to flow and lower diastolic velocities, so the RRI increases.
- RRI >0.7 is associated with high risk of developing AKI in septic patients.

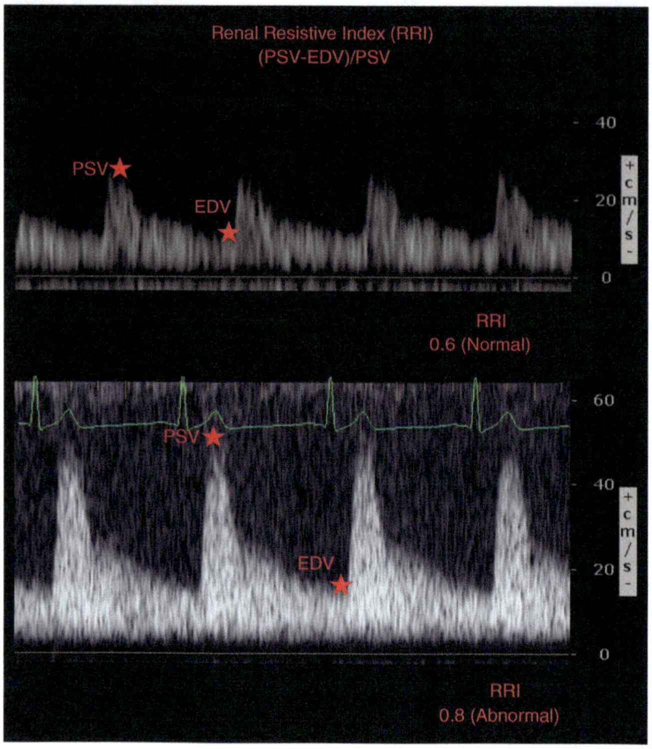

Fig. 4 Renal resistive index (RRI). Upper panel: Normal RRI. PSV peak systolic velocity, EDV end-diastolic velocity. Lower panel: High RRI

5 Troubleshooting and Pointers

- Patients with severe kidney injury or requiring renal replacement may not have measurable PWD waveform:
  - If unable to see CFD despite optimizing the scale or gain, then PWD cannot be assessed.
    - Color flow is a type of pulsed wave Doppler.
- Renal resistive index requires measurement of peak flow, which is dependent on the angle of acquisition and user experience:
  - Although it is an active area of research, there is no clear use for RRI in the management of shock.
- Visual assessments of renal venous flow pattern changes may be less dependent on obtaining ideal images:
  - May indicate when to transition from fluid resuscitation to diuresis

Suggested Reading

Beaubien-Souligny W, Benkreira A, Robillard P, et al. Alterations in portal vein flow and intrarenal venous flow are associated with acute kidney injury after cardiac surgery: a prospective observational cohort study. J Am Heart Assoc. 2018;7(19):e009961.

Haitsma Mulier JLG, Rozemeijer S, Röttgering JG, Spoelstra-de Man AME, Elbers PWG, Tuinman PR, de Waard MC, Oudemans-van Straaten HM. Renal resistive index as an early predictor and discriminator of acute kidney injury in critically ill patients; A prospective observational cohort study. PLoS One. 2018;13(6):e0197967. https://doi.org/10.1371/journal.pone.0197967. PMID: 29889830; PMCID: PMC5995360.

Husain-Syed F, Birk HW, Ronco C, Schörmann T, Tello K, Richter MJ, Wilhelm J, Sommer N, Steyerberg E, Bauer P, Walmrath HD, Seeger W, McCullough PA, Gall H, Ghofrani HA. Doppler-derived renal venous stasis index in the prognosis of right heart failure. J Am Heart Assoc. 2019;8(21):e013584. https://doi.org/10.1161/JAHA.119.013584. Epub 2019 Oct 19. PMID: 31630601; PMCID: PMC6898799.

Thoracic Ultrasound

Emily Hart and Sarah B. Murthi

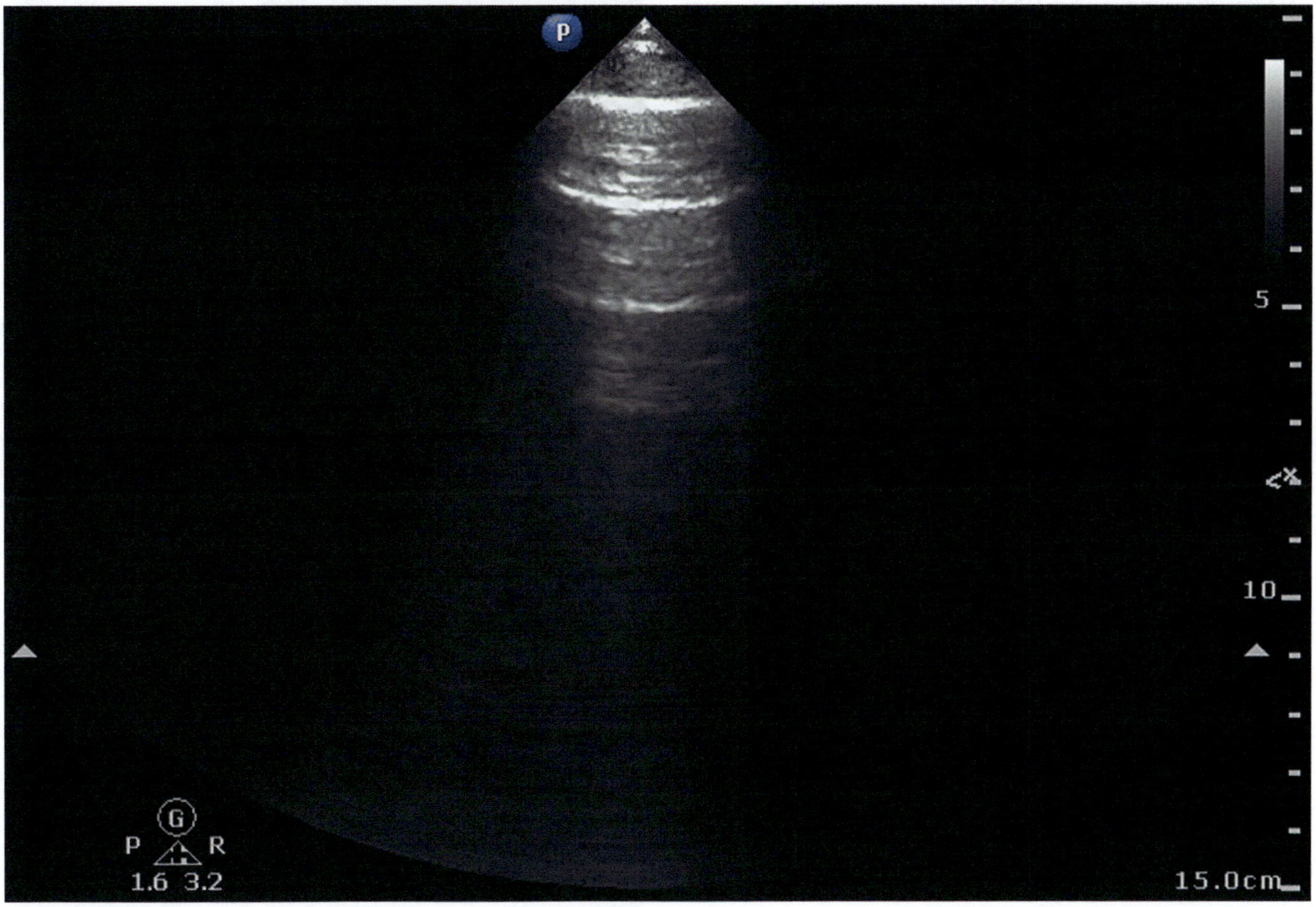

E. Hart
R. Adams Cowley Shock Trauma Center, University of Maryland, Baltimore, MD, USA

S. B. Murthi (✉)
Department of Surgery, Program in Trauma and Critical Care, R Adams Cowley Shock Trauma Center, University of Maryland School of Medicine, University of Maryland Medical Center, Baltimore, MD, USA
e-mail: smurthi@som.umaryland.edu

A. Salerno et al. (eds.), *Atlas of Critical Care Echocardiography*, https://doi.org/10.1007/978-3-030-74687-2_8

Abbreviations

FAST	Focused Assessment Sonogram for Trauma
FREE	Focused Rapid Echocardiographic Evaluation
POCUS	Point-of-Care Ultrasound
RUSH	Rapid Ultrasound for Hypotension

1 Introduction

Lung ultrasonography has gained popularity over the past decade among emergency and critical care providers. Point-of-care ultrasonography (POCUS) is a noninvasive, minimally disruptive bedside exam that provides real-time visualization of structures within the chest cavity including ribs, pleura, lung, heart, and great vessels. POCUS lung examinations are often used to help providers identify and differentiate the pathology of respiratory failure including pleural effusion and pneumothorax. It can also be a useful tool in evaluating for pulmonary edema from elevated left atrial pressure. Lung imaging is a standard part of the Focused Assessment Sonogram for Trauma (FAST), the Rapid Ultrasound for Hypotension (RUSH), and the Focused Rapid Echocardiographic Evaluation (FREE).

There is a growing body of literature on using lung ultrasound to diagnose consolidation and pneumonia, which is beyond the scope of this book. In this and related chapters, we focus on its role in diagnosing the etiology of shock, and in assessment of volume status when used in conjunction with echocardiography.

2 Uses for Thoracic Ultrasound in Shock

- Immediate information is available to help tailor a diagnosis and guide treatment for patients with hypotension.
- It allows for rapid, accurate diagnosis of pneumothorax with greater sensitivity and specificity then chest X-ray.
- It is faster, less expensive, and less radiation compared to conventional imaging.

3 Obtaining the Thoracic Views

- *Transducer selection* (Fig. 1)
  - Tailored to the purpose of the exam
  - Phased array transducer (Fig. 1a)
    - Small footprint
      - Only able to image one rib space at a time
    - Lower frequency, deeper imaging
    - Used for cardiac imaging and the FAST (by some providers)

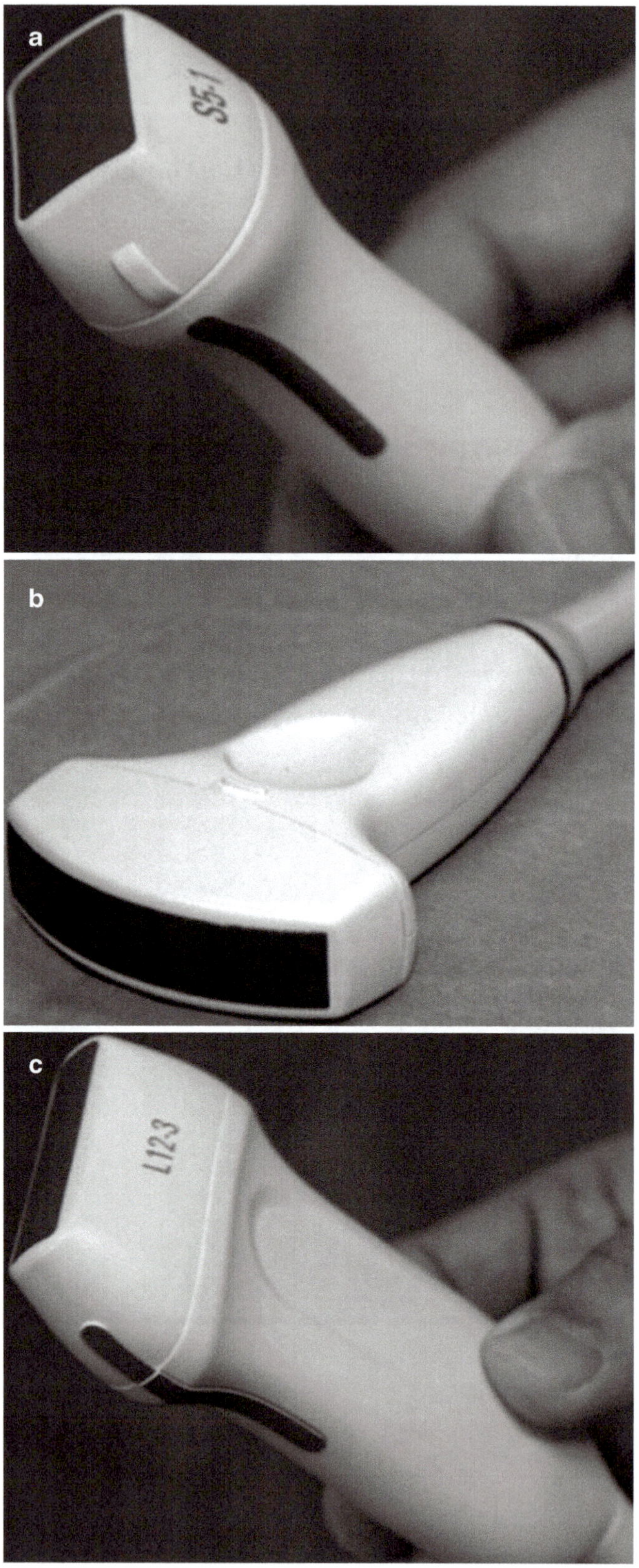

Fig. 1 Lung ultrasound transducers. **Panel A**, Phased array transducer; **Panel B**, Curvilinear transducer; **Panel C**, Linear high-frequency transducer

        - Often used when lung imaging is added to these assessments
    - *Primary use*: superficial, rapid assessment of pneumothorax and hemothorax
  - Curvilinear transducer (Fig. 1b)
    - Visualization of deeper structures
    - Covers a large surface area
        - Able to see multiple rib spaces
    - *Primary use*: thorough exam of the entire thorax
  - High-frequency linear transducer (Fig. 1c)
    - High-frequency, more superficial imaging
    - Able to see 1–2 rib spaces
    - *Primary use*: detailed examination of the pleura and confirmation and diagnosis of pneumothorax
- *Patient positioning*
  - Largely depends on the indication.
  - Allow gravity to work in your favor:
    - Fluid collects in the most dependent regions of the chest:
        - Inferiorly above the diaphragm
    - Air accumulates in the least dependent areas:
        - Apices of the lungs
  - Consider laying the patient flat to look for pneumothorax anteriorly.
  - Consider raising the head of the bed to evaluate for intrathoracic fluid.
  - Place the patient in the lateral decubitus position to allow imaging posterior, dorsal lung fields.
- *Imaging techniques*
  - Simplified rapid assessment (Fig. 2)
    - Lung imaging is an important part of the FAST, RUSH, and FREE protocols. The exams are described in detailed in their respective chapters.
    - Rapid 1–3-minute assessments.
    - RUSH and FAST
        1. Transducer and exam type/preset used for abdominal imaging.
        2. 1–2 cm off the sternum, around the 2–4th rib space.
        3. Adjust the depth to optimize pleural imaging:
            - Assessing the pleura for large pneumothorax causing hypotension
    - FAST
        1. As part of the right and left upper quadrant window, the transducer is fanned into the lower, posterior part of the chest.
            - Assessing for hemothorax from traumatic injury
    - FREE
        1. Change from cardiac to lung imaging presets/exam type
        2. Three anterior zones on each lung
            - Assessing for B-lines indicating pulmonary edema
  - Comprehensive dedicated lung evaluation (Fig. 3)
    - Dedicated lung exam, 10–15 minutes.
    - Divide each lung into six regions (anterior, lateral, and posterior; upper and lower) to total six zones in each lung. Every zone should be systematically examined to ensure comprehensive coverage of the entire thorax:
        1. Start with the probe placed perpendicular to the ribs and slide midline to the patient's lateral side. Repeat in each lung zone.
        2. Flip transducer 90° for parallel scanning in each zone.
        3. Move the probe to the right flank to examine the inferior thoracic space. In a coronal plane, tilt angle superiorly to visualize the diaphragm. Repeat on the left.

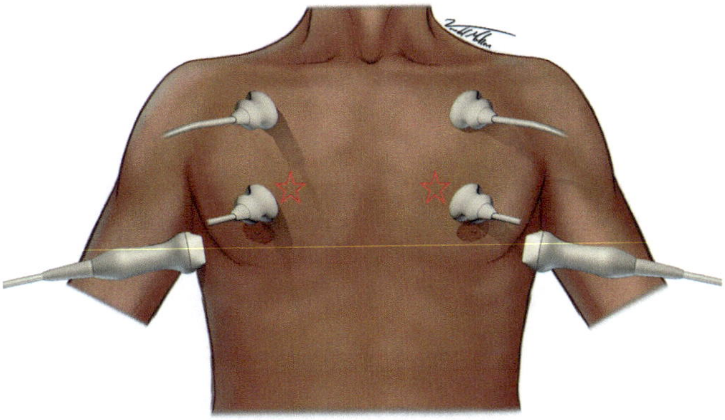

Fig. 2 Rapid lung ultrasound assessments. The anterior views displayed are part of the FREE exam. The stars indicate the fields in the FAST and RUSH exams

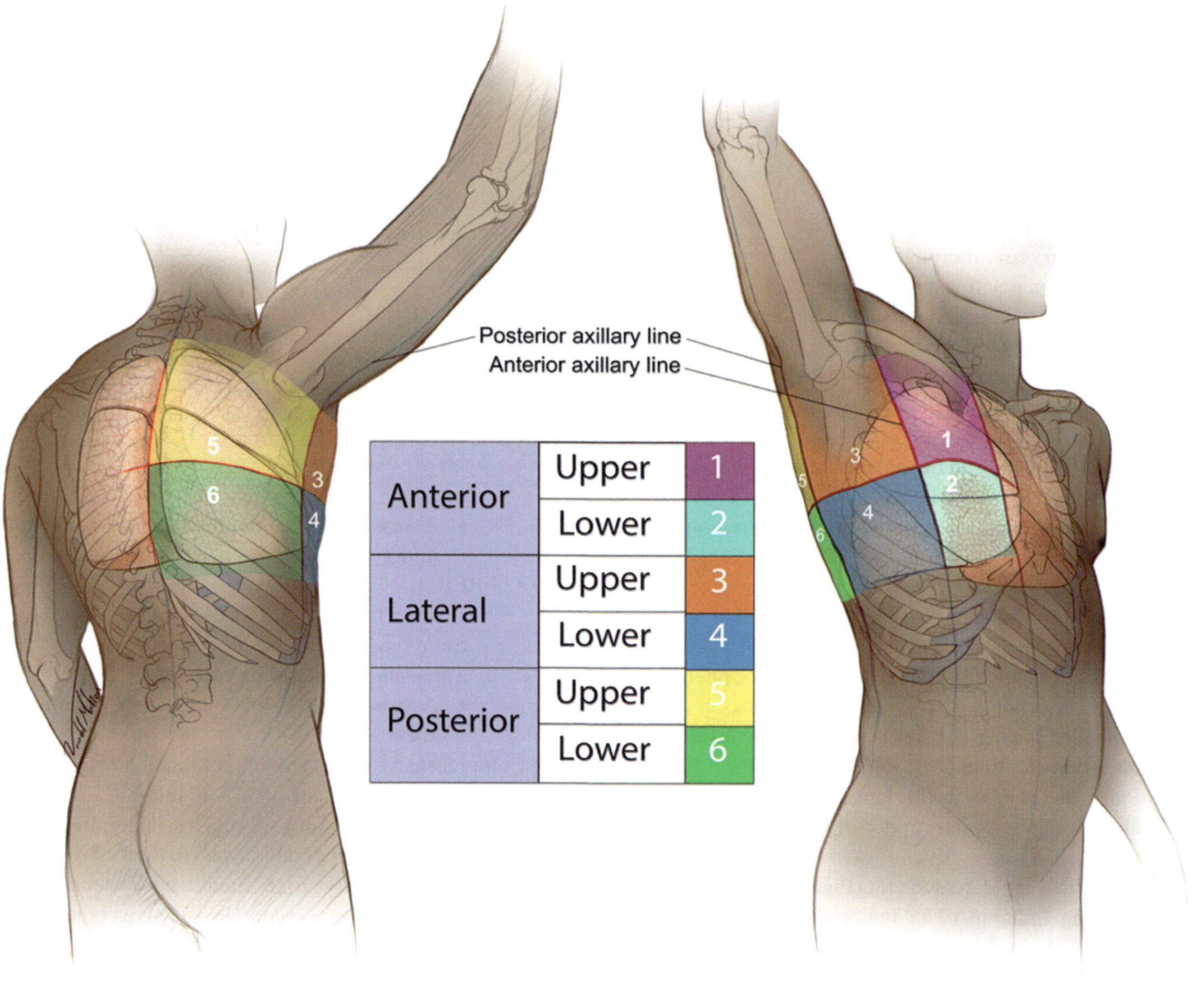

Fig. 3 Comprehensive lung exam. Displayed are the six zones of the right lung. A comprehensive exam is repeated on the left, for a total of 12 lung zones

4 Normal Anatomical Structures (Fig. 4)

- *Chest wall*
  - Echogenic soft tissue
- *Ribs*
  - Located just below the chest wall.
  - Hyperechoic continuous smooth line of the anterior cortex is seen in conjunction with posterior acoustic shadowing.
- *Pleura*
  - Hyperechoic horizontal line comprised of both the visceral and parietal portions of the pleura.
    - Located just below the ribs
  - The pleural line will slide back and forth synchronously with respiration and has been described as the bat sign with the pleural line moving in between the acoustic shadowing of two ribs.
  - Differentiation between the two pleural structures is challenging to visualize separately unless using a higher-frequency probe.

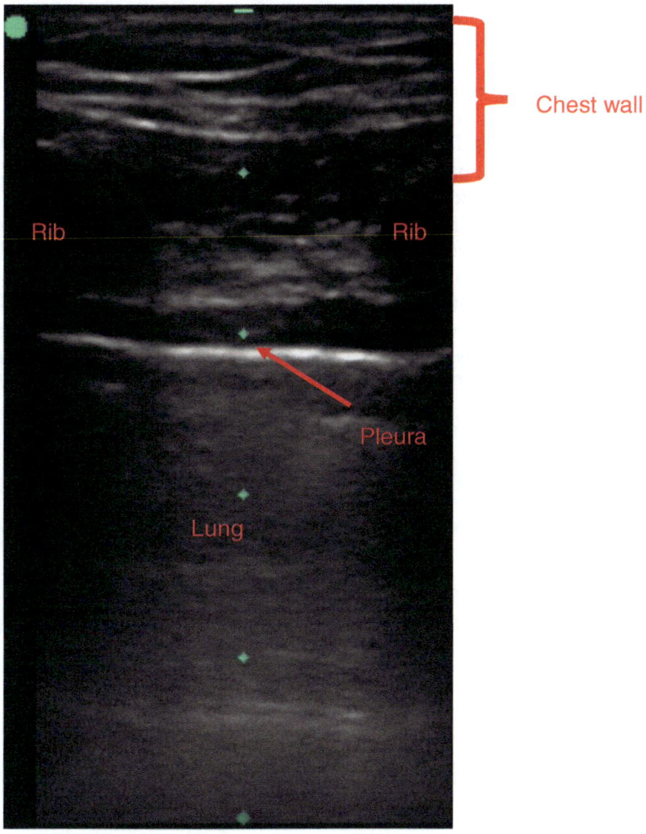

Fig. 4 Normal lung anatomy. This is an image of the lung acquired with a high-frequency linear transducer

5 Artifacts (Fig. 5)

- *A-lines* (see Fig. 4)
  - Normal lung parenchyma is air filled and therefore not visualized with ultrasound because the signal does not return to the transducer. A lines are a reverberation artifact that occur from the signal bouncing back and forth between the visceral and parietal pleura. A-lines are a normal finding and signify healthy open lung.
  - A-lines are horizontal, stationary, regularly spaced hyperechoic lines which represent reverberations of the pleura through a normal lung.
- *B-lines* (see Fig. 4)
  - Discrete hyperechoic reverberation artifacts that originate from the pleural line and extend toward the bottom of the ultrasound screen.
  - Evidence of three or more B-lines in multiple intercostal spaces bilaterally suggests lung interstitial fluid due to pulmonary edema or can be a sign of ARDS.
  - B-lines localized to one or two lung regions may be more consistent with pneumonia or other localized lung process such as pulmonary contusion.

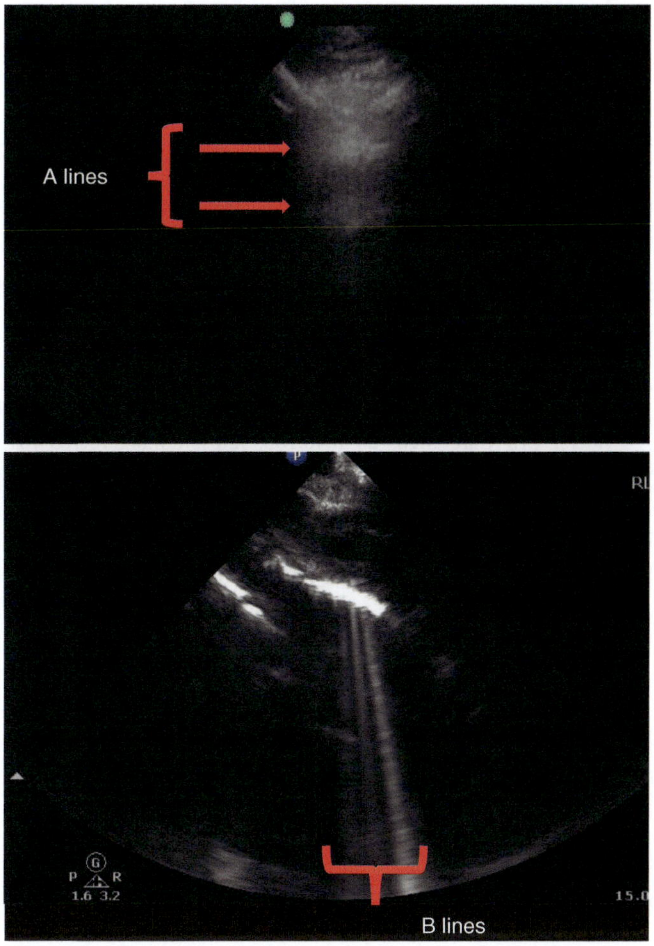

Fig. 5 Lung artifacts. Upper panel: Image of a normal lung with A-lines obtained with a low-frequency transducer. Lower panel: Pathologic B-lines

6 Tips and Pointers

- Obtain confirmatory imaging when time and patient stability allow it.
- Perform the exam the same way every time to make interpretation easier.
- Healthy individuals may have B-lines present in the lower lung portions.

7 Special Considerations

- Clinical context is important:
  - In the FAST pleural fluid is likely blood, whereas in an ICU patient, it is most often an effusion.
  - B-lines indicating lung interstitial fluid can be caused by various pathologies:

  - Interstitial pneumonia or pneumonitis
  - Diffuse parenchymal lung disease (i.e., pulmonary fibrosis)
  - Acute lung injury or acute respiratory distress syndrome (ARDS)
- This is a limited discussion of lung ultrasound in shock, not a comprehensive description of its utility in respiratory distress.

Suggested Reading

Acero NM, Quinn C, Mihm F, Hennessey E. 1127: Lung ultrasound. Crit Care Med. 2018;46:547. https://doi.org/10.1097/01.ccm.0000529132.11016.9e.

Chen L, Mead E, D'Agostino R, Halpern N. Point-of-care ultrasound training program for critical care medicine advanced practice providers. Crit Care Med. 2018;46:163. https://doi.org/10.1097/01.ccm.0000528380.35273.a9.

Irwin Z, Cook JO. Advances in point-of-care thoracic ultrasound. Emerg Med Clin N Am. 2016;34(1):151–7. http://ovidsp.ovid.com/ovidweb.cgi?&T=JS&PAGE=reference&MODE=ovidclassic&CSC=y&NEWS=n&D=mesx,prem,mesz,medp&SEARCH=26614246.ui. https://doi.org/10.1016/j.emc.2015.09.003.

Lichtenstein DA. BLUE-Protocol and FALLS-Protocol: two applications of lung ultrasound in the critically ill. Chest. 2015;147(6):1659–70. https://doi.org/10.1378/chest.14-1313.

Mojoli F, Bouhemad B, Mongodi S, Lichtenstein D. Lung ultrasound for critically ill patients. Am J Respir Crit Care Med. 2019;199(6):701–14. https://doi.org/10.1164/rccm.201802-0236CI.

Singh S, Kaur H, Singh S, Khawaja I. Basic insights of lung ultrasonography in critical care setting. Cureus. 2018;10(12):e3702. Published 2018 Dec 7. https://doi.org/10.7759/cureus.3702.

Volpicelli G. Point-of-care lung ultrasound. Praxis. 2014;103(12):711–6. http://ovidsp.ovid.com/ovidweb.cgi?&T=JS&PAGE=reference&MODE=ovidclassic&CSC=y&NEWS=n&D=mesx,prem,mesz,medp&SEARCH=24894615.ui. https://doi.org/10.1024/1661-8157/a001690.

Part II

Measurements and Interpretation

During and after cardiac imaging it is useful to do qualitative and quantitative assessments of volume status, cardiac function, and volume status. The measurements allow informed decision making about the cause of shock and can help guide resuscitation. Also learning how to do them will improve the quality of your global assessments. In this section we review how to do measurements and analysis relevant to acute and critical care medicine.

Measurement	Equation/method	Normal values
LVEF (%)	Visual estimation	50–70 %
LVOT (cm)	Measured 2D	1.7–2.3
LV VTI (cm)	Measured PW	18–25
Stroke Volume (mL/beat)	$3.14\ (LVOTD/2)^2 \times LV\ VTI$	70–140
Stoke Volume Index ($mL/m^2/beat$)	SV/BSA	34–47
Cardiac Output (L/min)	(SV × HR)/1000	4–7
Cardiac Index ($L/min/m^2$)	CO/BSA	2.8–4.2
SVR (dynes -sec/cm^5)	((MAP-RAP)/CO) × 80	800–1200
SVR Index (dynes -sec/cm^5/m^2)	((MAP-RAP)/CI) × 80	1970–2390
PASP (mmHg)	$4(TR\ V_{max})^2 + RAP$	5–25
EPSS (cm)	Measured M-mode	EF > 50% <0.7 EF < 30% > 1.8
TASPE (mm)	Measured M-mode	> 17 mm
Aortic root (cm)	Measured 2D	Women: 2.7–3.3 Men: 3.1–3.7
• Use 10 mmHg for RAP most cases, good enough for an estimate and easy to use		
• 5 very small underfilled RA, RV, IVC		
• 15 Dilated RA, RV, ICV		
• ASE guidelines 3, 8, 15 mmHg based on IVC and IVC sniff		
• Less accurate in ventilated patients and more complex		

Left Ventricular Ejection Fraction and E-point Septal Separation

Brandon Masi Parker

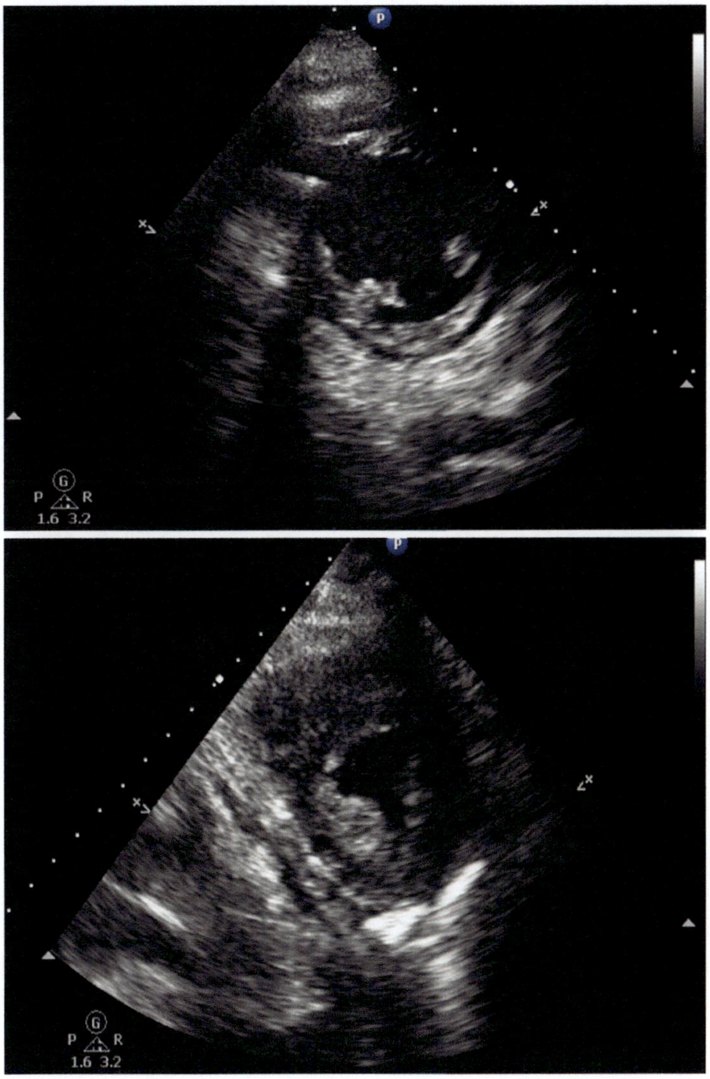

Supplementary Information The online version of this chapter (https://doi.org/10.1007/978-3-030-74687-2_9) contains supplementary material, which is available to authorized users.

B. M. Parker (✉)
Department of Surgery, University of Miami Miller School of Medicine, Miami, FL, USA
e-mail: bmp55@med.miami.edu

A. Salerno et al. (eds.), *Atlas of Critical Care Echocardiography*, https://doi.org/10.1007/978-3-030-74687-2_9

1 Introduction

One of the most important questions in complex shock is, "What is the function of the left heart?" This can be answered by assessment of the left ventricular ejection fraction (LVEF) and E-point septal separation (EPSS), which correlates with LVEF [1, 2]. One-third of ICU patients will have reduced LVEF during their ICU stay, and, therefore, assessment of LVEF is recommended by the Society of Critical Care Medicine in all ICU patients with pre-existing or hospital-acquired cardiac disease. We have also found LVEF assessment essential in *any* patient with complex shock to manage fluid and inotropic support during ongoing resuscitation.

2 LVEF and EPSS

Quantitative LVEF (i.e., Simpson method) is time-consuming and requires multiple views and calculations that can be difficult for busy providers. Also, it needs ideal images aligned along standard planes that are simply not possible in most mechanically ventilated ICU patients. Visual assessment, however, is reliable, is easy to do, and can be obtained in most ICU patients. Similarly, EPSS can be easily assessed in any patient with a reasonable parasternal long axis (PLA), and reliably detects severe LV dysfunction (EF < 30%).

2.1 Uses for LVEF and EPSS

1. Diagnosing primary cardiac shock
2. Understanding the cardiac component of complex shock
3. Indication for inotropic support (i.e., epinephrine)
4. Trending responses to an intervention
5. Helps guide fluid management

2.2 Obtaining the Views LVEF and EPSS

- LVEF is assessed in all windows. The most important views are the PLA and the apical four (AP 4) chamber:
  - Obtain a long clip (3–5 beats or 3–5 seconds).
  - Slow the clip down and assess the LV cavity at end diastole (when it is fattest diameter) and end systole (when it is at its smallest diameter) (Fig. 1).
  - Mentally trace the cavity at end systole and end diastole.
  - It is easier than it sounds, but it does take practice and training.
- The PLA is used to assess the EPSS.

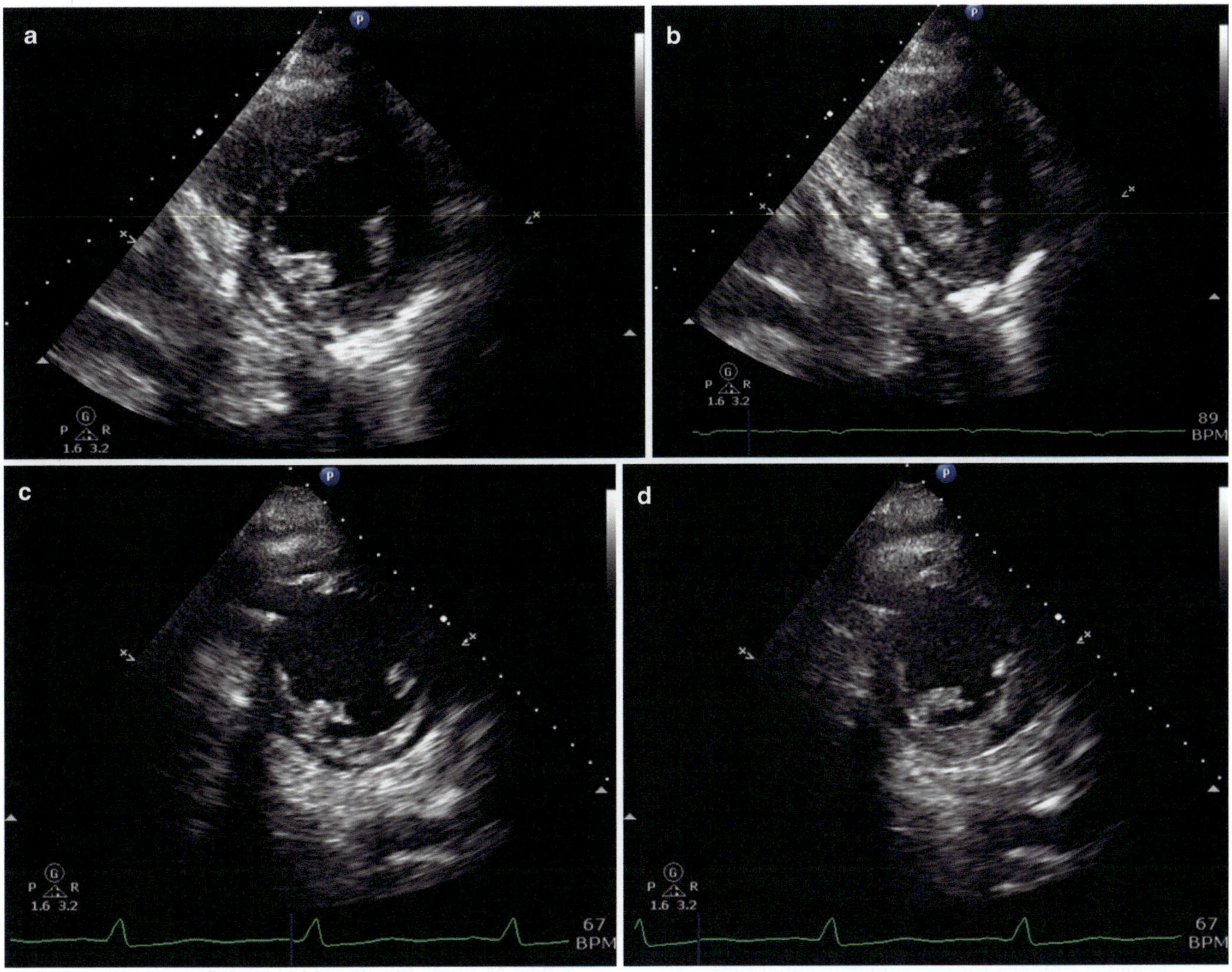

Fig. 1 Visual assessment of LVEF. When visually estimating the LVEF, you will need to compare the LV diameter in LV end diastole to LV end systole. (**a**) Normal EF in end diastole. (**b**) Normal EF in end systole. (**c**) Low LVEF in end diastole. (**d**), Low LVEF in end systole. Note that in panels (**c**) and (**d**), there is essentially no difference in LV cavity size (EF < 30%). In (**a**) and (**b**), there is a marked decrease in the LV cavity at end systole (EF 55–70%)

3 Visual Estimation of the LVEF

Visual assessment of LVEF becomes intuitive quickly. Studies have shown that trainees can reliably estimate LVEF after 10 hours of training. Assessing ejection fraction (EF) is simply assigning a numerical range to a global assessment. It may be easier to think of it as shockingly bad, some contraction but still terrible, not as good as it should be, good, and excellent. See below for a more scientific explanation (Video 1). Some physicians combine mild and moderate into one category (mild/moderate dysfunction).

- Window All
- Mode visual assessment
- Units %

- Normal 55–70%
- *Severe dysfunction*
  - EF < 30%.
  - Shockingly bad function.
  - In end systole the LV appears full; there is minimal change in cavity size from end diastole.
  - Very poor contraction, LV barely moving.
- *Moderate dysfunction*
  - EF 30–40%.
  - Poor function.
  - In end systole the left ventricle (LV) is smaller than end diastole, but still mostly full.
  - LV contracting, but poorly.
- *Mild dysfunction*
  - EF 40–55%.
  - Function is okay, but not great.

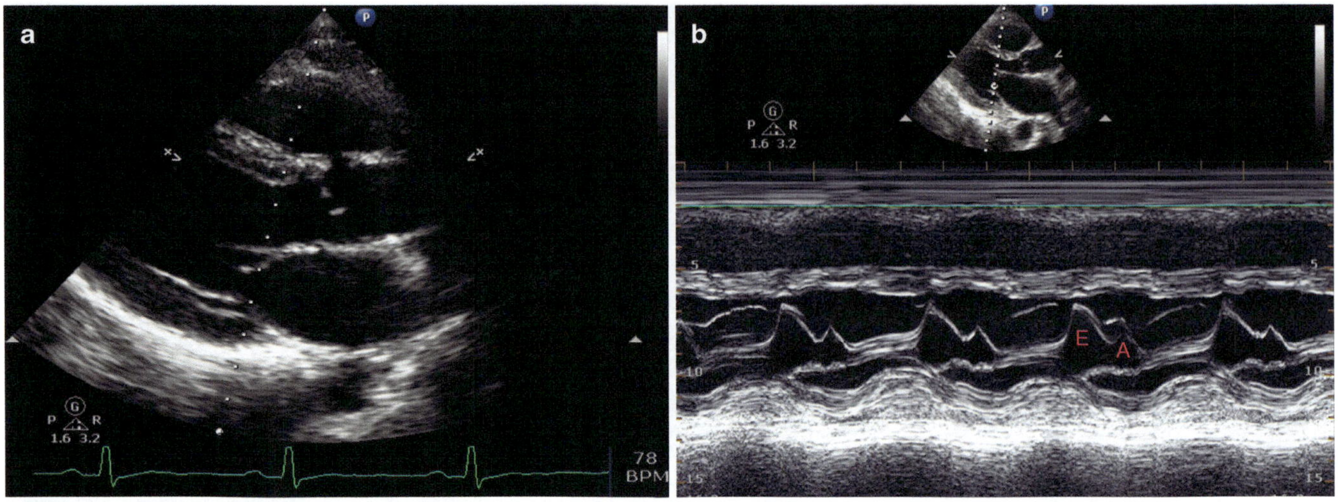

Fig. 2 How to measure EPSS: (**a**) PLA view with correct cursor placement (**b**) The mitral valve waveform has two waves the E-wave and the A-wave. EPSS is measured over the E-wave as illustrated

    - In end systole the LV is markedly smaller; blood remains in the chamber.
    - LV contracting, but not as well as it should.
- *Normal function*
    - 55–70%.
    - Function is good.
    - In end systole the LV is markedly smaller; some blood remains in the chamber.
    - LV contracting well.
- *Hyperdynamic*
    - EF > 70%.
    - Function is excellent.
    - In end systole the LV is completely collapsed.
    - LV contracting strongly and completely.

4 Measurement of EPSS

The LVEF is predicted to be normal as the anterior mitral leaflet approaches the interventricular septum during diastole in the cardiac cycle. The degree of mitral valve movement toward the interventricular septum while opening in diastole is dependent on a pressure differential between the left atrium (LA) and left ventricle. In the setting of decreased LVEF, a patient has a full left ventricle at the end of systole. Thus, with poor function, the pressure differential between the LA and LV is decreased, and the mitral leaflets will not open as vigorously [3].

- Window: PLA
- Mode: M-mode
- Units: mm
- Normal: <7 mm (EF 55–70%)
- *Mild/moderate dysfunction* >7 and <13 (EF 30–50%)
- *Severe dysfunction* > 13 EF <30%
- *Normal* <7 mm
- Obtain an ideal PLA view where the mitral leaflets are well visualized (Fig. 2).
- Select M-mode to activate the cursor.
- Align the cursor along the tip of the anterior leaflet of the mitral valve passing through the intraventricular septum. Select M-mode again to obtain the tracing.
    - (Fig. 2, Video 2)
- Two waves are present in the tracing during diastole (Fig. 2):
    - The first wave (E-wave) represents early filling.
    - The second wave (A-wave) represents the atrial kick.
    - The A-wave is usually smaller than the E-wave.
- EPSS is the distance from the peak to the valley of the E-wave (Fig. 2).
- EPSS >13 mm is consistent with an EF <30% (Fig. 3).

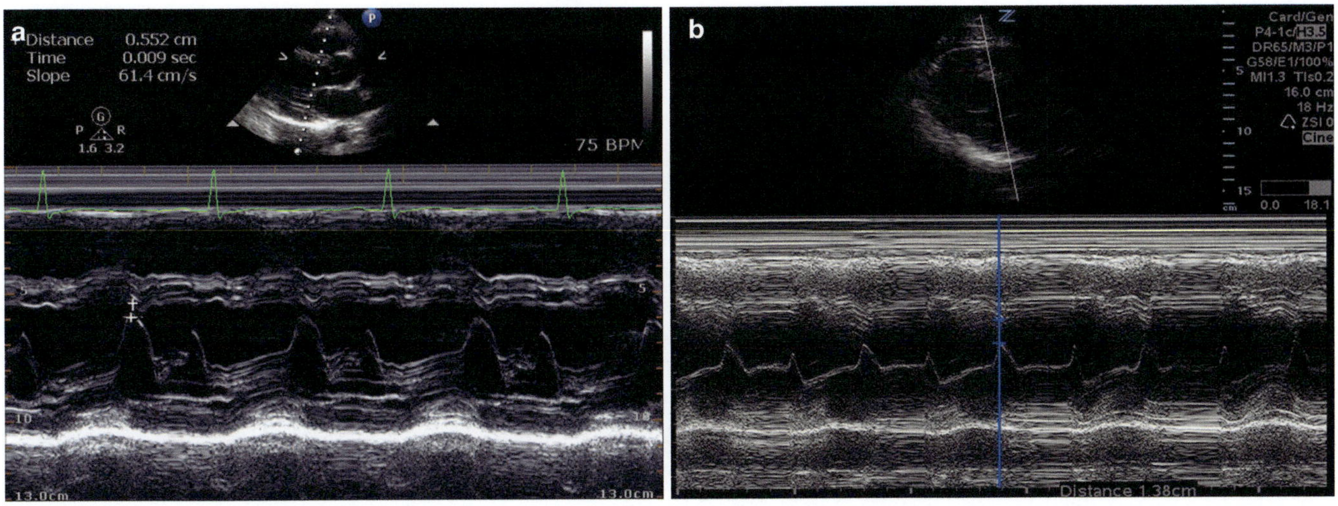

Fig. 3 Normal vs abnormal EPSS: (**a**) EPSS <7 mm, which correlates with normal EF. (**b**) EPSS >13 mm which correlates with severe LV dysfunction

5 Special Considerations

The EPSS has been shown to be predictive of LVEF, but attention should be paid to circumstances that can decrease reliability of this test.

- *Atrial fibrillation*
  There will be no A-wave. Also, the EPSS may be variable in different beats. There are average 3–5 measurements.
- *Valvular pathology*
  EPSS should not be used if significant valvular pathology is present, including aortic valve (AV) stenosis/regurgitation or mitral valve (MV) stenosis/regurgitation.
- *Prosthetic mitral valve*
  EPSS cannot be used with a prosthetic MV, as there are no valve leaflets.

References

1. Massie BM, Schiller NB, Ratshin RA, Parmley WW. Mitral-septal separation: new echocardiographic index of left ventricular function. Am J Cardiol. 1977;39(7):1008–16.
2. Lew W, Henning H, Schelbert H, Karliner JS. Assessment of mitral valve e point-septal separation as an index of left ventricular function in acute and chronic ischemic heart disease. Am J Cardiol. 1978;41(2):436.
3. Saul T, Siadecki SD, Berkowitz R, Rose G, Matilsky D, Sauler A. M-mode ultrasound applications for the emergency medicine physician. J Emerg Med. 2015;49(5):686–92.

Stroke Volume, Cardiac Output, and Systemic Vascular Resistance

Sarah B. Murthi and Syeda Fatima

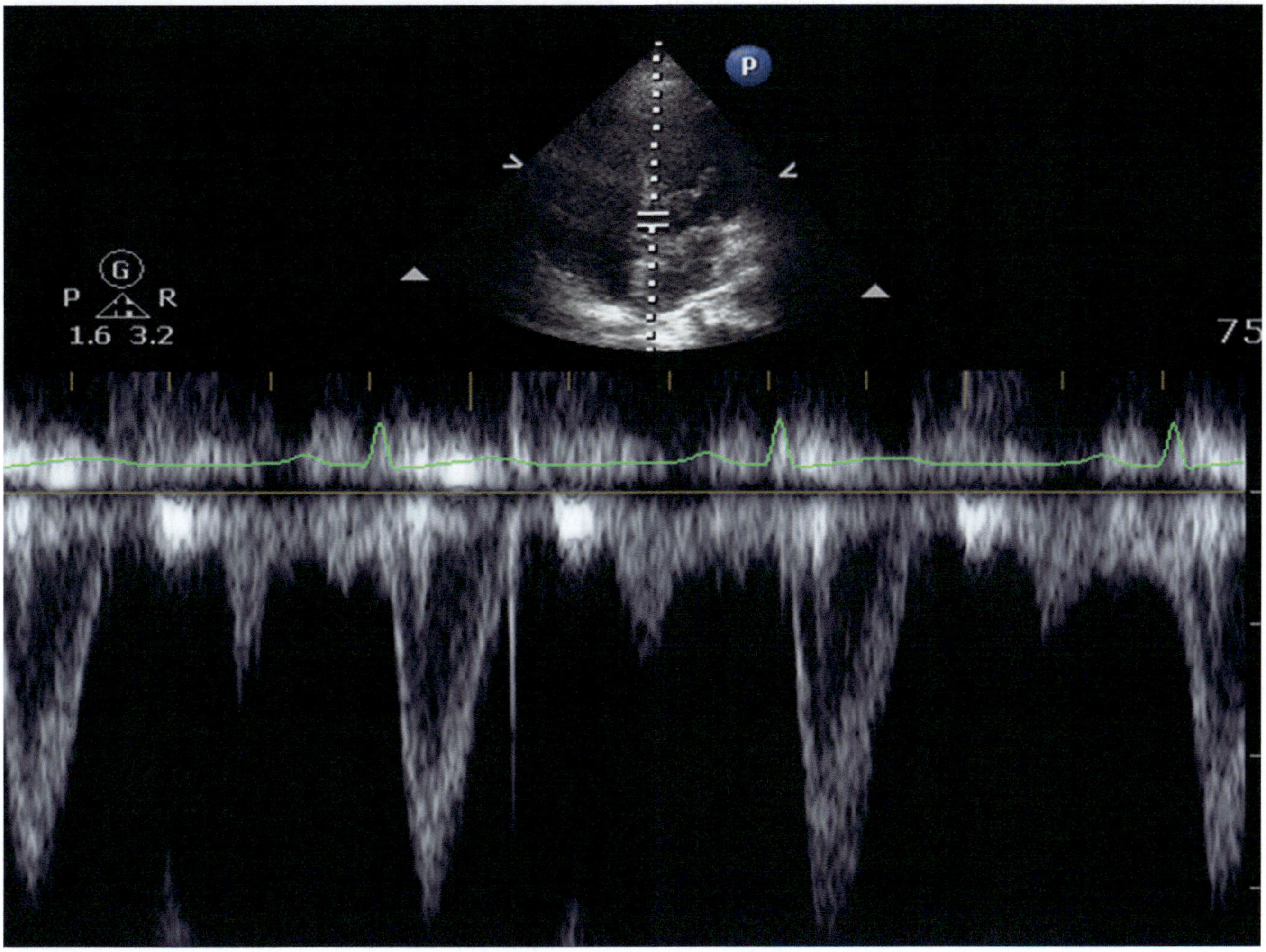

S. B. Murthi (✉)
Department of Surgery, Program in Trauma and Critical Care,
R Adams Cowley Shock Trauma Center, University of Maryland
School of Medicine, University of Maryland Medical Center,
Baltimore, MD, USA
e-mail: smurthi@som.umaryland.edu

S. Fatima
R. Adams Cowley Shock Trauma Center, University of Maryland,
Baltimore, MD, USA

A. Salerno et al. (eds.), *Atlas of Critical Care Echocardiography*, https://doi.org/10.1007/978-3-030-74687-2_10

1 Introduction

The stroke volume (SV), cardiac output (CO), and systemic vascular resistance (SVR) are all derived from two ultrasound measurements: the left ventricular outflow tract diameter (LVOTD) and the left ventricular outflow tract velocity time integral (LVOT VTI). The SV is the root measurement, which is simply multiplied by the heart rate (HR) to obtain the cardiac output. The systemic vascular resistance (SVR) can be calculated using patient's mean arterial blood pressure (MAP) and CO. Most ultrasound systems have software to automatically calculate the SV once the LVOTD and LVOT VTI are entered. However, few will have the CO and SVR calculations. These values can be calculated either using the formulas below or with the help of online or phone applications.

2 SV and SV Index (SVI)

Stroke volume and stroke volume index are very useful indicators of cardiac volume and function. The LVOTD and the LVOT VTI are used in the calculation. The LVOTD is related to the patient's size and is relatively fixed in an adult. It does not change in the short term. The VTI will change with variations in cardiac function and preload. Therefore, changes in the VTI can be used to trend changes in the stroke volume. So, when obtaining serial assessments in a patient, consider using the original LVOTD and not remeasuring it every time the patient is being assessed. This will improve accuracy while making it easier to obtain the SV. The LVOTD can be difficult to obtain, and it is squared as part of the stroke volume assessment, so it is the primary source of error and the primary reason the SV cannot be obtained. The VTI is a more reliable metric.

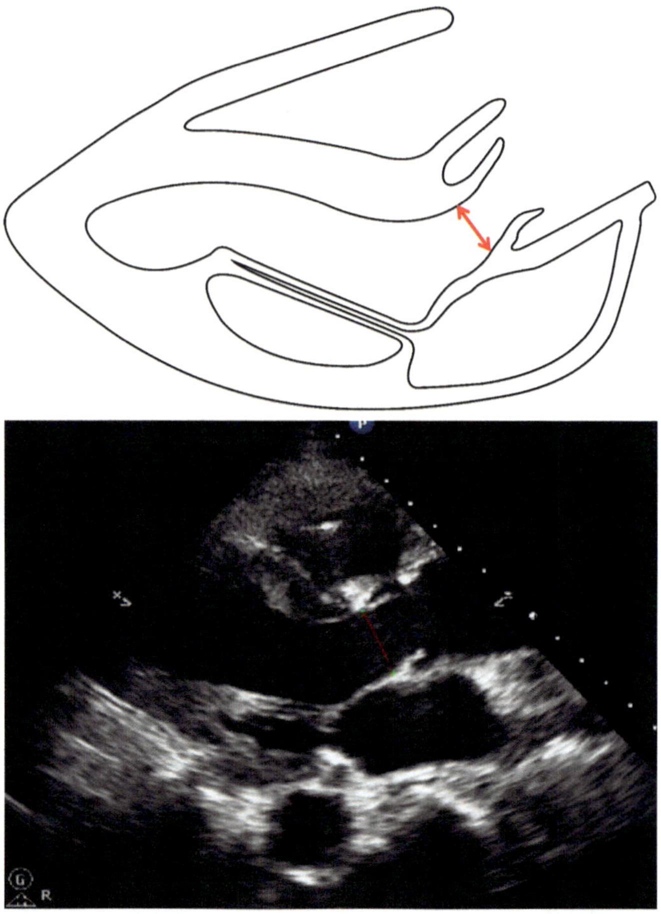

Fig. 1 Obtaining the LVOTD: From the PLA, freeze the image in systole, with the aortic valve completely open. Measure just inside the LVOT at the base of the AV. Often the leaflets can be seen inserting at the AV base

Table 1 Normal and reference values

Metric	Units	Normal
LVOTD	cm	1.7–2.3
LV VTI	cm	18–25
SV	mL/beat	70–140
SVI	mL/m²/beat	35–45
CO	L/min	4–7
CI	L/m²/beat	2.5–4.5
SVR	dynes –sec/cm⁵	800–1200
SVRI	dynes –sec/cm⁵/m²	1970–2390

2.1 Uses for SV

1. The root measurement for cardiac output
2. Measure of volume status
3. Compliments EF in assessing function
4. Used to calculate stroke volume variation

2.2 Measurement of SV

- *LVOTD* (Fig. 1)
  - Window: Parasternal long axis (PLA; chapter "Parasternal Long Axis")
  - Mode: 2D measurement
  - Units: cm
  - Normal: 1.7–2.3 (Table 1)
- *LVOT VTI* (Fig. 2)
  - Window: Apical five chamber (AP 5; chapter "Apical 4 Chamber and Apical 5 Chamber")
  - Mode: Pulsed wave Doppler
  - Units: cm
  - Normal: 18–25 (Table 1)

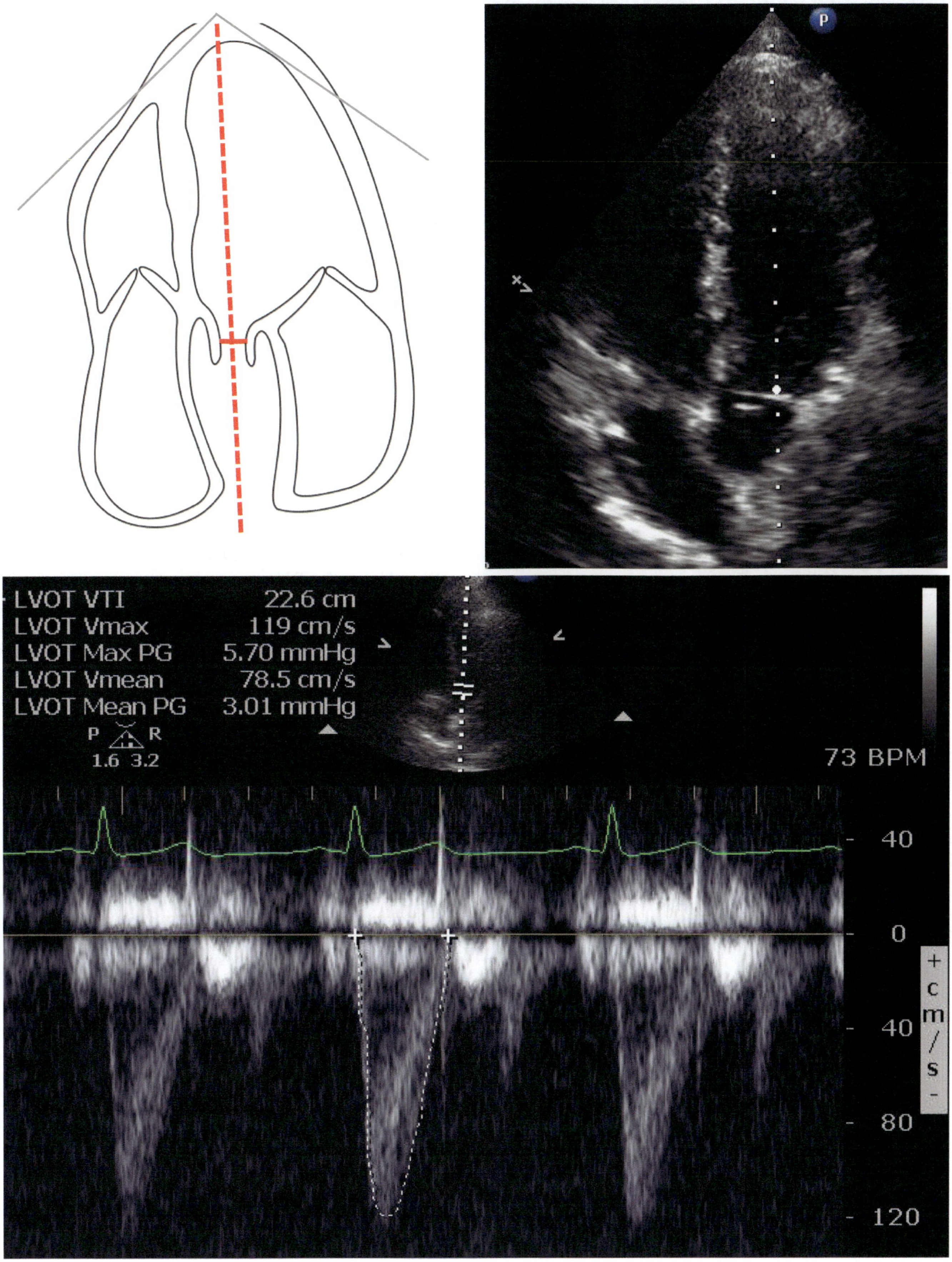

Fig. 2 Obtaining the LVOT VTI: From the AP place the cursor so that it is passing through the AV. Place the PW sample volume indicator, larger ball in the cursor, just inside the AV valve (upper right and upper left panels) in approximately the same place the LVOTD is measured in the PLA. Select PW to get the LVOT VTI tracing (lower panel)

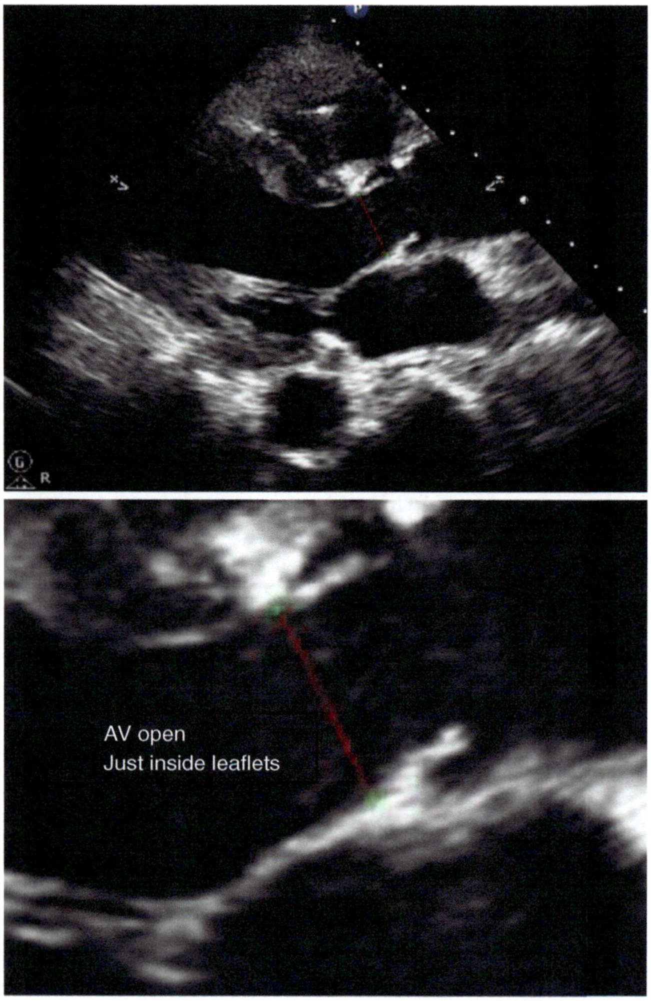

Fig. 3 Correct measurement of the LVOTD: Use active zoom if available to enlarge the AV valve (lower panel). Select LVOTD measurement in the calculations. Measure from inner edge to inner edge just inside the LVOTD, immediately proximal to the AV valve leaflet insertion

2.3 Tips and Pointers

- *Measuring LVOTD* (Fig. 3)
  - In the PLA moving clip, closely examine the opening of the AV.
    - Look for aortic stenosis:
      - Make sure the leaflets are opening well.
  - Stay inside the left ventricular outflow tract, just at the base leaflet insertion (Fig. 4):
    - AV open.
    - Do not measure inside the aortic valve.
    - Do not measure inside the left ventricle.
  - Measure leading edge-to-leading edge.
- *LVOTD can be estimated*
  - Accuracy is still under investigation.
  - Measure whenever possible:
    - If the patient's BSA <1.8 cm, use an LVOTD 1.8 cm.
    - If the patient's BSA is 1.8–2.2 cm, use BSA in cm.
    - If the patient's BSA is >2.2, use 2.2 cm.
- *Acquiring the LVOT VTI* (Fig. 5)
  - In the five-chamber view, align the cursor parallel to the flow through the AV.
  - Color flow Doppler can be used to locate the AV blood flow.
  - Place the PW sample volume just above the AV leaflets.
  - Select PW again to obtain the VTI tracing.
  - Do not measure if the cursor passes through the ventricular septum.
- *Measuring LVOT VTI*
  - Stay tight to the envelope of flow.
  - In atrial fibrillation and other arrhythmias:
    - Measure 3–5 beats and average the VTI.
  - If the baseline is noisy:
    - Use ECG; systole is from the mid-QRS to the end of the T-wave (Fig. 6).
    - If no ECG identify the tip of the waveform, and follow the trajectory of the envelope all the way to the baseline (Fig. 7).
    - Do not measure if poor signal or high flow causes aliasing (Fig. 8).
- *Using the VTI as a clinical tool*
  We calculate the SV because it is a common metric familiar to everyone who takes care of sick patients. However, it requires measurement of the LVOTD which can be difficult and inaccurate. The VTI is the value which changes over time and it is less prone to error. Once familiar with the VTI, it can be used on its own as measure of volume and function.

2.4 Equation for SV

- *Formula for the volume of a cylinder*
  - The base is the LVOTD; the height is the LVOT VTI.
- $SV = \pi(LVOTD/2)^2 \times LVOT\ VTI$
  - Units: mL/beat
  - Normal: 70–140 (Table 1)
- SV index (SVI) = SV/body surface area
  - Units: mL/m^2/beat
  - Normal: 35–45 (Table 1)

2.5 Special Considerations

- *LVOTD is a squared value*
  - Source of error.
  - Most people are between 1.7 and 2.3 cm.
  - Larger people will have bigger outflow tracts.
- *Anatomic measurement does not change*
  - Only need to measure once.
  - Use changes in VTI to trend SV and CO/CI.

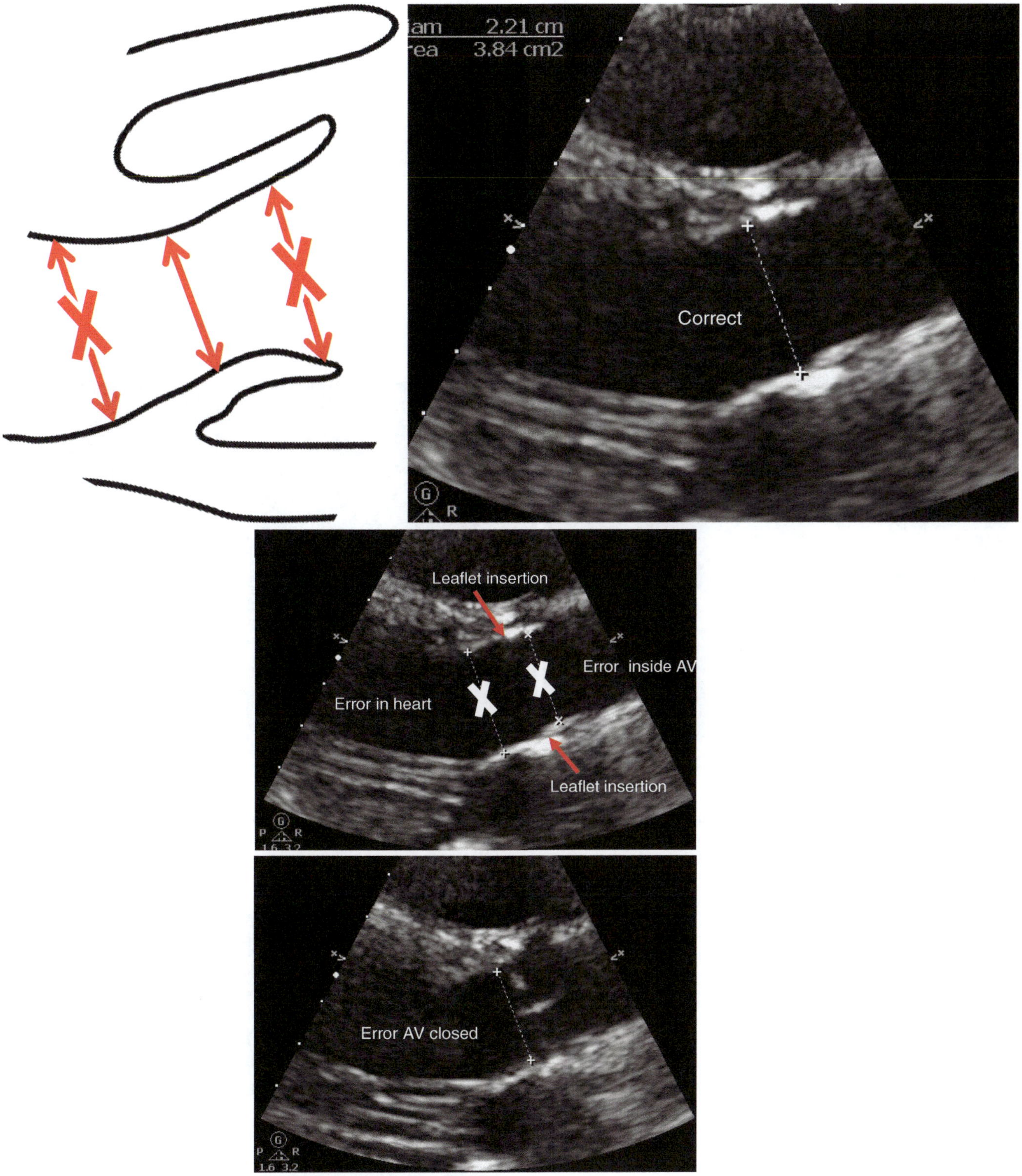

Fig. 4 Errors in LVOTD: Upper panels show correct measurement; just inside the open AV. Middle panel shows the LVOT being measured too far in the heart and too far out in aortic valve. The bottom panel shows incorrect measurement with the AV closed

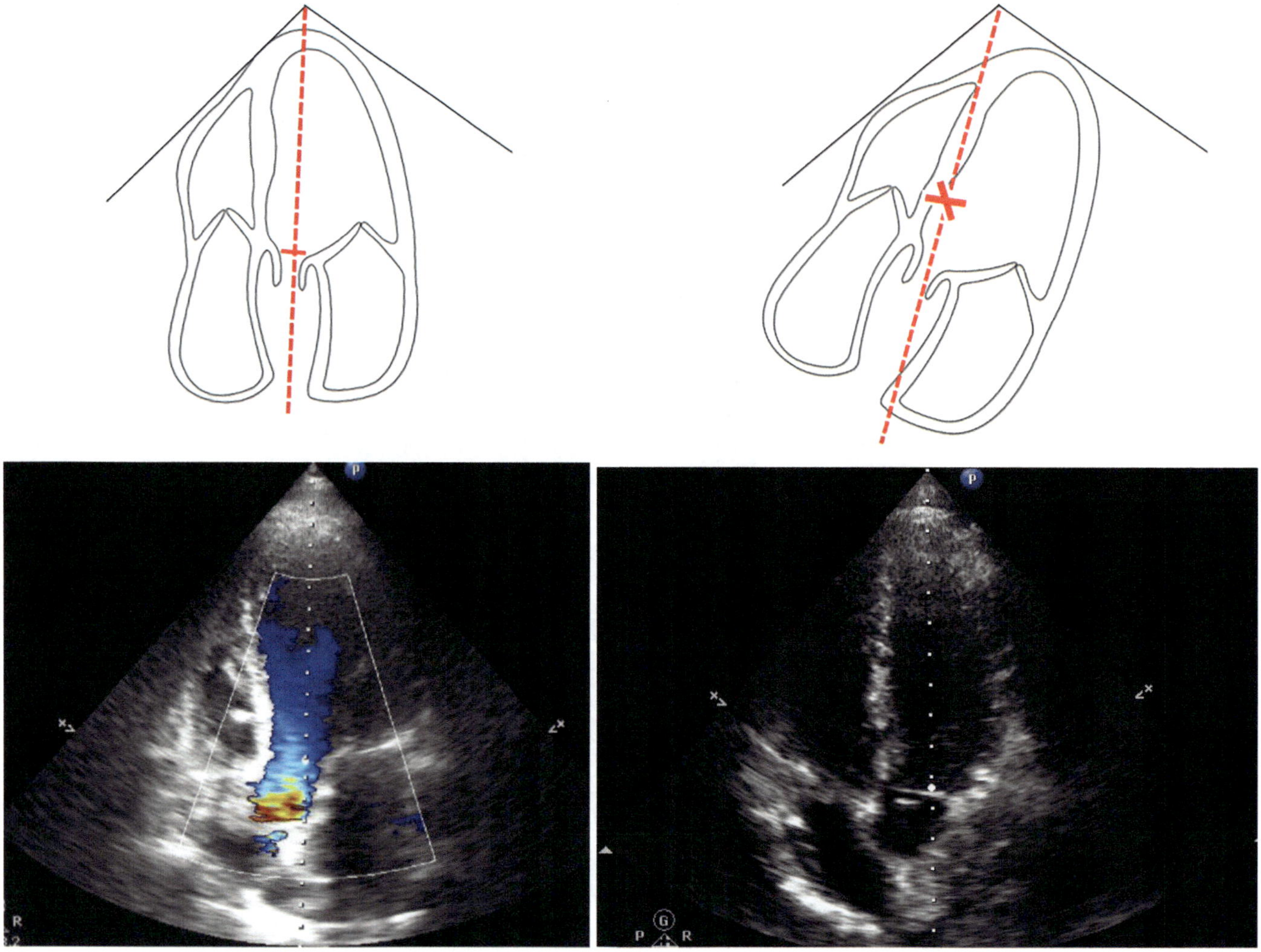

Fig. 5 Correct LVOT VTI: The left upper panel shows correct PW cursor placement, parallel to flow, through the AV. The right upper panel shows incorrect placement with the cursor passing through the septum. The lower left panel shows color flow to help identify the area of maximum blood flow. The lower right panel shows correct placement of the PW cursor on an echo image

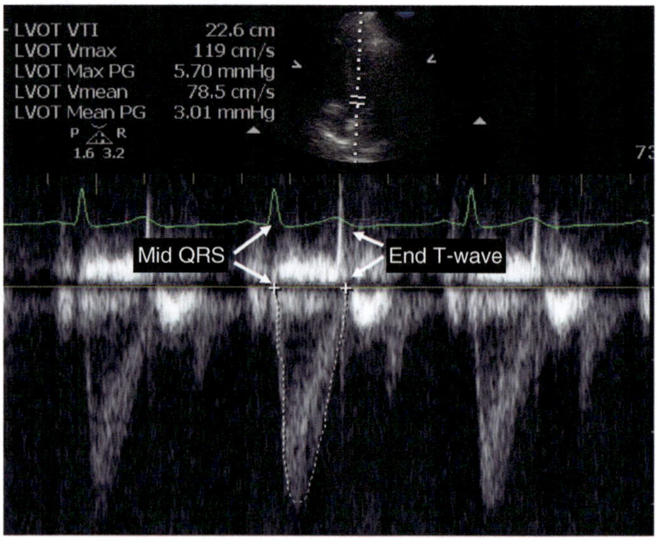

Fig. 6 ECG to measure the VTI: Ventricular systole starts in the middle of the QRS wave and continues to the end of the T-wave. Start the tracing at the baseline, and continue around the waveform along the VTI signal and back to the baseline

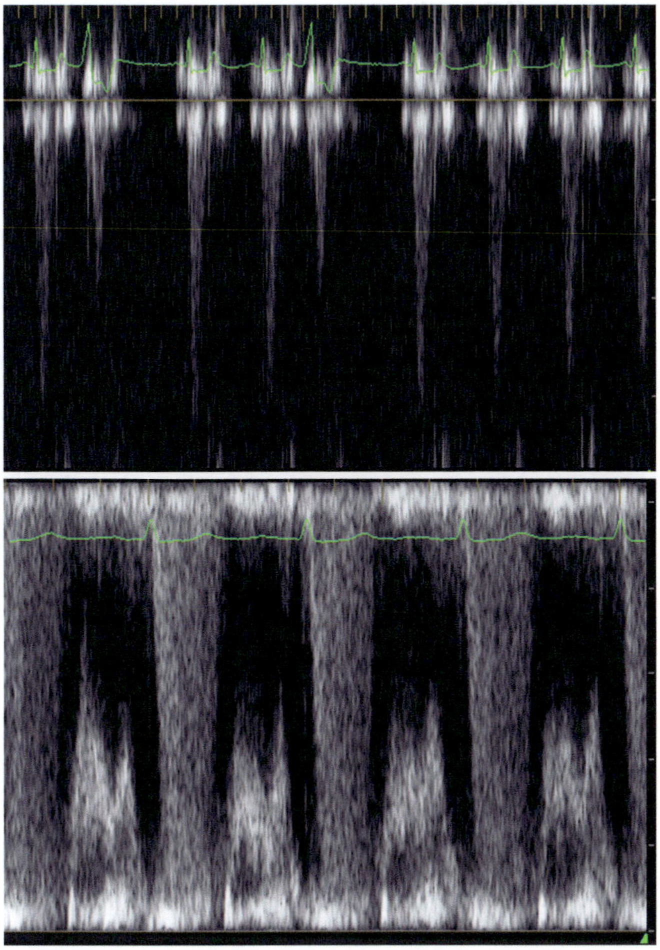

Fig. 7 Tip tracing of the VTI without the ECG: Locate the tip of the VTI signal; mentally follow the line to the baseline. Start the tracing at the baseline, and continue around the tip and back down to the baseline on the other side of the envelope

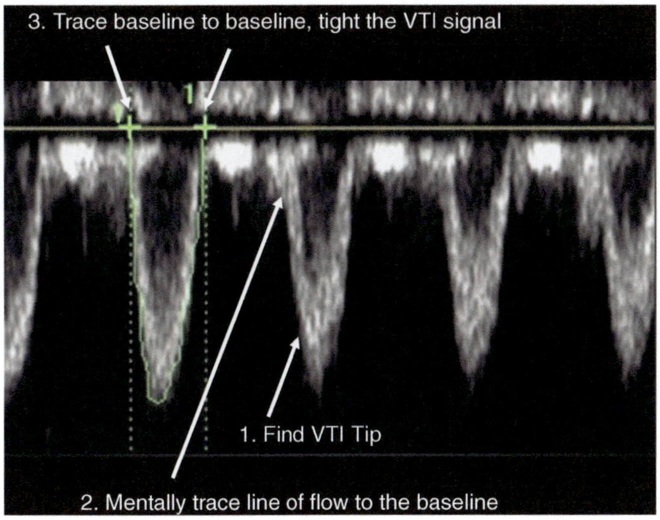

Fig. 8 Poor VTI tracing: The VTI should not be used to estimate the stroke volume if there is a bad signal. In the upper panel, the signal is poor because the PW cursor could not be aligned with flow. In the lower panel, the PW signal is aliasing from high flow, and the tip cannot be identified. In both examples the VTI should not be used to estimate stroke volume

3 Cardiac Output and Cardiac Index (CO and CI)

Cardiac output and index are measures of cardiac function. If the CO and MAP are known, the SVR can be calculated.

3.1 Uses for CO

1. Compliments EF in assessing function
2. Used to calculate the SVR

3.2 Measurement of CO

- Calculated from the SV

3.3 Equations for CO and CI

- CO = SV × HR
- CI = CO/BSA

4 Systemic Vascular Resistance (SVR) and SVR Index (SVRI)

4.1 Uses for SVR

1. Helpful in deciding when to use a vasopressor
2. Helpful in deciding when to use a vasodilator

4.2 Measurement of SVR

- Window: None
- Mode: None
- Units: dynes -sec/cm^5
- Normal: 800–1200 (Table 1)
- *Calculated from the CO*
- *Need to estimate the central venous pressure*
  - 5, 10, and 15 mmHg
    - Generally select 10 mmHg, trying to get a rough estimate.
    - If small underfilled heart, select 5.
    - If large and overloaded, select 15.

4.3 Equation for SVR

- SVR = ((MAP – CVP)/CO) × 80
  - Estimate CVP as 5, 10, or 15 mmHg

4.4 Measurement of SVRI

- Window: None
- Mode: None
- Units: dynes -sec/cm^5/m^2
- Normal: 1970–2390 (Table 1)
- *Calculated from the CI*

4.5 Special Considerations

- *SVR and SVRI are calculated value from the CO:*
  - If the CO is wrong, the SVR will also be wrong.
  - SVRI may be useful in obese patients.

Suggested Reading

American Society of Echocardiography. Assessment of structure and function. http://asecho.org/assessment-of-structure-and-function/

Orde S, Slama M, Hilton A, Yastrebov K, McLean A. Pearls and pitfalls in comprehensive critical care echocardiography. Crit Care. 2017;21:279.

Quinones MA, Otto CM, Stoddard M, Waggoner A, Zoghbi WA, Doppler Quantification Task Force of the Nomenclature and Standards Committee of the American Society of Echocardiography. Recommendations for quantification of Doppler echocardiography: a report from the Doppler Quantification Task Force of the American Society of Echocardiography. Am Soc Echocardiogr. 2002;15(2):167–84. https://doi.org/10.1067/mje.2002.120202. PMID: 11836492.

Diastolic Function

Alexis Salerno and Sarah B. Murthi

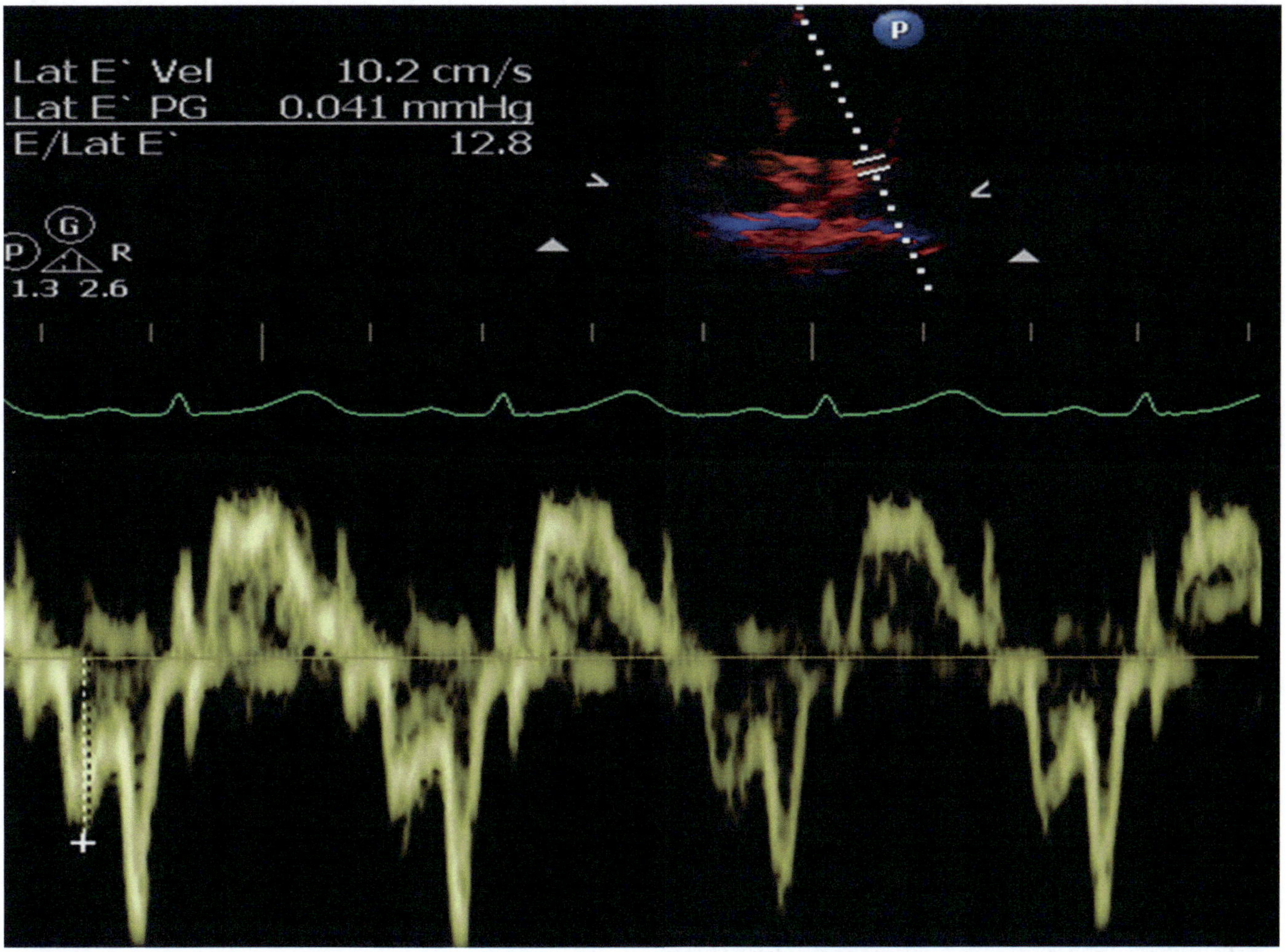

A. Salerno
Department of Emergency Medicine, University of Maryland School of Medicine, Baltimore, MD, USA

S. B. Murthi (✉)
Department of Surgery, Program in Trauma and Critical Care, R Adams Cowley Shock Trauma Center, University of Maryland School of Medicine, University of Maryland Medical Center, Baltimore, MD, USA
e-mail: smurthi@som.umaryland.edu

A. Salerno et al. (eds.), *Atlas of Critical Care Echocardiography*, https://doi.org/10.1007/978-3-030-74687-2_11

Abbreviations

A	Atrial contraction pulsed wave Doppler
a′	Atrial contraction tissue Doppler
a'_{TRV}	Atrial contraction ventricular movement in diastole with Tissue Doppler Imaging
A_{TRV}	Atrial contraction flow velocity through the tricuspid valve with pulsed wave Doppler
E	Early mitral pulsed wave Doppler
e′	Early mitral annulus tissue Doppler
e'_{TRV}	Early ventricular movement in diastole with Tissue Doppler Imaging
ECG	Electrocardiogram
EF	Ejection Fraction
E_{TRV}	Early diastolic flow velocity through the tricuspid valve with pulsed wave Doppler
LAP	Left atrial pressure
LV	Left Ventricle
MV	Mitral valve
MV	Mitral Valve
PWD	Pulsed wave Doppler
RAP	Right Atrial Pressure
RV	Right ventricle
TDI	Tissue Doppler Imaging
TRV	Tricuspid Valve

1 Introduction

Assessment of cardiac relaxation is an important part of critical care. With echocardiography, we can evaluate diastolic function rapidly and noninvasively. The most recent algorithm from the American Society of Echocardiology for assessing left ventricular (LV) diastolic dysfunction is complex. While it may be suitable for outpatient assessments in people with long-standing dysfunction, it cannot be used in critically ill patients. Therefore, a simplified method looking at the mitral valve inflow with pulse wave Doppler (PWD) and tissue Doppler imaging (TDI) is used by most intensivists. While assessments of right ventricular (RV) diastolic function are not commonplace yet, they are potentially important in detecting elevated right atrial pressure.

2 Diastolic Function

Diastole is an active energy requiring process. It is not a passive filling of the heart. The ventricle relaxes, untwists, and rapidly descends pulling in blood. With age and in critical illness, the ventricle stiffens. Impaired relaxation causes increased atrial pressure and decreased ventricular filling. High venous pressure is needed to fill a stiff atria and ventricle. This results in venous congestion and low stroke volume, placing patient at risk for both pulmonary edema and hypoperfusion.

Diastolic dysfunction is a normal part aging. It is found in patients with a low LV ejection fraction (EF). But it can also exist in patients with normal systolic function. Acute dysfunction is increasingly recognized in sepsis and other types of shock. Because cardiac ultrasound is the only way to detect it noninvasively and more advanced point-of-care echocardiography is new, the importance of acute diastolic dysfunction is a source of active research.

There are no pharmacologic treatments for diastolic dysfunction, but therapies including lower volume fluid boluses and measures to control heart rate may be beneficial. Diastolic function is not improved and may be worsened with alpha and beta agonists like norepinephrine, epinephrine, and dobutamine.

3 Obtaining the Measurements LV Diastolic Function

Left ventricular diastolic function is assessed with PWD through the MV and TDI at the mitral valve (MV) annulus. PWD measures velocity of blood flow through the valve into LV during diastolic filling. TDI measures how rapidly the ventricle muscle itself is moving down to allow filling. TDI can be assessed at either the lateral or medial aspect of the MV annulus, but most commonly at the lateral annulus.

The nomenclature for diastolic function is somewhat confusing. Early diastolic PWD flow is termed E and flow resulting from atrial contraction late in diastole is A. Early TDI diastolic movement is e′, and movement with atrial contraction a′. Patients with atrial fibrillation will not have an A or a′ wave, but they will still have E and e′ so diastolic function can still be assessed. In general, E/e′ is the most reliable metric.

3.1 Pulsed Wave Doppler Through the Mitral Valve: E and A (Fig. 1)

- Obtain the Apical 4 Chamber View (*see* Chap. 4).
- Place the pulse wave Doppler cursor through the MV.
  - Set the marker within the tip MV leaflets.
- Acquire the waveform and save the image.
- Identify the E wave and the A wave above the baseline.
  - Use the electrocardiogram (ECG).
    - The E wave occurs between the T wave and the QRS.
    - The A wave occurs just before or on the QRS.
      - It is easiest to find the A wave first, the other wave is the E.
      - In atrial fibrillation there is no A wave, only the E wave is present.
- Measure the peak velocity of the E wave and the A wave, save the measurement.

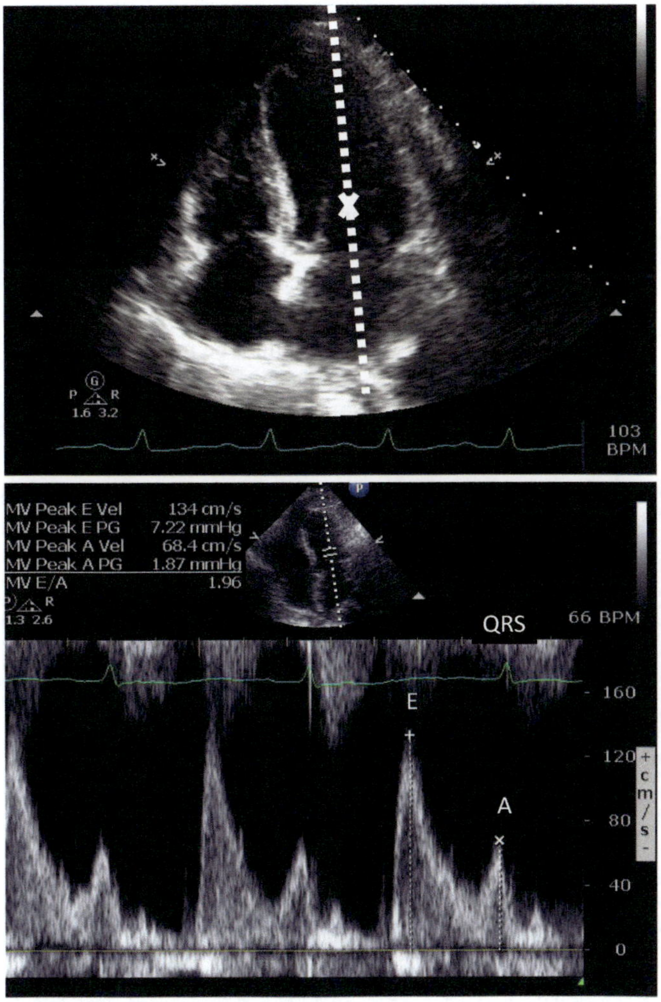

Fig. 1 Obtaining E and A with pulsed wave Doppler. Upper panel demonstrates correct placement of the PWD cursor; X marks the correct placement of the marker. Lower panel normal E and A wave form. Note the A wave occurs just before the QRS

3.2 Tissue Doppler at the Lateral Mitral Valve Annulus: e′ and a′ (Fig. 2)

- Obtain the same view and angle used for PWD.
- Select tissue Doppler imaging
- Place the cursor through the lateral annulus of the mitral valve.
  - Set the marker in the thickest part of the annulus
- Obtain the TDI waveform, save the image
- Identify the e′ wave and the a′ wave
  - Use the ECG tracing
  - The a′ wave occurs right before the QRS.
- Measure the e′ peak, save the measurement.

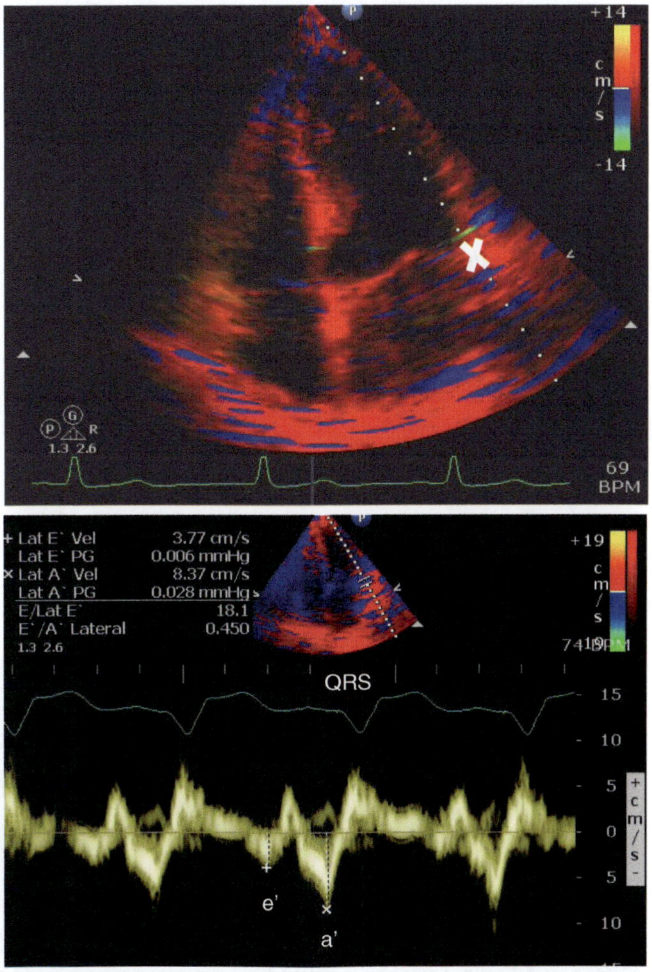

Fig. 2 Obtaining the e′ and a′ with tissue Doppler. Upper panel shows correct cursor placement. The marker (white X) should be placed in the middle of the LV in the mitral annuls. This patient has grade 3 diastolic dysfunction. Note the a′ wave occurs just before the QRS

4 Interpreting Measurements: Grading LV Diastolic Function (Figs. 3 and 4)

- If the e′ is <10 cm/sec and/or the LV EF is <55% ,diastolic dysfunction is present.
- *Normal*
  - e′ > 10 cm/sec
    - Rapid descent of ventricle
    - Often >15 or 20 cm/sec in young hyperdynamic hearts
    - Usually e′ > a′
  - E/e′ < 10
    - Normal fast diastolic flow (E) from rapid descent of the ventricle (e′)
  - E > A
    - Rapid early flow, marginal increase from atrial kick
    - Sometimes see E < A in underfilled, hyperdynamic hearts
      - If this is the case, the LV appears underfilled, high EF, and e >> 10 cm/sec
- *Dysfunction is present*
  - e′ < 10 m/s and/or EF < 55%
  - Usually, E/A 0.8–2.0.
- *Grade 1*
  - e′ < 10 cm/sec
    - Slow decent of the ventricle, often just below 10 cm/sec
    - Often e′ < a′
  - E/e′ < 10
    - Left atrial pressure (LAP) is normal.
    - Filling is from ventricular decent.
  - E < A (ratio ≤ 0.8)
    - Also called E/A reversal
    - Impaired LV relaxation with normal LAP, decreases early diastolic flow (E)
    - Flow into the ventricle is more rapid with the atrial kick.
- *Grade 2*
  - e′ < 10 cm/sec
    - Slow decent of the ventricle, usually clearly below 10
    - Often e′ = a′
  - E/e′ 10–14
    - Increased LAP
    - Filling is from increased atrial pressure as LV becomes less complaint.
  - E = A or E > A (0.8-2.0)
    - Increased atrial pressure results in pseudo-normalization of the E/A ratio.
- *Grade 3*
  - e′ < 10 cm/sec, usually less than 6
    - Often e′ = a′ or e′ < a′
  - E/e′ > 14
    - High left atrial pressure
    - Rapid inflow is from increased pressure, not rapid decent of the LV.
  - E >> A (≥2)
    - Stiff, high pressure left atria and ventricle result in high velocity flow.

The ASE guidelines for grading include assessment of left atrial size and presence of elevated tricuspid peak velocity as evidence of long-standing dysfunction causing other findings. With acute dysfunction, these findings would not be expected. Also, the area of the LA usually cannot be measured, and the tricuspid jet can be hard to detect in intubated patients. We propose and alternative simplified method in Fig. 5.

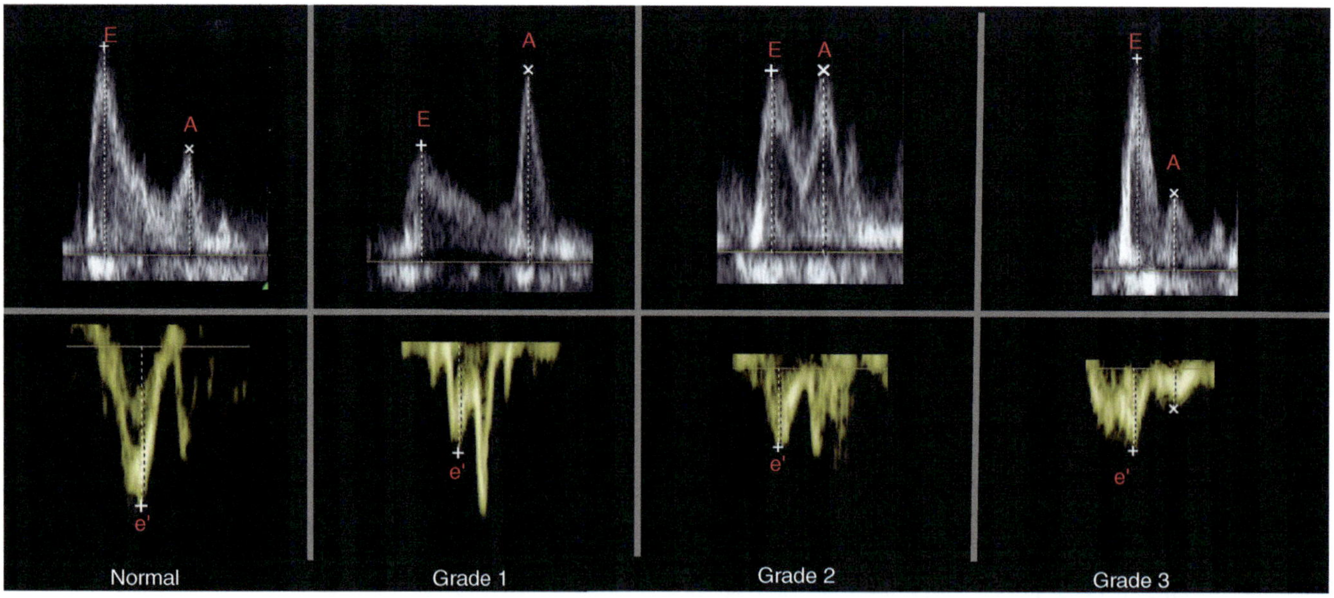

Fig. 3 Pulsed wave and tissue Doppler changes with diastolic dysfunction. Top panels: E and A waves with PWD. Bottom panels: e′ and a′ changes with TD

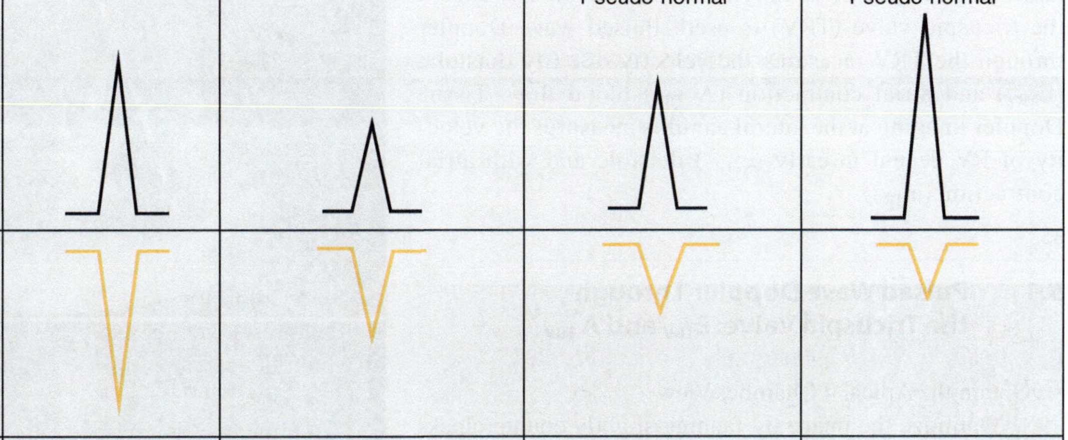

	Normal	Grade 1	Grade 2	Grade 3-4
PW Miltral Value (Blood flow)			Pseudo-normal	Pseudo-normal
TDI Lateral Annulus (LV movement)				
E/e′	< 10	< 10	10-14	> 14
Left Atrial Pressure (LAP)	Normal	Normal	↑↑	↑↑↑↑

Fig. 4 Ratio of E/e′ in LV diastolic dysfunction. TDI tissue Doppler imaging

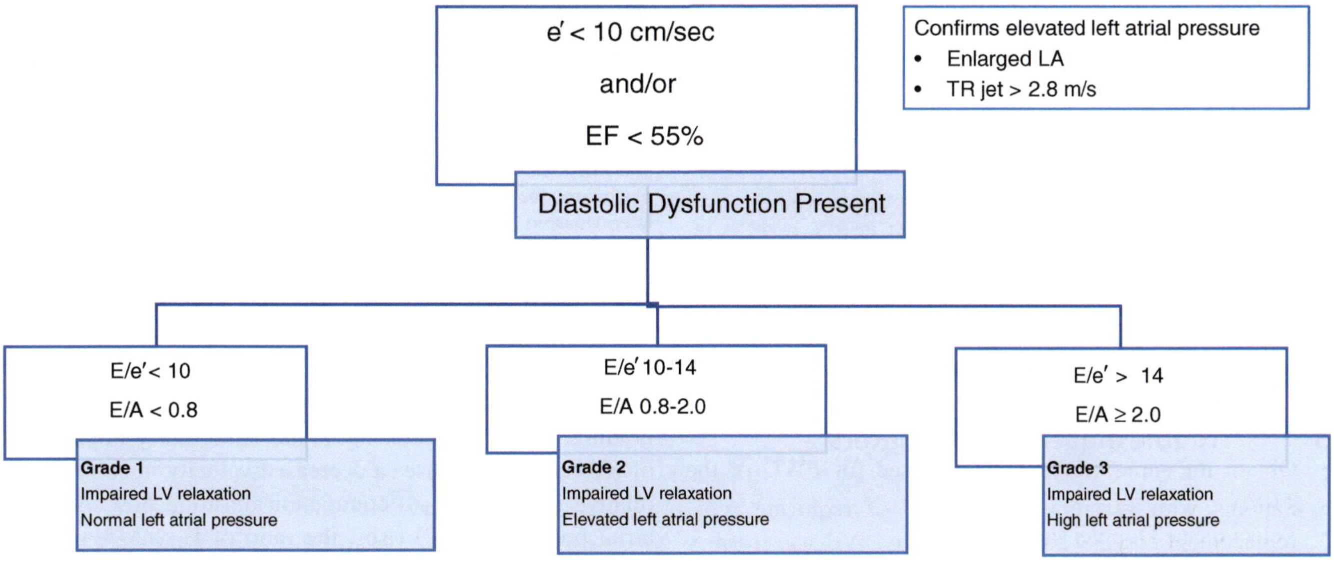

If mixed findings; combination grade, Grade 1-2 (mild to moderate) or Grade 2-3 (moderate to severe)
Modification of ASE guidelines for POCUS, may over or underestimate
Do not assess if poor quality waveforms

Fig. 5 Grading of LV diastolic dysfunction for critical illness

5 Obtaining Measurements of RV Diastolic Function

Assessing RV diastolic function is similar to LV, except the tricuspid valve (TRV) is used. Pulsed wave Doppler through the TRV measures the velocity of early diastolic (E_{TRV}) and atrial contraction (A_{TRV}) blood flow. Tissue Doppler imaging at the lateral annulus measures the velocity of RV decent in early (e'_{TRV}) diastole and with atrial contraction (a'_{TRV}).

5.1 Pulsed Wave Doppler Through the Tricuspid Valve: E_{TRV} and A_{TRV}

- Obtain the Apical 4 Chamber View
  - Optimize the image by fanning slightly counterclockwise to bring the RV free wall into focus.
  - Sometimes moving the transducer medially toward the sternum brings the TRV and RV free wall into the image.
- Place the PWD cursor through the tricuspid valve.
  - Set the marker within the tip TRV leaflets (Fig. 6, upper panel).
- Select PWD again to acquire the waveform, save the image.
- Identify E_{TRV} and the A_{TRV} above the baseline (Fig. 7, upper panel).
  - Use the ECG as described for LV assessment to identify the waves
    - The A_{TRV} will be on or just after the QRS; the other wave is E_{TRV}.
    - In atrial fibrillation. there is no A_{TRV} wave.
- Measure the peak velocity of E_{TRV} and A_{TRV}.
  - Save the measurement.

5.2 Tissue Doppler Imaging at the Lateral Mitral Annulus: e'_{TRV} and a'_{TRV}

- Obtain the same view and angle used for PWD of the TRV.
- Select tissue Doppler imaging.
- Place the cursor through the lateral annulus of the TRV (Fig. 6, lower panel).
  - Set the marker in the thickest part of the annulus.
- Obtain the TDI waveform; save the image.
- Identify the e'_{TRV} and the a'_{TRV} (Fig. 7, lower panel).
- Measure the e'_{TRV} peak velocity.
  - Save the measurement.
- Interestingly, the peak of the systolic wave (S'_{TRV}) is a measure of RV systolic function which is discussed in Chap. 12.

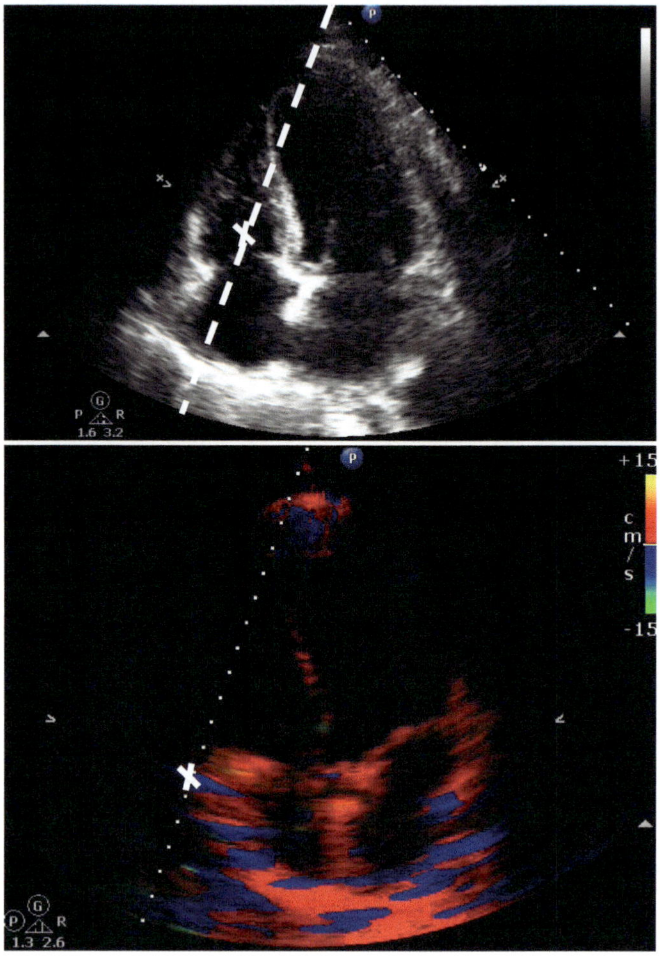

Fig. 6 Right ventricular pulsed wave and tissue Doppler placement. Upper Panel: PWD cursor placement; the marker (X) shows correct placement just inside the tricuspid leaflets. Lower Panel: TDI cursor placement; the marker (X) shows correct placement in the middle of the later tricuspid annulus

5.3 Interpreting RV Diastolic Dysfunction Measurements

Assessing RV diastolic function is less complicated than LV grading. The overall concept is the same. Early impairment of RV relaxation causes a decreased velocity in early (E_{TRV}) relative to atrial (A_{TRV}) contraction diastolic flow. As right atrial pressure (RAP) rises, the ratio of E_{TRV}/A_{TRV} pseudonormalizes, detected by an increase in the E/e′ or a decrease in how rapidly the RV relaxes (e′) relative to the speed of blood inflow (E) (Table 1).

Elevations in right atrial pressure can lead to increased visceral venous congestion, discussed in detail in Chap. 16. In a direct comparison between echo and pulmonary artery catheter derived RAP, $E_{TRV}/e'_{TRV} \geq 4$ predicts right atrial pressure >10 mmHg with a high sensitivity and specificity in non-cardiac surgery patients.

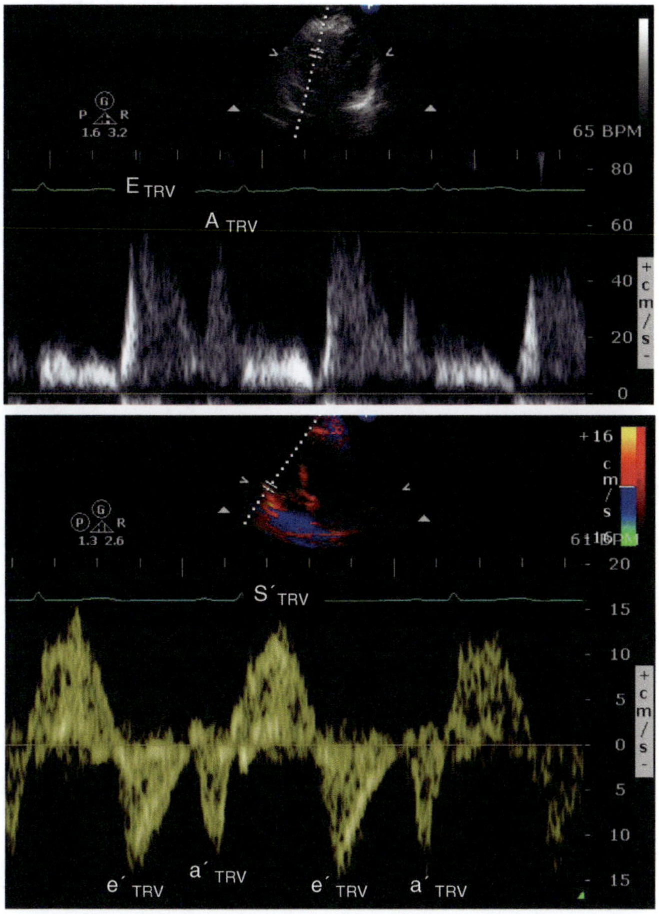

Fig. 7 Right ventricular pulsed wave and tissue Doppler waveforms. Upper Panel: PWD waveform. E_{TRV}; velocity of early blood flow through the tricuspid valve. A_{TRV} velocity of blood flow from atrial contraction. Lower Panel: TDI Waveform. e'_{TRV}; velocity of early RV movement in diastole. a'_{TRV}; velocity of RV movement with the atrial contraction. S'_{TRV}; RV movement with systolic contraction

Table 1 Interpreting RV diastolic dysfunction measurements

	Normal	Impaired	Impaired with elevated RAP (Pseudo-normalization E/A)
E_{TRV}/A_{TRV}	0.8-2.1	<0.8	0.8–2.1
E_{TRV}/e'_{TRV}	<6	<6	>6
Hepatic flow	S > D	S ≥ D	S < D or S above the baseline

6 Tips and Pitfalls

- Obtain the E, A, and e′ measurements from the same view and angle. Save the images and do the measurements after both tracings have been obtained.
- Obtain E_{TRV}, A_{TRV}, e'_{TRV} from the same view and angle. Save the images and do the measurements after both tracings have been obtained.
- Not valid in patients with valve pathology
- It can be difficult to tell E (and e′) from the atrial waves
  - Easiest to find A (and a′) on or just before the QRS
- In tachycardic, the E and the A wave may fuse making it difficult to distinguish
- E/A ratio is not reliable in atrial fibrillation.
- E/A ratio is affected by volume status and cannot be used alone.
- E/e′ and E_{TRV}/e'_{TRV} are the most reliable metrics.

Suggested Reading

Greenstein YY, Mayo PH. Evaluation of left ventricular diastolic function by the intensivist. Chest. 2018;153(3):723–32.

Rudski LG, Lai WW, Afilalo J, Hua L, Handschumacher MD, Chandrasekaran K, Solomon SD, Louie EK, Schiller NB. Guidelines for the echocardiographic assessment of the right heart in adults: a report from the American Society of Echocardiography endorsed by the European Association of Echocardiography, a registered branch of the European Society of Cardiology, and the Canadian Society of Echocardiography. J Am Soc Echocardiogr. 2010;23(7):685–713; quiz 786–8.

Sade LE, Gulmez O, Eroglu S, Sezgin A, Muderrisoglu H. Noninvasive estimation of right ventricular filling pressure by ratio of early tricuspid inflow to annular diastolic velocity in patients with and without recent cardiac surgery. J Am Soc Echocardiogr. 2007;20:982–8.

Walley KR. Sepsis-induced myocardial dysfunction. Curr Opin Crit Care. 2018;24(4):292–9.

Right Ventricular Systolic Function

Alexis Salerno

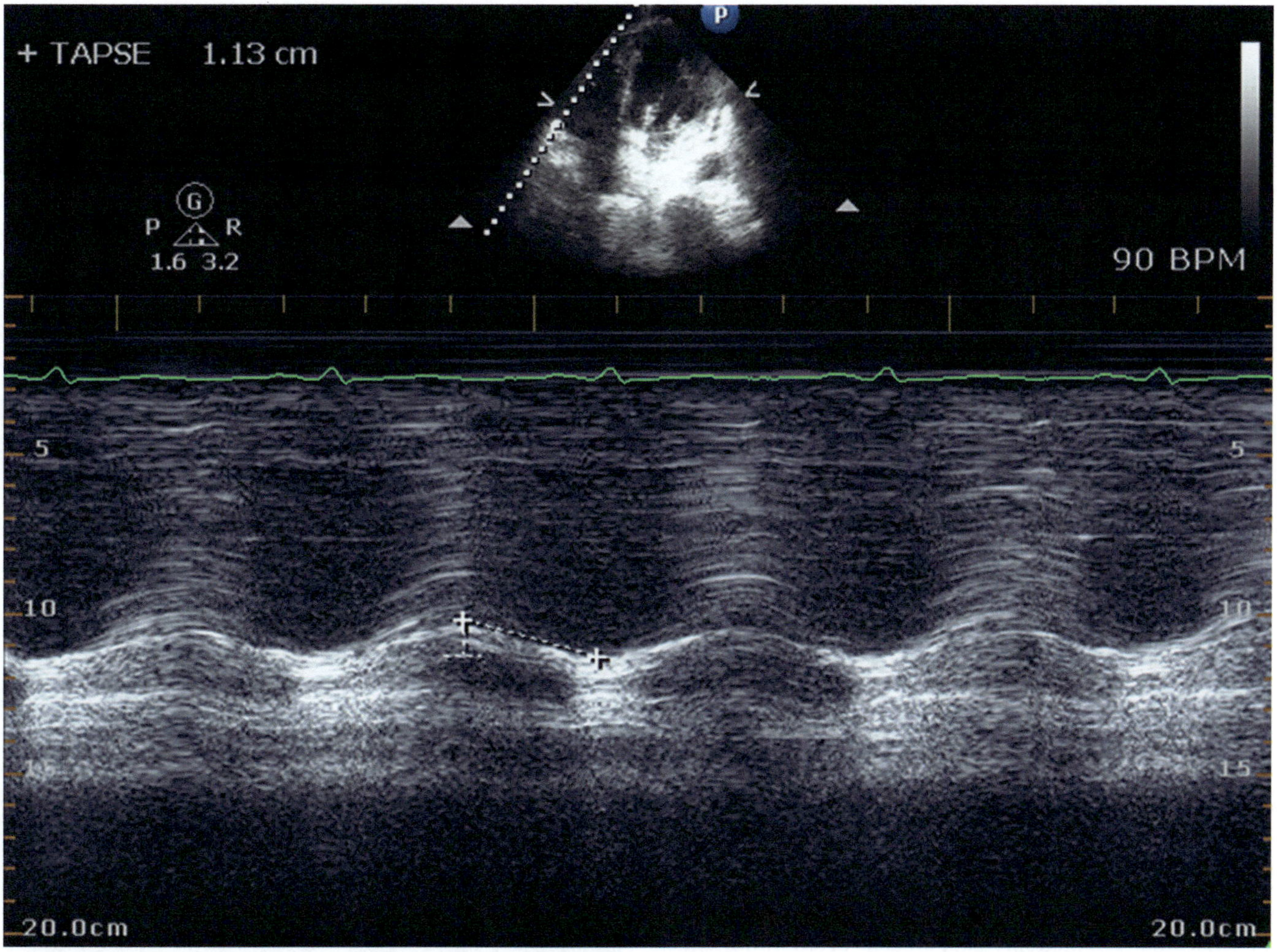

Supplementary Information The online version of this chapter (https://doi.org/10.1007/978-3-030-74687-2_12) contains supplementary material, which is available to authorized users.

A. Salerno (✉)
Department of Emergency Medicine, University of Maryland School of Medicine, Baltimore, MD, USA
e-mail: Alexis.Salerno@som.umaryland.edu

A. Salerno et al. (eds.), *Atlas of Critical Care Echocardiography*, https://doi.org/10.1007/978-3-030-74687-2_12

Abbreviations

AP 4	Apical 4 Chamber View
IC	Isovolumetric contraction
LV	Left ventricle
PSA	Parasternal Short Axis View
PSL	Parasternal Long Axis View
RV	Right ventricle
S′	Systolic wave with tissue Doppler imaging
TAPSE	Tricuspid annular plane systolic excursion
TDI	Tissue Doppler imaging

1 Introduction

The right ventricle (RV) is no longer the forgotten chamber as studies have shown that critically ill patients with RV dysfunction are at high risk for mortality. Right ventricular failure can result from elevated pulmonary pressures, excessive preload, and myocardial dysfunction. In this chapter, we discuss measures of systolic function. In Chap. 11, assessments of diastolic function are described. There are several easy ways to evaluate RV systolic function from transannular plane systolic excursion (TAPSE) with M-mode to systolic velocity with tissue Doppler imaging (TDI) and simply systematically visualizing the RV in different windows.

2 RV Dysfunction

Outside of echo, RV dysfunction is hard to diagnose. There are few physical exam or laboratory findings that are present until severe dysfunction occurs. Additionally, many of the interventions in shock management worsen RV function including aggressive fluid resuscitation and positive pressure mechanical ventilation.

3 Uses for RV Assessment

1. Diagnosing primary cardiac shock
2. Understanding the cardiac component of complex shock
3. Indication for inotropic support and determining which inotrope is most likely beneficial (i.e., epinephrine, milrinone) (*see* Chaps. 22 and 23)
4. Diagnosis and management of Pulmonary Embolus (*see* Chap. 17)
5. Assessing cardiac function in severe hypoxic respiratory failure
6. Guiding fluid management (*see* Chaps. 22 and 24)

4 Obtaining Views

- It is important to examine the RV in all 4 windows:
  - The most important views are the parasternal short axis (PSA) and the apical 4 (AP 4) chamber view.
- In the PSA look for (Fig. 1 and Video 1):
  - Septal flattening and D-shaped LV
  - Enlarged RV
  - Best seen at the papillary level
- In the AP 4 look for (Fig. 1 and Video 2):
  - Enlargement of the RV relative to the LV
    - The RV should be 1/3 the LV
    - Often closer to equal in intubated patients
  - Anterior motion of the RV at the tricuspid valve
    - Basis of TAPSE, but can be assessed visually

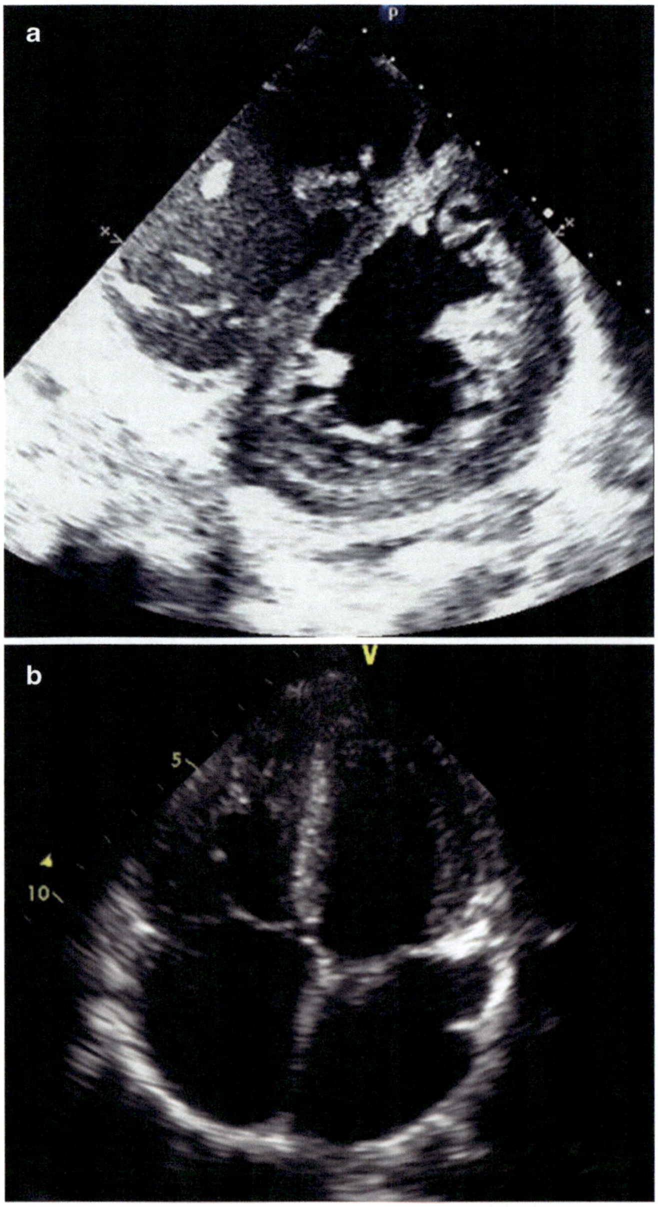

Fig. 1 Ultrasound images of RV dysfunction. (**a**) Dilated RV on PSA. (**b**) Dilated RV on A4C

4.1 Visual Estimation of the RV

- The RV can be graded as normal function or mild, moderate, and severe dysfunction. It may also be easier to think of it as fine, not great and terrible.
  - Progression of RV dysfunction (Video 3)

4.2 Tips and Pointers

- Make sure to use cardiac exam or presets. If using abdominal imaging, the heart will look dysfunctional.
- If the RV is foreshortened (looks more like a softball, then a football), it may look dysfunctional when function is normal.

4.3 Measurement of Transannular Plane Systolic Excursion (TAPSE) (Figs. 2 and 3)

- TAPSE measures the longitudinal movement of the lateral tricuspid annular plane during systole (Fig. 2). Obtain an AP 4 view (*see* Chap. 4).
  - To better visualize the RV, consider fanning slightly counterclockwise or moving the transducer more medially until the RV free wall and the septum are parallel to the transducer.
  - Window: AP 4, RV
  - Mode: M-mode
  - Units: mm
  - Severe dysfunction: <16
- Select M-mode to activate cursor.
- Align the cursor along the lateral tricuspid annulus. Select M-mode again to get the tracing (see Fig. 3 and Video 4).
  - Measure the peak distance of the tricuspid annulus at end-diastole and end- systole.
- A TAPSE less than 17 mm suggests decreased RV systolic function.

4.4 Measurement of Peak Systolic Velocity at the Tricuspid Valve (S'_{TRV})

S′ measures the myocardial velocity if the RV at the tricuspid annulus using TDI (Fig. 4). While it requires a US system capable of doing TDI it is not difficult to preform and it has been validated in large patient cohorts. As described above, obtain an AP 4 window which focuses on the RV.

  - Window: AP 4, RV
  - Mode: TDI
  - Units: cm/s
  - Severe dysfunction: <10
- Select TDI to activate cursor.
- Align the cursor along the lateral tricuspid annulus. Select TDI again to get the tracing.
  - Measure the peak systolic velocity of the tricuspid annulus, above the baseline.

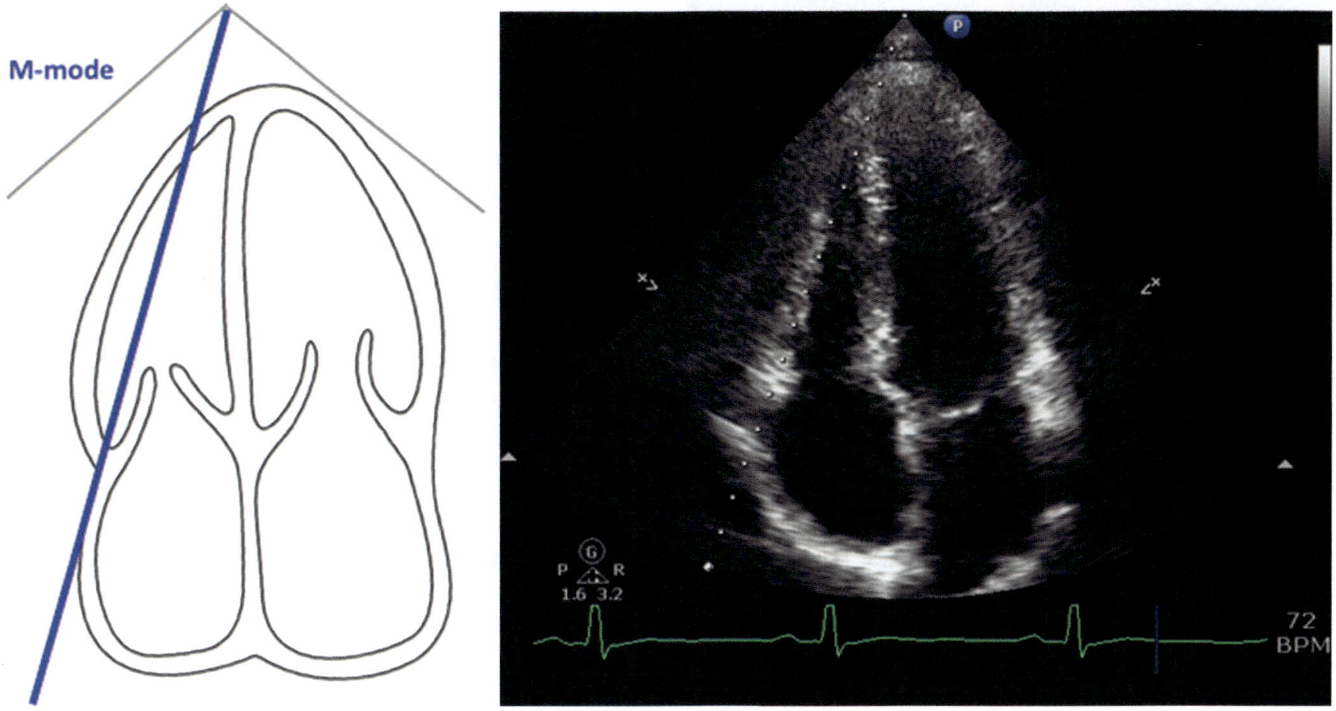

Fig. 2 How to measure TAPSE. (**a**) Schematic view of obtaining TAPSE. (**b**) US view of obtaining TAPSE

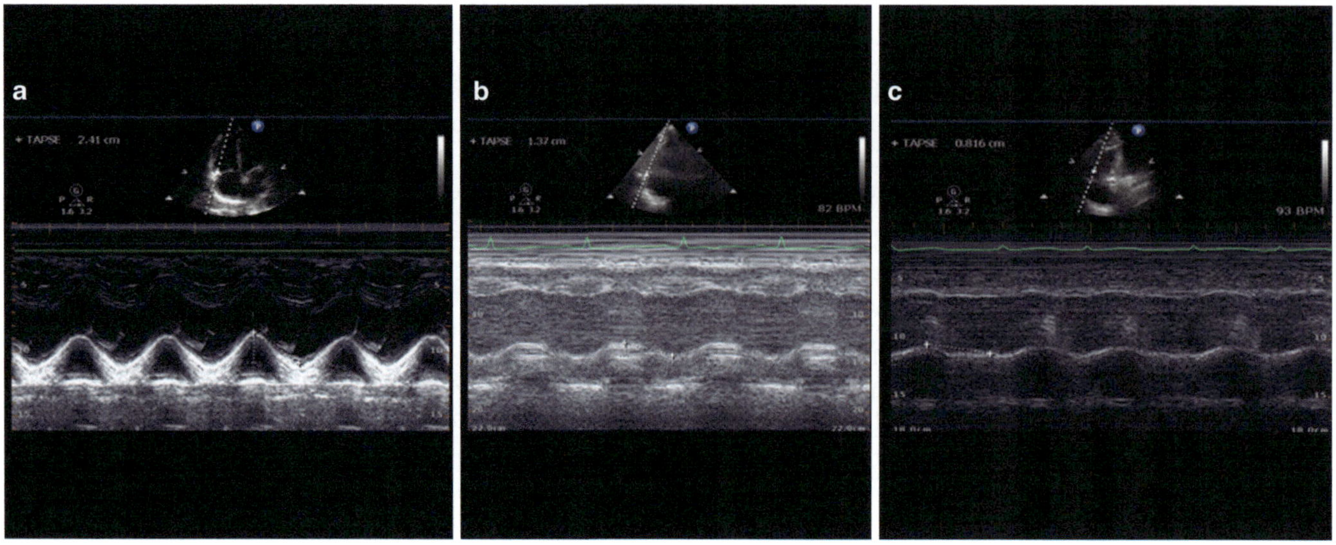

Fig. 3 TAPSE measurements. (**a**) Normal TAPSE. (**b**) Moderate RV dysfunction on TAPSE. (**c**) Severe RV dysfunction on TAPSE

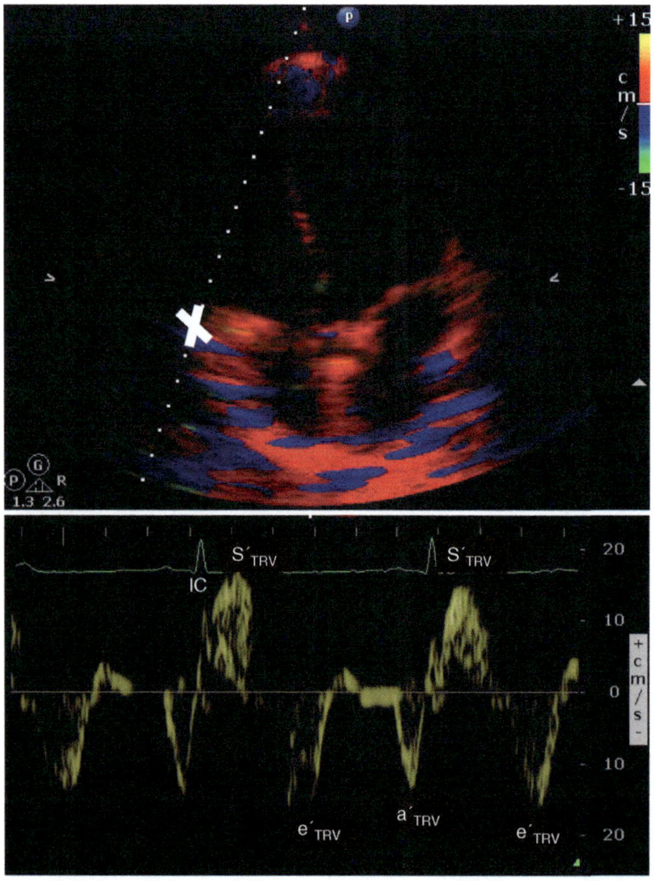

Fig. 4 TDI of the tricuspid annulus. Upper Panel, TDI cursor placement. X marks the correct placement of the indicator at the lateral tricuspid annulus in the thickest part of the muscle. Lower panel, TDI waveform. IC isovolumetric contraction, S'_{TRV} systolic velocity, e'_{TRV} early diastolic velocity, a'_{TRV} atrial contraction velocity

  - A S'_{TRV} less than 10 cm/s suggests severely decreased RV systolic function.
  - e'_{TRV} and a'_{TRV} are used in assessment of RV diastolic dysfunction described in Chap. 11.

5 Tips and Pointers for TAPSE and S′

- Do not use TAPSE with poor 2D visualization of the right heart as M-Mode and TDI depend on good 2D images.
  - Check the TASPE and S′ against your visual estimate of RV function.
  - Poor cursor alignment causes falsely low values.
- It is very important to align the cursor properly with the annular longitudinal excursion as TAPSE is angle dependent.
- Compare at least 5 cardiac cycles for the most accurate measurement.

6 Special Considerations

- On a ventilator, the right heart is often dilated to equal the size of the LV.
- Patients with chronic pulmonary disease or pulmonary hypertension often have dilated right hearts.

7 Normal and Reference Values

- Abnormal TAPSE <17 mm
- Abnormal S′ < 10 cm/s

Suggested Reading

Aloia E, Cameli M, et al. TAPSE: an old but useful tool in different diseases. Int J Cardiol. 2016;225:177–83.

Hori Y, Kano T, Hoshi F, Higuchi S. Relationship between tissue Doppler-derived RV systolic function and invasive hemodynamic measurements. Am J Physiol Heart Circ Physiol. 2007;293(1):H120–5. https://doi.org/10.1152/ajpheart.00097.2007. Epub 2007 Feb 23.

Lang RM, Badano LP, et al. Recommendations for cardiac chamber quantification by echocardiography in adults: an update from the American Society of Echocardiography and the European Association of Cardiovascular Imaging. J Am Soc Echocardiogr. 2015;28(1):1–39.e12.

Rudski LG, Lai WW, Afilalo J, Hua L, Handschumacher MD, Chandrasekaran K, Solomon SD, Louie EK, Schiller NB. Guidelines for the echocardiographic assessment of the right heart in adults: a report from the American Society of Echocardiography endorsed by the European Association of Echocardiography, a registered branch of the European Society of Cardiology, and the Canadian Society of Echocardiography. J Am Soc Echocardiogr. 2010;23(7):685–713; quiz 786-8. https://doi.org/10.1016/j.echo.2010.05.010.

Pulmonary Hypertension

Alexis Salerno, Allison Lankford, and Sarah B. Murthi

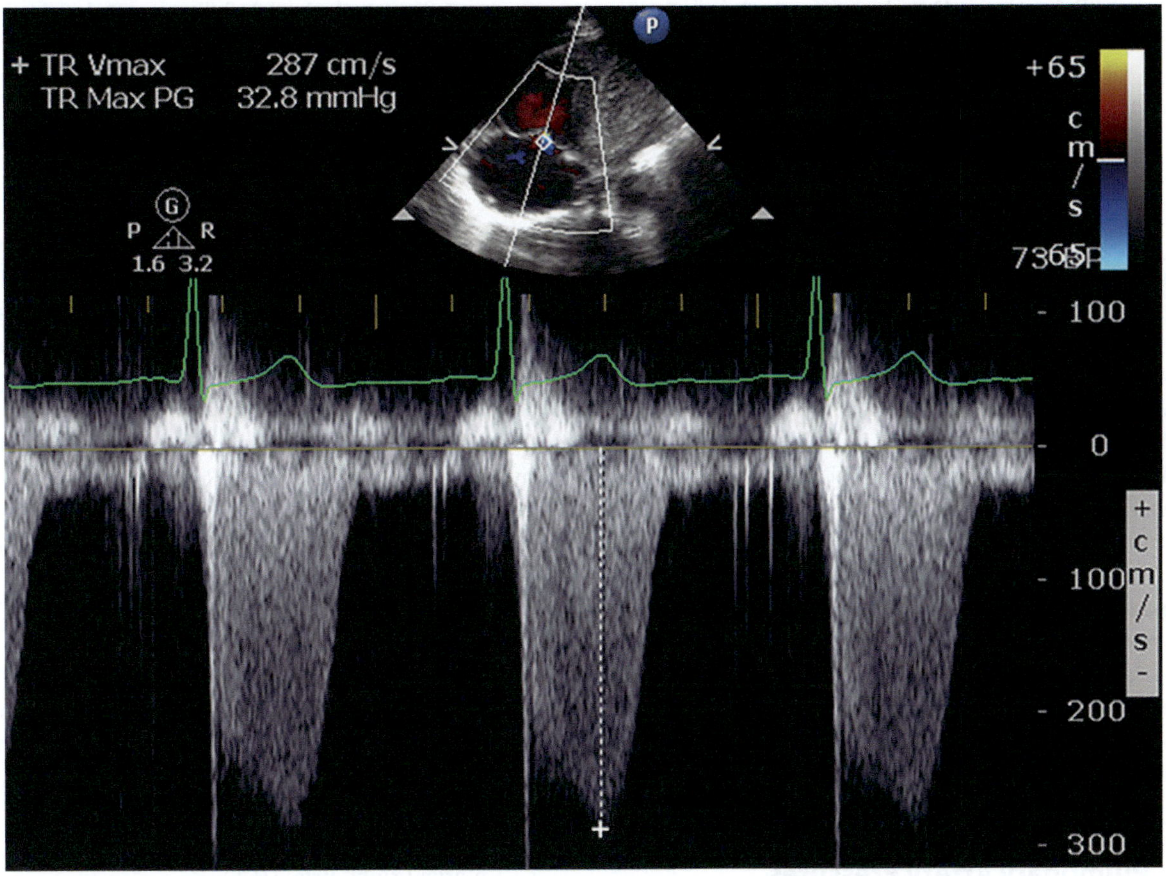

Supplementary Information The online version of this chapter (https://doi.org/10.1007/978-3-030-74687-2_13) contains supplementary material, which is available to authorized users.

A. Salerno
Department of Emergency Medicine, University of Maryland School of Medicine, Baltimore, MD, USA

A. Lankford
Department of Obstetrics and Gynecology and Reproductive Surgery, Division of Maternal Fetal Medicine, Anesthesia Critical Care, University of Maryland School of Medicine, R Adams Cowley Shock Trauma Center, Baltimore, MD, USA

S. B. Murthi (✉)
Department of Surgery, Program in Trauma and Critical Care, R Adams Cowley Shock Trauma Center, University of Maryland School of Medicine, University of Maryland Medical Center, Baltimore, MD, USA
e-mail: smurthi@som.umaryland.edu

A. Salerno et al. (eds.), *Atlas of Critical Care Echocardiography*, https://doi.org/10.1007/978-3-030-74687-2_13

Abbreviations

ARDS	Adult respiratory distress syndrome
AV	Aortic valve
CWD	Continuous wave Doppler
IVC	Inferior vena cava
LV	Left ventricle
ms	Milliseconds
PASP	Pulmonary artery systolic pressure
PAT	Pulmonary acceleration time
PE	Pulmonary embolus
PHTN	Pulmonary hypertension
PLA	Parasternal long axis
PV	Pulmonic valve
PWD	Pulsed wave Doppler
RA	Right atria
RAP	Right atrial pressure
RV	Right ventricle
RVOT	Right ventricular outflow tract
RVSP	Right ventricular systolic pressure
TR maxPG	Tricuspid regurgitant maximum pressure gradient
TR Vmax	Tricuspid regurgitant velocity maximum
TR	Tricuspid regurgitation

1 Introduction

Pulmonary artery hypertension (PHTN) is defined as a mean pulmonary artery pressure of >25 mmHg at rest. A complication of cardiac and pulmonary disease, pulmonary hypertension causes right ventricular (RV) dysfunction. Those with it are at greater risk of death. Also, pulmonary embolus (PE) and hypoxia from adult respiratory distress syndrome (ARDS) can cause acute PHTN leading to right heart dysfunction. Traditionally, it is diagnosed with right heart catherization. Echocardiography is a noninvasive, minimal risk, method of identifying patients.

2 Pulmonary Artery Pressures

The pulmonary artery pressure can be assessed by continuous wave Doppler (CWD) through the tricuspid regurgitant (TR) jet or pulsed wave Doppler (PWD) through the pulmonic valve (PV).

Clinical Relevance

- Diagnosis of pulmonary hypertension
- Defining a group of patients with ARDS who may benefit from pulmonary vasodilators (i.e., inhaled prostaglandins, nitric oxide)
  - Dilated right ventricle (RV) with evidence of pressure volume overload combined with a small underfilled left ventricle (LV)
  - Trend changes with therapeutic interventions
- Diagnosis of PE
  - The 60/60 sign is supportive of PE (see Chap. 18)
    - Tricuspid regurgitant jet maximum gradient >60 mmHg
    - Pulmonary acceleration time <60 milliseconds (ms)
      - Assessed via the right ventricular outflow tract (RVOT)

3 Visual Inspection the RV and LV in All Windows (Fig. 1)

The most important finding of pulmonary hypertension is evidence of RV pressure volume overload and a small underfilled LV. Depending on the clinical scenario, this suggests that reducing PA pressure with vasodilators may improve RV function and LV filling.

- Primary goal is detecting moderate and severe pulmonary hypertension contributing to RV dysfunction.
  - Less concerned with mild PHTN
- *The most important tool is visual inspection of all windows* (Fig. 1).
  - The RV is bigger than the LV in the Apical 4 Chamber (AP 4).
    - RV/LV base diameter is measurement >1.
      - Most useful on initial assessment prior to intubation because this is a common finding in mechanically ventilated patients
  - Flattened intraventricular septum
    - Often causing a D-shaped left ventricle
  - Enlarged right atrial (RA)
  - Dilated inferior vena cava (IVC)
    - Most important on initial presentation
    - Common finding in mechanically ventilated patients

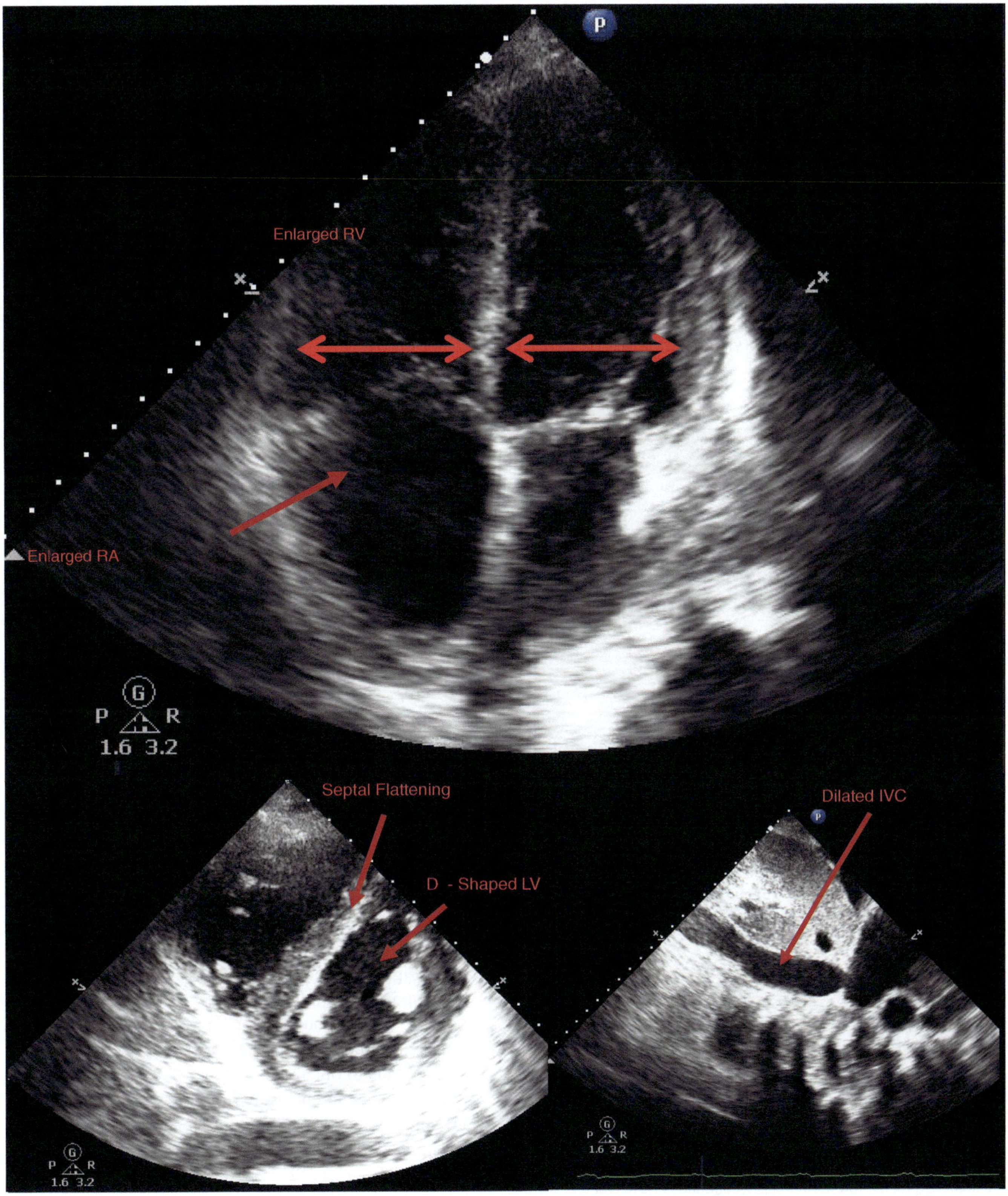

Fig. 1 Common findings with severe pulmonary hypertension. Upper panel; RV/LV ≥ 1 in the Apical 4 Chamber. The diameter is measured at the base of the LV and RV just proximal to the tricuspid and mitral valves. Lower left panel: Septal flattening in the parasternal short axis. Note the D-shaped LV. Lower right panel: Dilated non-collapsing IVC

4 Assessment with the Tricuspid Regurgitant Jet (Fig. 2)

As the RV contracts against increasing pulmonary resistance, a small amount of retrograde flow forms a measurable TR jet. The jet shoots from the RV back into the RA through the closed tricuspid valve. The velocity of TR increases as pulmonary artery systolic pressure (PASP) rises. The maximum pressure gradient of the jet and the estimated right atrial pressure (RAP) are used to estimate the PASP, also called the right ventricular systolic pressure (RVSP).

- Window: Apical 4-Chamber, Parasternal short axis (PSA) at the aortic valve (AV)
  - Any window that allows visualization of TR can be used.

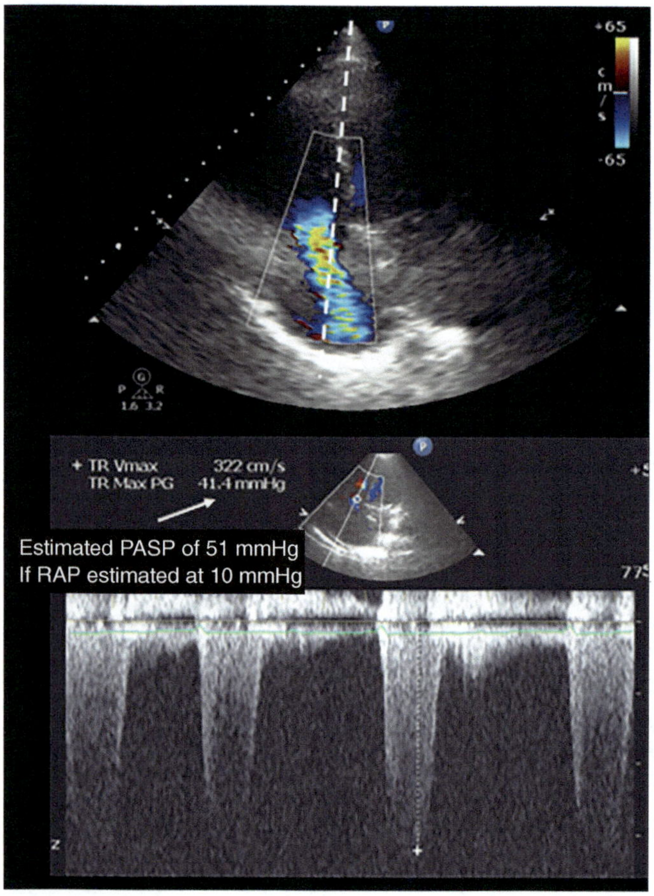

Fig. 2 Tricuspid regurgitant jet in assessment of pulmonary hypertension. Upper panel: color flow Doppler through TR jet. Dotted line is the continuous wave Doppler (CWD) cursor. Note how it is placed through the highest velocity flow. Lower panel: continuous wave Doppler waveform; TR Vmax tricuspid regurgitant velocity maximum, TR Max PG tricuspid maximum pressure gradient, PASP pulmonary artery systolic pressure, RAP right atrial pressure. The dotted line is measuring TR Vmax, the TR MAX PG is calculated. The estimated RAP is added to the TR Max PG to estimate the PASP. See the text for details on estimating the RAP

  - The Apical 4 provides the best parallel alignment with flow.
  - Often the jet can be seen in the PSA to patient's right and lower than the AV.
  - Sometimes the jet is seen in the parasternal long axis or the subxiphoid window.
    - Angle the face of the transducer up from the PLA to open up the RV and the tricuspid valve (TV)
- Mode: Color flow Doppler, continuous wave Doppler (CWD)
  - CWD is used because the jet velocity is high and flow cannot be accurately measured with pulsed wave Doppler.
- Units: mmHg
- Reference Values PASP
  - Normal <25
  - Mild 35–45
  - Moderate 45–60
  - High >60
- Rather than a specific value for PASP, think in terms of categories; likely severe pulmonary hypertension is present rather than as a precise numeric measurement (i.e., 67 vs 73 mmHg).
  - Most patients will have confirmatory findings, as described above
    - RV/LV ratio > 1 in the AP 4, septal flattening with a D-shaped LV, large RV with a small underfilled LV
- Trending changes with interventions are reasonable, for example, TR velocity changes after starting a pulmonary vasodilator in a patient with ARDS.

Measuring the Peak Velocity of the Tricuspid Regurgitation Jet (Fig. 2)

- Obtain an image of the tricuspid valve.
- Place the color flow Doppler box over the valve.
- Observe for tricuspid regurgitation. Place CWD cursor through the regurgitant jet.
  - A bright blue jet will flow back into the RA when the valve is closed (Video 1).
  - Place cursor though highest velocity TR jet flow.
  - Line the cursor up so that it is parallel with flow.
- Select CWD to obtain the tracing.
  - Save image and measure peak flow.
- TR velocity max (TR Vmax) reference values
  - High: TR >3.4 m/s
    - Likely severe PHTN
  - Intermediate: TR 2.8—3.4 m/s
    - Indeterminant
    - Assess for confirmatory findings
  - Low: TR < 2.8 m/s
    - Likely normal pulmonary arterial pressure

Calculating Right Ventricular/Pulmonary Artery Systolic Pressure

- Referred to as the PASP or the right ventricular systolic pressure (RVSP)
- The TR max pressure gradient (TR maxPG) and the estimated RAP are used to assess PASP or RVSP.
  - TR maxPG = 4 × [TR Vmax]^2
    - Automatically calculated when the peak is measured in most packages
    - The pressure gradient is used in the 60/60 sign for PE.
  - PASP = (4 × [TR Vmax]^2) + RAP
- Estimating the RAP
  - The American Society of Echocardiography recommends using the IVC diameter and collapsibility to estimate the RAP as 3, 8, or 15 mmHg
    - Not feasible in critically ill patients, it involves a sniff maneuver
    - Also, mechanical ventilation and thoracoabdominal surgery cause a dilated IVC which does not accurately reflect RAP
  - We recommend a simplified method:
    - Small, underfilled RA and RV
      - 5 mmHg
    - Normal RA/RV
      - 10 mmHg
    - Dilated RA/RV
      - 15 mmHg
    - We use 10 mmHg most of the time, simply getting an estimate.
- Simplified method (Fig. 1 lower panel)
  - Measure the velocity of the TR Vmax.
  - Just add 10 mmHg (or 15 if the RA/RV are enlarged) to the TR maxPG automatically calculated and displayed on the screen.

5 Assessment of Flow Through the Right Ventricular Outflow Tract

Blood passes out of the RVOT into the pulmonary artery. As pulmonary artery pressure increases, pulmonary acceleration time (PAT) decreases and the pattern of systolic flow changes.

- Window: Parasternal short axis at the aortic valve
- Mode: Color flow Doppler, pulsed wave Doppler (PWD)
- Units: milliseconds (ms)

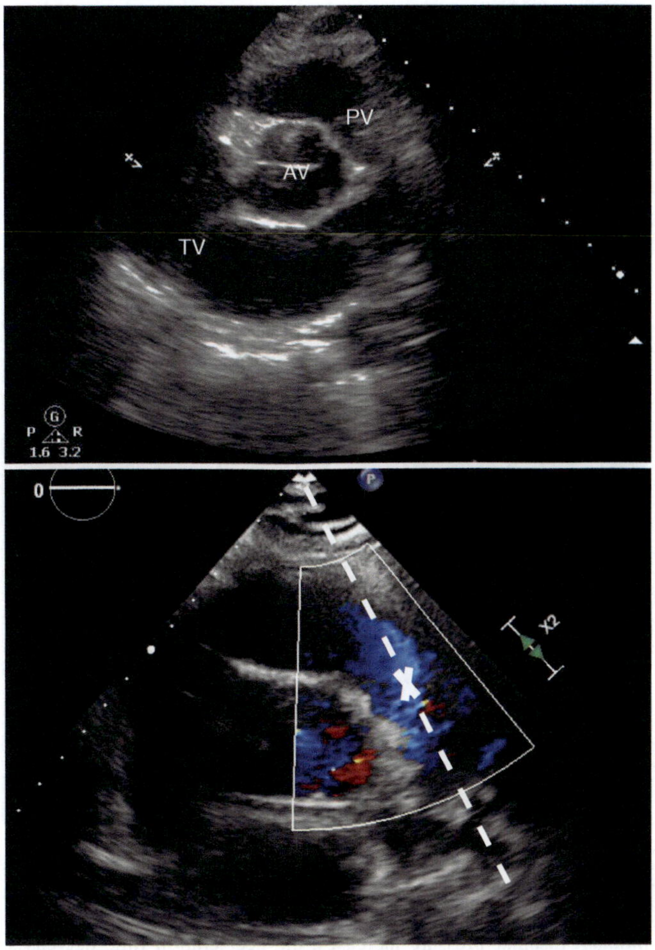

Fig. 3 Color flow Doppler through the pulmonic valve. Upper panel: parasternal short axis at the aortic valve. TV tricuspid valve, AV aortic valve, PV pulmonic valve. Lower Panel: color flow Doppler through the PV. The dotted line is the cursor for pulsed wave Doppler. The white X demonstrates the sample volume taken just inside the valve

• Reference Values	*PAT*	*Waveform*
Normal:	>130 msec	normal parabola
Severe PHTN:	<80 msec	mid-systolic notch
PE	<60 msec	mid-systolic notch

Pulmonary Acceleration Time (PAT) (Figs. 3 and 4)

- Apply ECG leads.
- Obtain the parasternal short axis view at the aortic valve.
- Optimize the view of the pulmonic valve.
  - Superior and to the patient's left
  - Color flow Doppler can help identify the valve (Video 2)
- Place indicator/sample just proximal to the pulmonic valve.

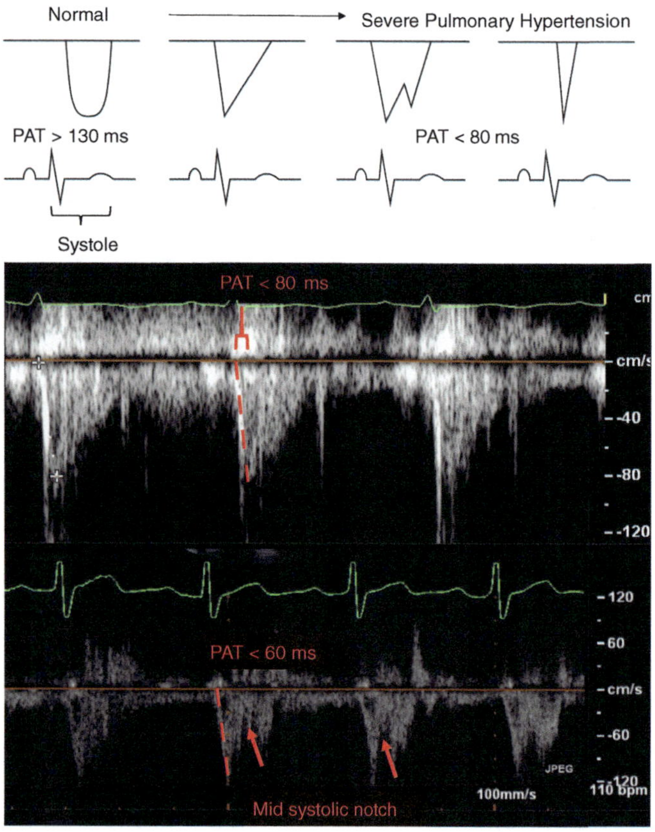

Fig. 4 Changes in right ventricular outflow tract (RVOT) velocities with severe pulmonary hypertension (PHTN). Upper panel: illustration of RVOT velocity changes. PAT: pulmonary acceleration time. As pulmonary vascular pressure increases, the acceleration time decreases. Middle panel: pulsed wave Doppler through the RVOT in a patient with severe PHTN. The dotted line is the velocity used to measure the PAT. Lower Panel: systolic notching in severe pulmonary hypertension. The red arrow is pointing to mid-systolic notching

- Select PWD to obtain the tracing.
  - If possible, adjust the image so that the signal has a closing snap but not an opening snap.
  - Save the tracing.
- Measure the time from onset of flow to the peak flow in systole. Time is displayed on the x-axis.

Pulmonary Artery Systolic Flow Patterns (Fig. 4)

- Dome-shape with no notching
  - Normal pulmonary vascular resistance
- Mid-systolic notch
  - Severely elevated pulmonary vascular resistance
  - Low pulmonary artery compliance
  - Found in acute PE

Suggested Reading

Arkles JS, Opotowsky AR, Ojeda J, Rogers F, Liu T, Prassana V, et al. Shape of the right ventricular Doppler envelope predicts hemodynamics and right heart function in pulmonary hypertension. Am J Respir Crit Care Med. 2011;183(2):268–76. https://doi.org/10.1164/rccm.201004-0601OC. Epub 2010 Aug 13.

Lopez-Candales A, Edelman K. Shape of the right ventricular outflow Doppler envelope and severity of pulmonary hypertension. Eur Heart J Cardiovasc Imaging. 2012;13:309–16. https://doi.org/10.1093/ejechocard/jer235.

Parasuraman S, Walker S, Loudon BL, et al. Assessment of pulmonary artery pressure by echocardiography-a comprehensive review. Int J Cardiol Heart Vasc. 2016;12:45–51. Published 2016 Jul 4. https://doi.org/10.1016/j.ijcha.2016.05.011.

Widrich J, Shetty M. Physiology, pulmonary vascular resistance. [Updated 2020 May 29]. In: StatPearls [Internet]. Treasure Island: StatPearls Publishing; 2020. Available from: https://www.ncbi.nlm.nih.gov/books/NBK554380/.

Inferior Vena Cava Respiratory Variation

Shannon Gaasch and Alexis Salerno

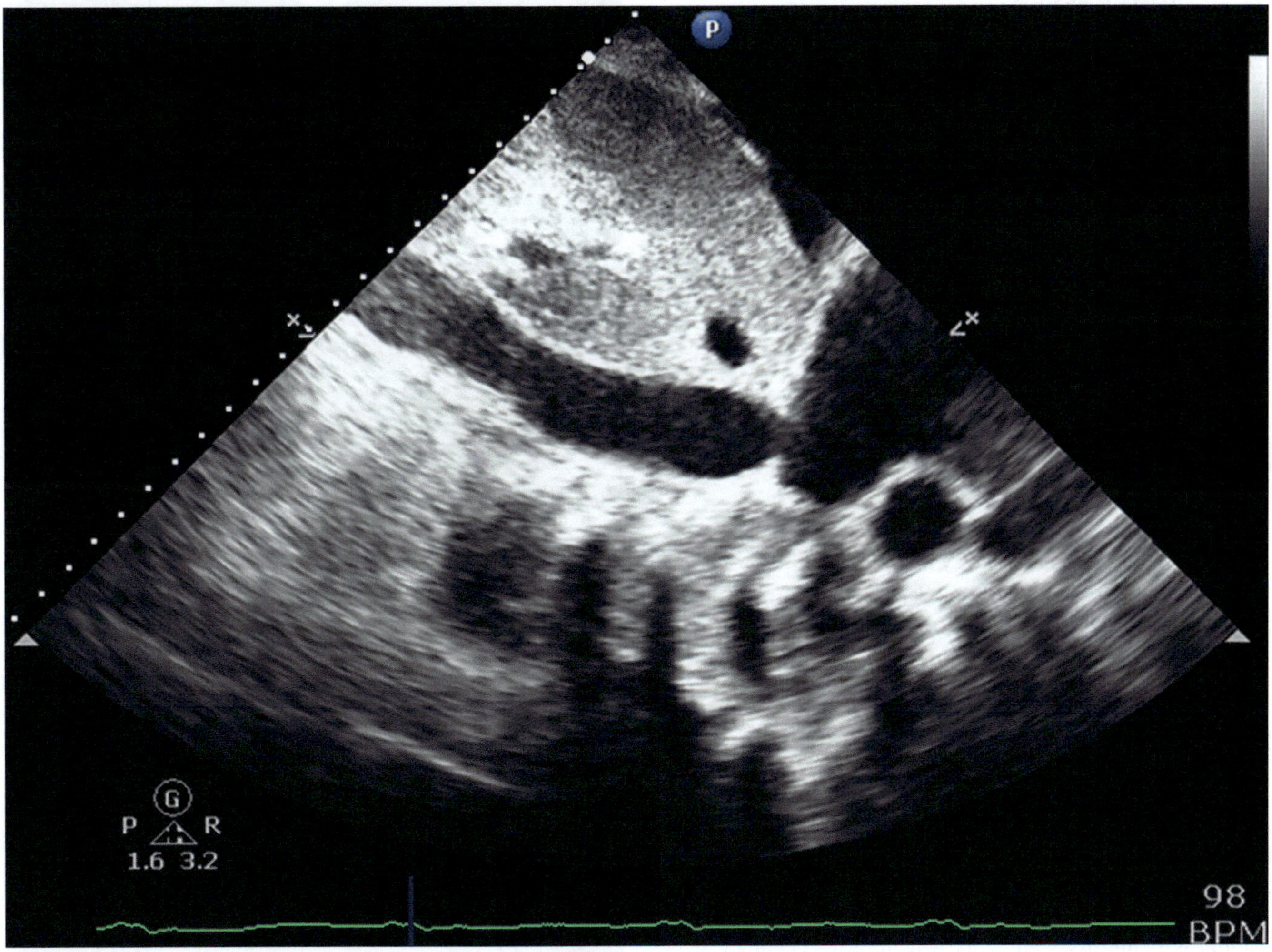

Supplementary Information The online version of this chapter (https://doi.org/10.1007/978-3-030-74687-2_14) contains supplementary material, which is available to authorized users.

S. Gaasch
R. Adams Cowley Shock Trauma Center, University of Maryland, Baltimore, MD, USA

A. Salerno (✉)
Department of Emergency Medicine, University of Maryland School of Medicine, Baltimore, MD, USA
e-mail: Alexis.Salerno@som.umaryland.edu

A. Salerno et al. (eds.), *Atlas of Critical Care Echocardiography*, https://doi.org/10.1007/978-3-030-74687-2_14

Abbreviations

2D	Two-dimensional
IVC	Inferior vena cava
RA	Right atria
SV	Stroke volume

1 Introduction

Previous studies have shown that the change in the diameter of the inferior vena cava (IVC) during the respiratory cycle correlates with volume responsiveness. Volume responsiveness (VR) is the likelihood the cardiac stroke volume (SV) will increase with a fluid bolus. In a spontaneously breathing patient, the IVC collapses with inspiration. In a passively ventilated patient, the IVC expands during inspiration. Both the Feissel and the Barbier methods described below have been shown to predict VR in mechanically ventilated patients on a set tidal volume. The data are mixed on the accuracy of using delta IVC to measure VR, so it should not be used alone to direct fluid management. We have found it especially problematic in patients who have undergone torso surgery or who have been vented using high mean airway pressure.

2 Obtaining the Views and Calculating Measurements

Obtain the IVC image

- Curvilinear or a phased array transducer
- Abdominal or cardiac presets (Fig. 1)
  - Abdominal
    - Transducer indicator will be displayed on the left of the screen
    - The right atria (RA), and hepatic veins will also be on the left.
  - Cardiac
    - The transducer will be displayed on the right of the screen.
    - The RA and hepatic veins will also be on the right.
- Obtain the view of the IVC entering the RA from the subxiphoid widow.
  - Place the M mode cursor 2 cm from the RA.
    - At the entrance of the hepatic vein into the IVC (Fig. 1)
    - Optimize the image and cursor placement so that it drops perpendicular to the IVC
    - Can use the 2D image for measurement if unable to line-up the cursor correctly
  - Obtain and save M mode tracing.
  - Measure the diameter of the IVC at the maximum and minimum (Fig. 2).

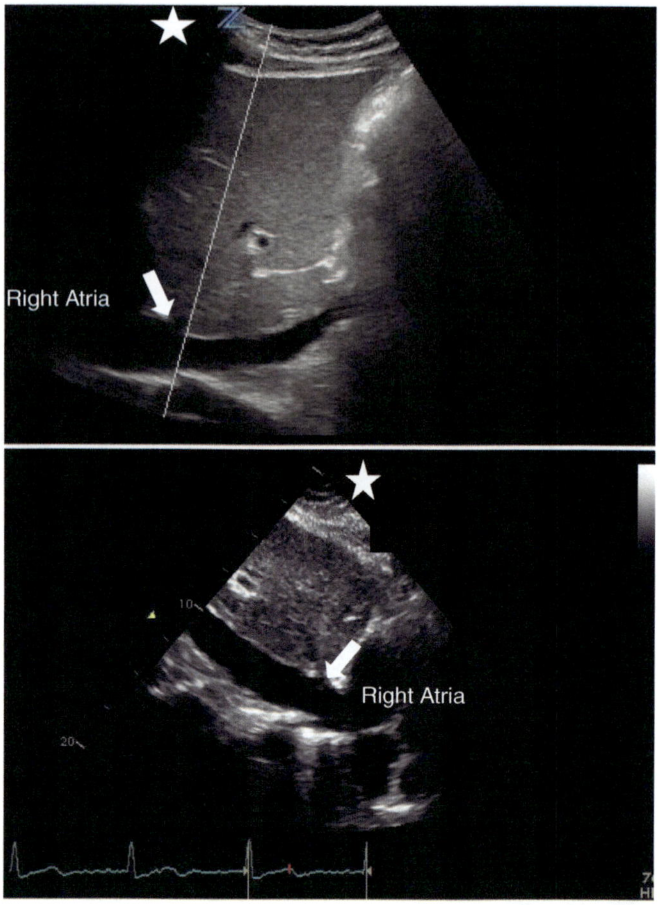

Fig. 1 IVC in abdominal and cardiac presets/exam type. Upper panel: Abdominal presets. Lower panel: Cardiac presets. Star: transducer indicator orientation. Arrow: hepatic vein

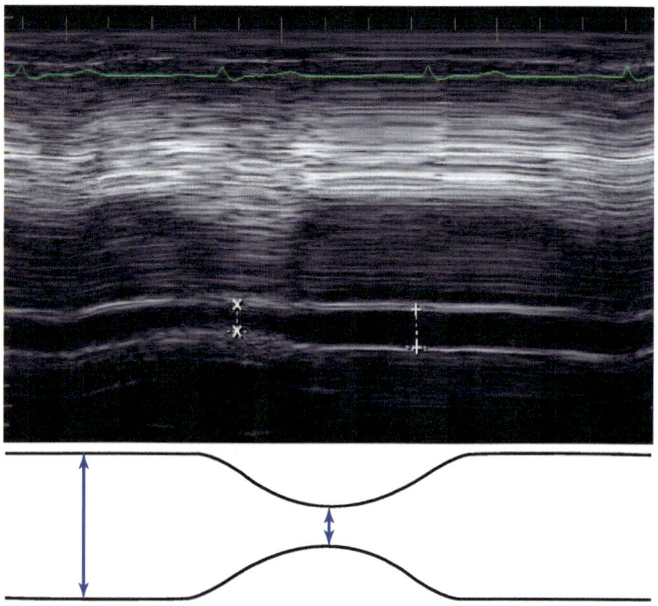

Fig. 2 IVC delta measurement. Measure leading edge to leading edge, just inside the white vessel wall

    - Leading edge to leading edge, just inside the vessel walls
  - It is important not to have the patient sniff or take a deep breath in while performing this measurement.
  - Or assess while the ventilator is delivering a volume control breath, also called passively ventilated.

Feissel Method

- Δ IVC = (IVC max − IVC min)/((IVC max + IVC min) × 0.5) × 100

Barbier Method

- Δ IVC = (IVC max − IVC min)/IVC min) × 100

3 Interpreting Measurements

- The values for change in diameter of the IVC are interpreted differently for passively ventilated patients as compared to spontaneously breathing patients.
  - *For Passively Ventilated Patients*
    - > 18% likely represents volume responsive
  - *For Spontaneously Breathing Patients*
    - > 25% likely represents fluid responsiveness
- These are cut off values based on retrospective interpretation of prospectively collected databases, usually from a single center.
- In ultrasound, precise cut off values are not reproducible, especially for an imprecise metric like volume responsiveness.
- We recommend using rounded numbers and a categorical interpretation of ultrasound measurements whenever possible.
- For the focused rapid echocardiographic evaluation (FREE), we use less likely VR, indeterminant, and more likely VR (Fig. 3; Videos 1, 2, and 3)
  - *Passively ventilated*
    - < 10% less likely volume responsive
    - 10–20% indeterminate
    - > 20% more likely volume responsive
  - *Spontaneously breathing*
    - < 25% less likely volume responsive
    - 25–50% indeterminate
    - >50% more likely volume responsive

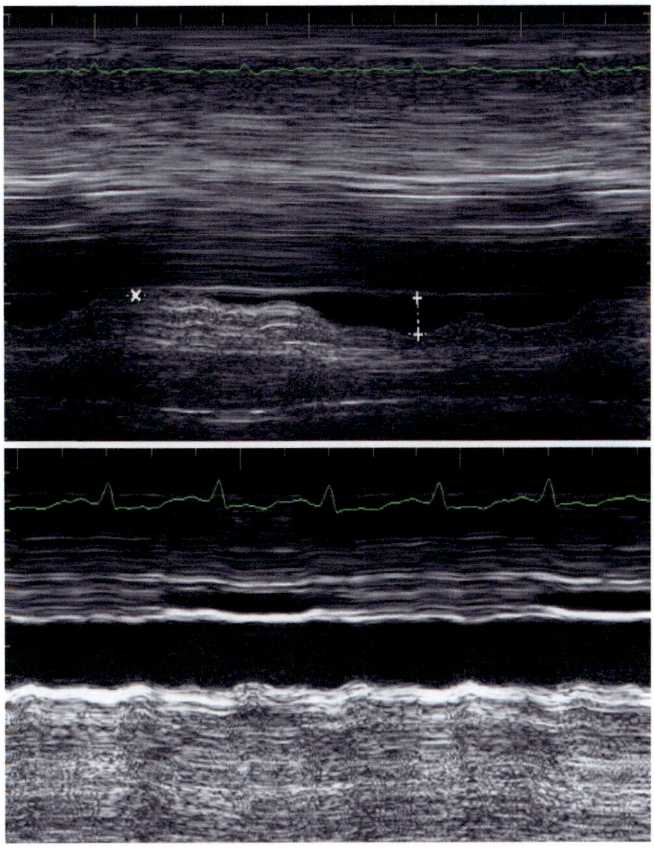

Fig. 3 IVC with and without variation. Upper panel: Complete collapse. Lower panel no collapse

4 Tips and Pitfalls

- Can confuse aorta for IVC, make sure to see hepatic veins coming into the vessel.
- IVC diameter and degree of collapse are influenced by an awake patient's respiratory effort.
- The amount of pressure support from a ventilator can impact IVC variation.
- Patients with chronic lung hyperinflation, right heart failure, increased intra-abdominal pressure will have an inaccurate IVC collapsibility.
- Since there are many situations where delta IVC may fail to predict fluid responsiveness, delta IVC should be used in context with other volume measurements.

Suggested Reading

Lee CW, Kory PD, Arntfield RT. Development of a fluid resuscitation protocol using inferior vena cava and lung ultrasound. J Crit Care. 2016;31(1):96–100.

Via G, Tavazzi G, Price S. Ten situations where inferior vena cava ultrasound may fail to accurately predict fluid responsiveness: a physiologically based point of view. Intensive Care Med. 2016;42(7):1164–7.

Stroke Volume Variation

Michelle F. Dawson and Alexis Salerno

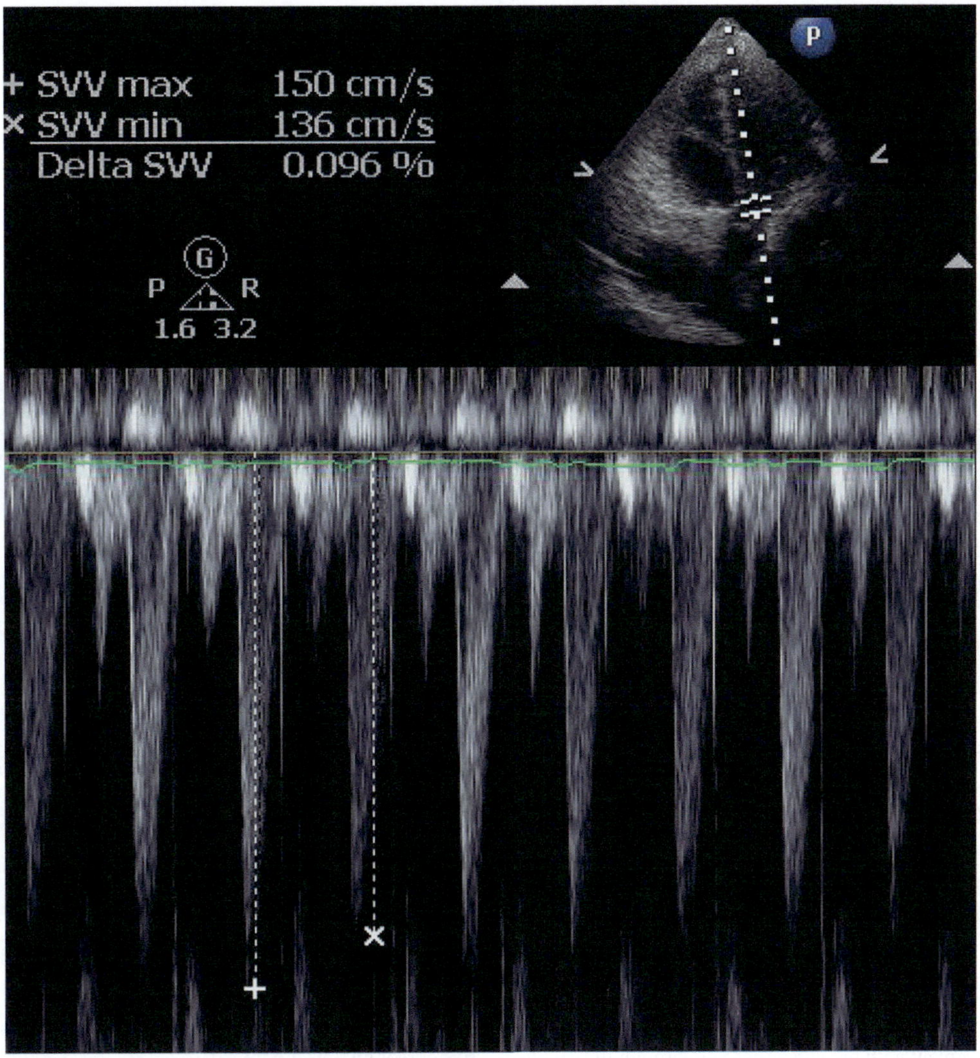

M. F. Dawson
University of Virginal Medical Center, Charlottesville, VA, USA

A. Salerno (✉)
Department of Emergency Medicine, University of Maryland
School of Medicine, Baltimore, MD, USA
e-mail: Alexis.Salerno@som.umaryland.edu

A. Salerno et al. (eds.), *Atlas of Critical Care Echocardiography*, https://doi.org/10.1007/978-3-030-74687-2_15

Abbreviations

AP 5	Apical Five Chamber
ICU	Intensive care unit
LV	Left ventricle
LVOTD	Left ventricular outflow tract diameter
PLR	Passive Leg Raise
RV	Right ventricle
SV	Stroke Volume
SVV	Stroke Volume Variation
Vpk	Peak Velocity
VR	Volume Responsiveness
VTI_{RV}	Velocity Time Integral Respiratory Variation
$VTI_{vpk\ max}$	Velocity Time Integral Peak Velocity Maximum
$VTI_{vpk\ min}$	Velocity Time Integral Peak Velocity Minimum
VTI	Velocity Time Integral

1 Introduction

Assessment of fluid responsiveness can be challenging. The primary goal of a fluid bolus is an increase in stroke volume (SV). However, repeated fluid challenges to assess volume responsiveness (VR) serve no benefit if your patient is on the flat portion of the Frank-Starling curve. Moreover, additional fluid could be harmful if it results in elevated atrial pressure and venous congestion.

An important assessment of intravascular volume status is the likelihood the SV will increase after a fluid bolus, also called volume responsiveness (VR). The stroke volume (SV) alone does not reflect VR. However, a respiratory stroke volume variation (SVV) of >12% accurately predicts fluid responsiveness. There are several useful methods in point-of-care echocardiography that can assist the clinician in evaluating SVV to guide fluid management.

2 SVV with Respiratory Peak Velocity Variation

- Stroke volume is assessed by the LV outflow tract diameter (LVOTD) and the LV velocity time integral (VTI) measured through the aortic valve (AV) with Doppler, details in Chap. 10.
- The LVOTD is a fixed anatomic measurement that does not change in adulthood
- So, changes in SV can be assessed by changes in the VTI.
  - Either peak velocity (Vpk) or the VTI envelope
    - Vpk
      - Easier to measure
    - VTI envelope
      - More difficult, harder to define max and min
- VTI variability during the respiratory cycle (VTI_{RV}) is a marker of volume responsiveness.

3 Uses VTI_{RV}

1. Measurement of volume responsiveness
2. Helps determine when a fluid bolus is likely to be beneficial

4 Window and Mode

- Window: Apical 5 Chamber (AP 5)
  - Mode: Pulsed Wave Doppler (PWD)

5 How to Measure SVV with VTI Vpk Variation

- Obtain the AP 5 view.
- Select PWD.
- Obtain VTI just inside the AV leaflets.
  - The same method as measuring SV
- Decrease sweep speed (Fig. 1).

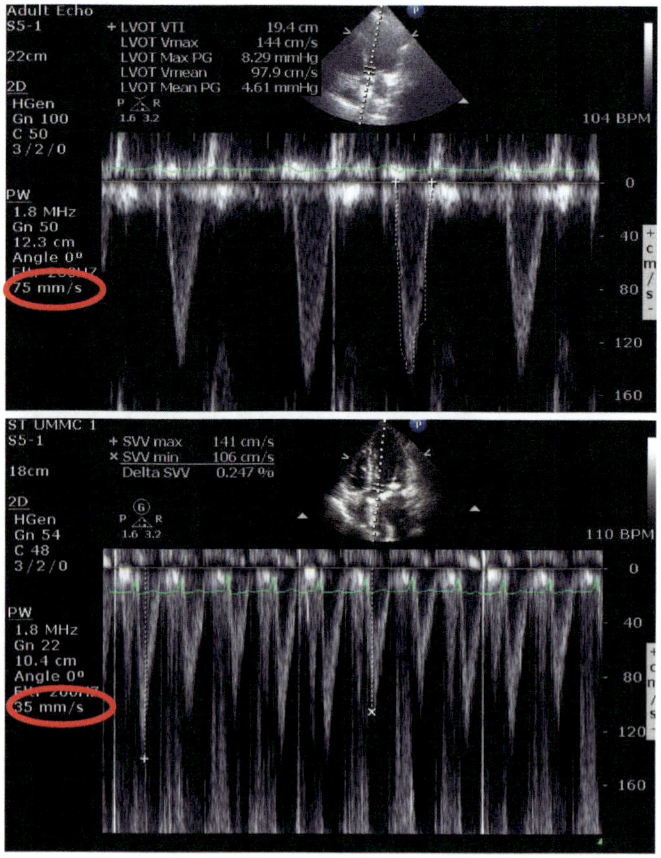

Fig. 1 Sweep speed. *Upper panel*, normal sweep speed of 75 mm/s (*red circle*). Lower panel, lower sweep speed for peak velocity measurement 35 mm/s (*red circle*)

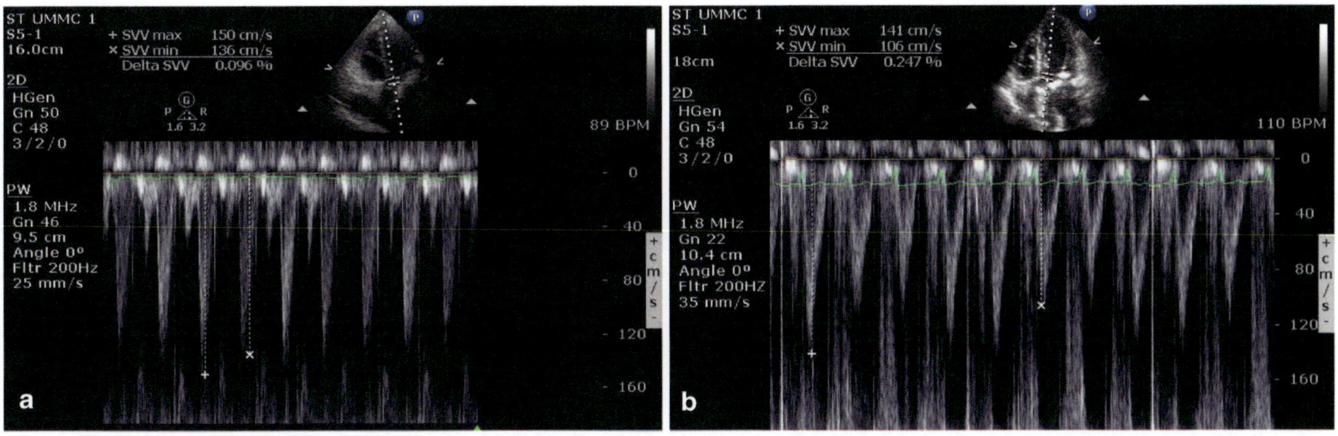

Fig. 2 Stroke volume variation measurement. (**a**) has a change less than 12%, indicating the patient may not be fluid responsive. (**b**) has a change greater than 12%, indicating the patient may be fluid responsive

  - < 50 mm/s
  - Pulse wave narrows to approximately 20 beats in view on the display
  - Able to see sinusoidal respiratory changes
  - Save image
- Measure highest peak velocity ($VTI_{pk\ max}$)
- Measure lowest peak velocity ($VTI_{pk\ min}$)
  $VTI_{RV} = (VTI_{vpk\ max} - VTI_{vpk\ min})/[(VTI_{vpk\ max} + VTI_{vpk\ min}) \times 0.5] \times 100$
  - 12% predicts volume responsiveness (Fig. 2)
    - Probably not reproducible
    - Too fine a line for repeated ultrasound measurements
      - See last paragraph in Chap. 1
  - Like more accurate
    - ≤ 10% Less Likely not volume responsive
    - >10, <15% Indeterminant
    - ≥15% More likely volume responsive

6 Special Considerations When Using APV and VTI Variation for SVV Assessment

Valid under the following conditions:

- Normal sinus rhythm
- Normal intra-abdominal pressure
- The patient's chest must be closed

7 SVV with Passive Leg Raise

There is data to support the use of SVV with passive leg raise (PLR) to determine VR. In our practices in the Emergency Department and Surgical ICU, we have found it impractical. A large portion of patients are unable to have PLR due to diagnosis such as leg fractures, pelvic fractures, or morbid obesity. For patients who can, a few staff members need to be available to hold up the leg while the tracing is obtained. Also, it is difficult to identify when to measure the change in the VTI.

Suggested Reading

De Backer D, Fagnoul D. Intensive care ultrasound: VI. Fluid responsiveness and shock assessment. ATS Seminars. 2014;11(1):129–36.

Ferrada P, Murthi S, Anand RJ, Bochicchio GV, Scalea T. Transthoracic focused rapid echocardiography examination: real-time evaluation of fluid status in critically ill trauma patients. J Trauma. 2011;70(1):56–62; discussion 62-4. https://doi.org/10.1097/TA.0b013e318207e6ee.

Levitov A, Marik PE. Echocardiographic assessment of preload responsiveness in critically ill patients. Cardiol Res Pract. 2012;2012:819696. https://doi.org/10.1155/2012/819696. Epub 2011 Sep 12

Miller A, Mandeville J. Predicting and measuring fluid responsiveness with echocardiography. Echo Res Pract. 2016;3(2):G1–G12. https://doi.org/10.1530/ERP-16-0008. Epub 2016 May 24

Pulmonary Findings

Alexis Salerno and Sarah B. Murthi

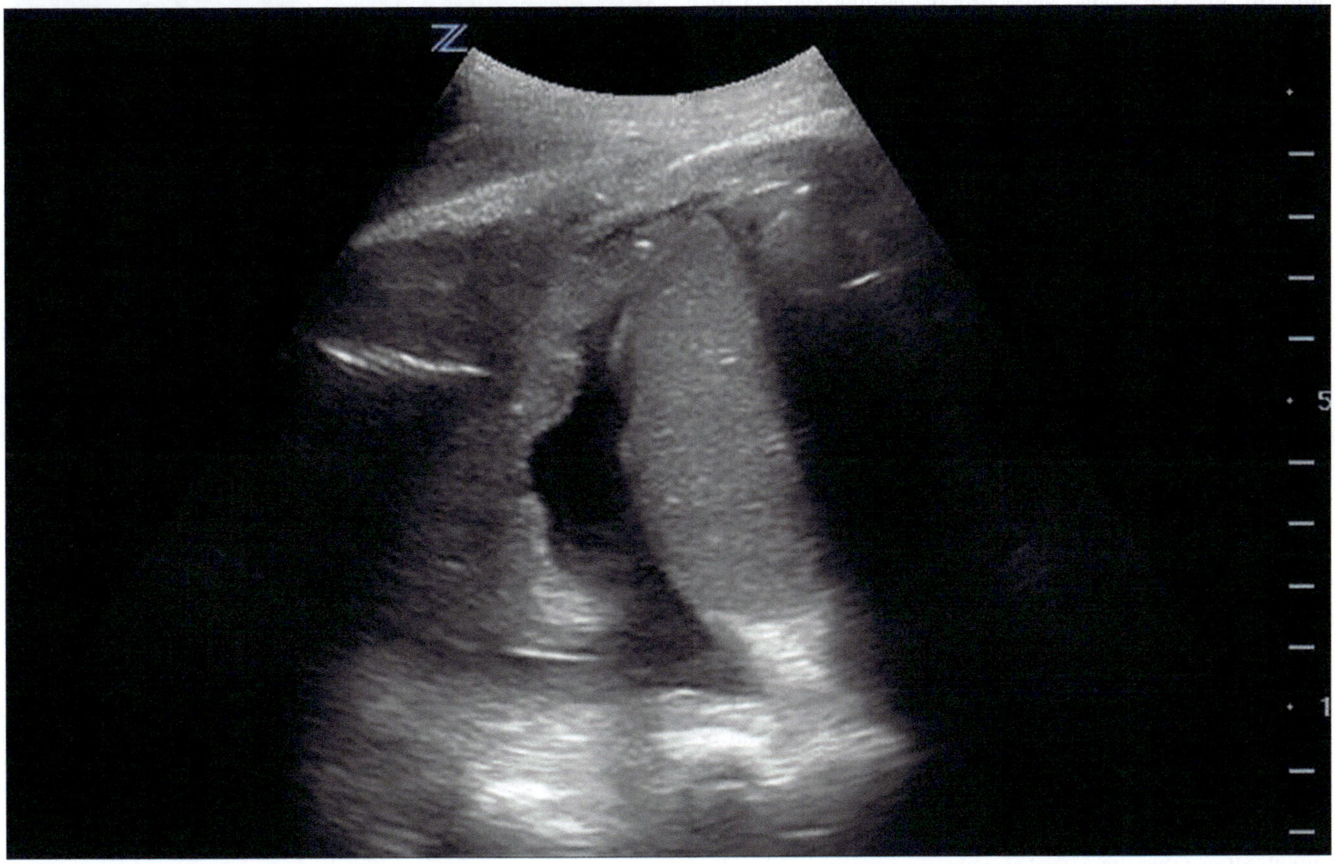

Supplementary Information The online version of this chapter (https://doi.org/10.1007/978-3-030-74687-2_16) contains supplementary material, which is available to authorized users.

A. Salerno
Department of Emergency Medicine, University of Maryland School of Medicine, Baltimore, MD, USA

S. B. Murthi (✉)
Department of Surgery, Program in Trauma and Critical Care, R Adams Cowley Shock Trauma Center, University of Maryland School of Medicine, University of Maryland Medical Center, Baltimore, MD, USA
e-mail: smurthi@som.umaryland.edu

A. Salerno et al. (eds.), *Atlas of Critical Care Echocardiography*, https://doi.org/10.1007/978-3-030-74687-2_16

Abbreviation

2D Two dimensional

1 Introduction

Lung ultrasound is an essential tool to differentiate between causes of dyspnea. It can also be helpful in guiding fluid resuscitation and diagnosing the cause of shock. A full discussion of pulmonary findings in point-of-care ultrasound is beyond the scope of this book, but we have summarized some of the finding relevant to management of shock in critically ill patients. Please see Chap. 8 for a summary of how to preform lung ultrasound and normal findings and the final sections of the book to understand how to include it with other forms of ultrasound assessment.

2 Uses for Lung Assessment

1. Diagnosis of Pulmonary Edema
2. Fluid Intolerance Monitoring
3. Diagnosis of Pleural Effusion
4. Diagnosis of Lung Collapse and Consolidation
5. Diagnosis of Pneumothorax

3 B-Lines as Evidence of Pulmonary Edema

In patients with severe pulmonary edema, B-lines are found bilaterally in multiple lung fields. Elevated left atrial pressure from fluid resuscitation results in increased intestinal fluid causing pulmonary edema. With aggressive resuscitation, re-evaluate for new or increased B-lines as a sign of fluid intolerance perhaps indicating diuresis is beneficial.

Normally air in expanded alveoli prevents transmission of the ultrasound signal. A uniform gray hum is seen below the pleural line. B-lines occur when interstitial fluid around the alveoli allows the ultrasound signal to pass between the alveolar walls where it bounces back and forth before the returns to the transducer (Fig. 1)

- Discrete hyperechoic reverberation artifacts
- Originate from the pleural line and extend toward the bottom of the ultrasound screen
  - Window: Upper, Middle, Lower Lung
  - Presets/Exam type: Lung or Abdominal (not Cardiac)
  - Mode: 2D
  - Units: none
  - Normal <3 B-lines
- Phased array or curvilinear transducer in abdominal or lung presets/exam type
- Indicator up toward the head

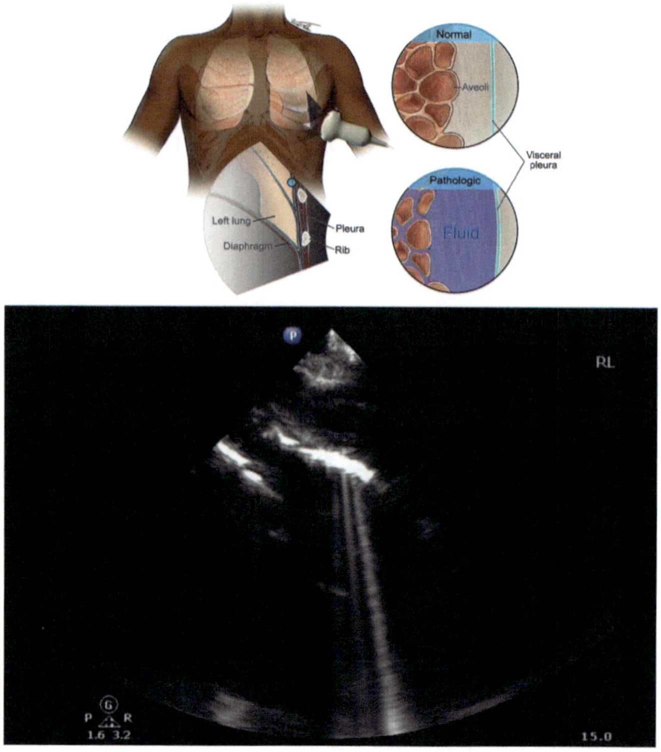

Fig. 1 B-lines: Upper panel: Normal lung and pulmonary fluid. The fluid between alveoli allows transmission of the ultrasound signal, which bounces back and forth forming the B-line reverberation artifact. Lower Panel: 2D image with a phased array transducer showing 3 discrete B-lines

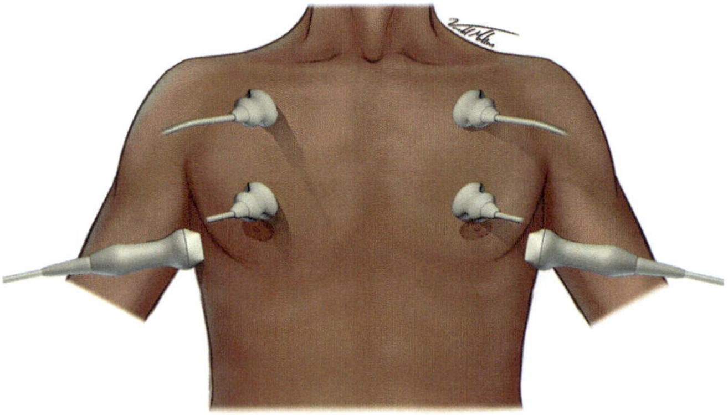

Fig. 2 Rapid lung ultrasound to assess for pulmonary edema. The transducers are place in the upper, middle, and lower fields

- Obtain views of the upper, middle, and lower sections of the lungs bilaterally (Fig. 2)
  - Easily incorporated into a hemodynamic echo assessment
- Evidence of 3 or more B-lines in multiple intercostal spaces bilaterally suggests lung interstitial fluid due to pulmonary edema
- B-lines localized to one or two lung regions may be more consistent with a pneumonia or other localized lung process

4 Tips and Pointers

- Perform the exam the same way every time (Left: upper, middle, lower and then Right: upper, middle, lower) to make interpretation easier
  - Save a clip from each section
- Healthy individuals can have B-lines present in the lower lung portions
  - Especially if mechanically ventilated and lying supine in a bed

5 Special Considerations

- Clinical context is important. B-lines indicating lung interstitial fluid can be caused by various pathologies
  - Interstitial pneumonia or pneumonitis
  - Diffuse parenchymal lung disease for example pulmonary fibrosis
  - Acute lung injury or acute respiratory distress syndrome
- Even if B-lines are from a pulmonary source, rather than an indication of elevated left atrial pressure from fluid administration, they may indicate a patient in whom a more fluid conservative strategy is reasonable
- We find trending B-lines especially useful in patients without preexisting lung pathology who have shock from a non-lung source (i.e., abdominal sepsis, post-op from major surgery)

6 Pleural Effusion, Consolidation, and Collapse

Chest X-ray is the most common form of lung imaging in critically ill patients, but differentiating between effusion, collapse, and consolidation can be difficult. These pathologies are managed very differently; effusions are often drained, collapse is treated with positioning and ventilatory changes, and consolidation helps detect pneumonia. Ultrasound makes diagnosis easier and faster (Fig. 3)

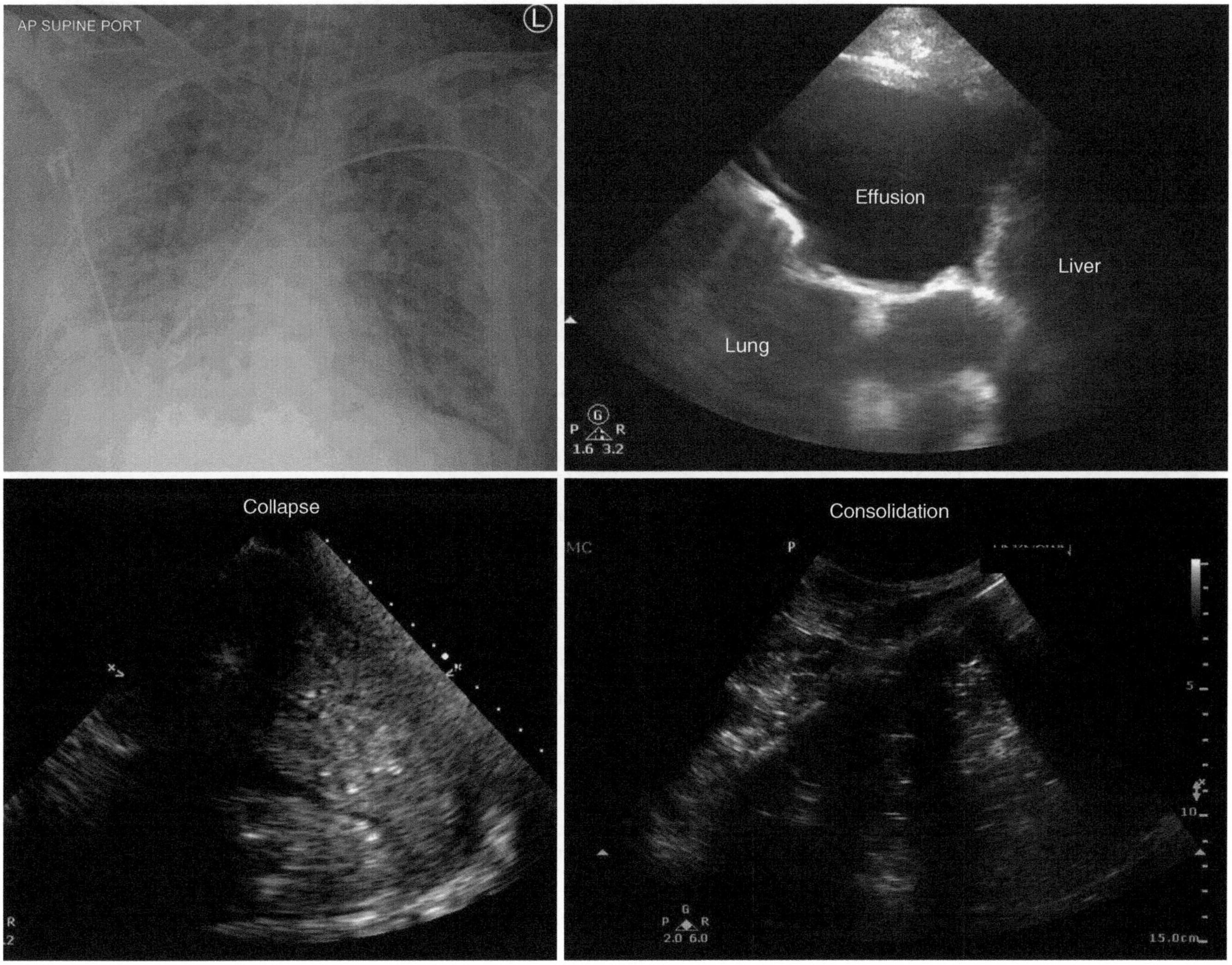

Fig. 3 Pleural effusion, collapse, and consolidation. Upper left: Classic chest x-ray in a critically ill patient. Upper right: effusion. Lower left: complete collapse of the left upper lobe. Lower left: consolidation of the right lower lobe with pneumonia

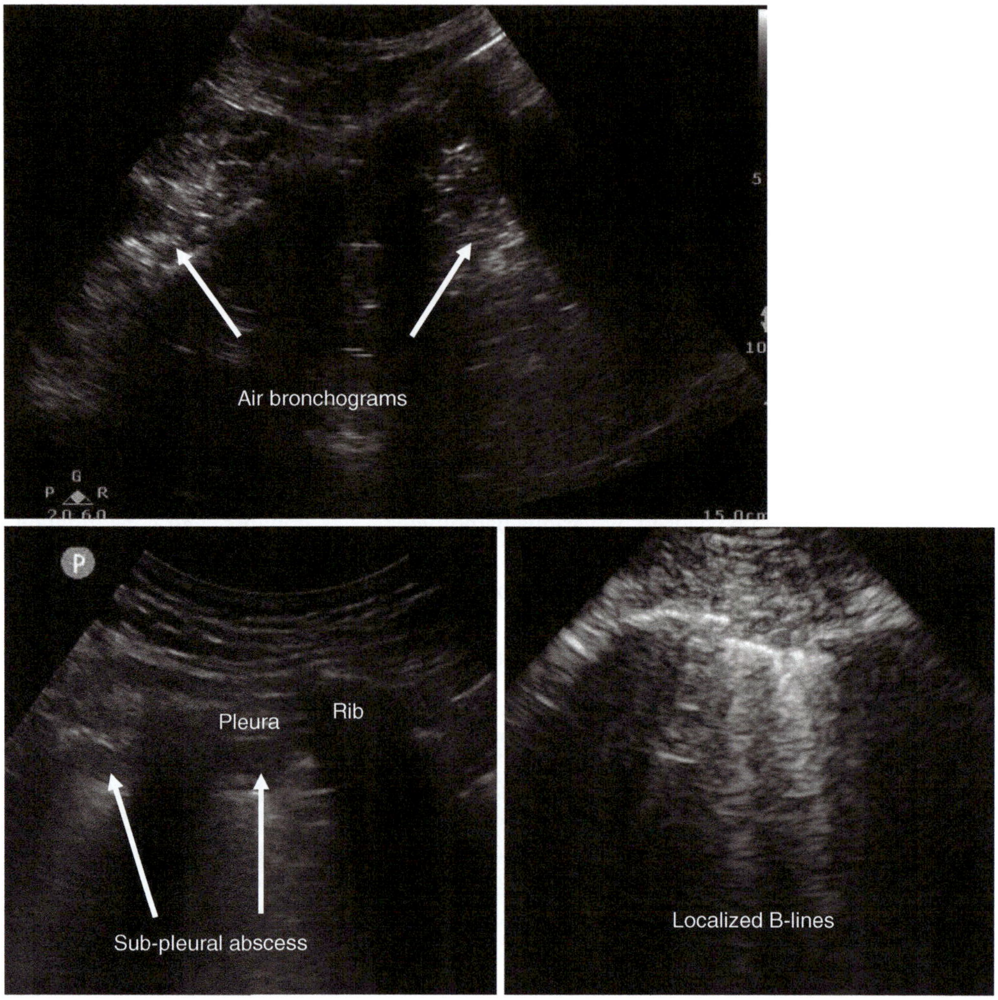

Fig. 4 Classic ultrasound findings in consolidation and pneumonia. Series of images in patients with consolidated pneumonia

- Windows: Anterior and posterior windows in the right and left lung fields
- Mode: 2D
- Units: none
- Phased array or curvilinear probe in abdominal or lung mode
- Indicator up toward the head
- The more lung fields imaged, the more complete the exam
- The posterior lung fields are especially important in differentiating between collapse and effusion
- Save a representative clip of each lung field

Pleural Effusion
- A pleural effusion will appear as anechoic area between the lung and the diaphragm (Fig. 3 upper right panel).

Lung Collapse
- Dense lung that transmits ultrasound signal (Fig. 3 lower left panel, Video 1)
  - Lung volume is reduced
  - More homogenous then with consolidation
- Improves with recruitment maneuvers, positional changes
- Effusion is often present

Consolidation (Fig. 4 and Video 2)
- Findings can be widespread, patchy, or lobar
- B-lines are localized to the area of interest
- Sub-pleural consolidations and small fluid collections (abscesses)
  - Scalloped pleural boarder
- Lung tissue is more dense and less uniform than with simple collapse
  - Lung volume may be increased
- Dynamic air bronchograms are present
  - Bubbles can be seen traveling in collapsed bronchioles
- Pulmonary vasculature can be seen in collapsed lung with color flow Doppler

7 Pneumothorax

Pneumothorax can occur spontaneously, from a mechanical ventilation, or from procedures. Pneumothorax can be visually identified as no movement along the pleural line. M-Mode over the pleural line to help identify movement.

- Window: Superior, Anterior, Lateral Lung
- Mode: 2D
- Units: none
- Use a linear ultrasound prove
- Place the indicator up toward the head, and place the probe in between two rib spaces.
- Visualize the movement of the pleural line which has been characterized as ants along a string or string of pearls (Fig. 4 and Video 3).
- If there is no movement, consider pneumothorax (Video 4).
- A lung point is highly specific for a partial pneumothorax (Video 5).
  - Transition point between pneumothorax and open expanded lung
    - Area where both sliding and no sliding can be seen

8 Evaluation of Pneumothorax by M-Mode

- Window: Anterior, Lateral Lung
- Mode: M-Mode
- Units: none
- Use a linear ultrasound probe.
- Place the indicator up towards the head and place the probe in between two rib spaces.
- Select M-mode to activate the M-Mode cursor, place the cursor through the pleural line.
- Select M-mode again to visualize the M-mode tracing (Fig. 5)
- A normal M-mode tracing is characterized as a sandy beach sign (Fig. 6).
- A pneumothorax is characterized as a barcode sign.

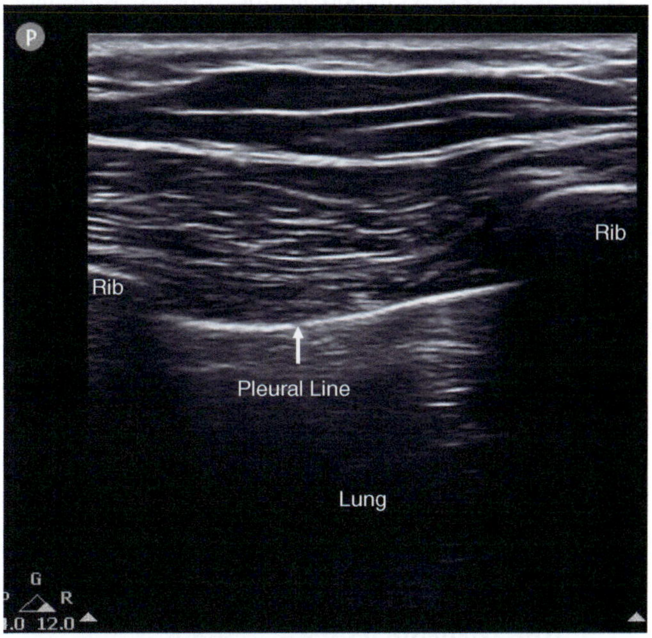

Fig. 5 Normal view of the pleural line. Normal view of the pleural line with a high-frequency transducer

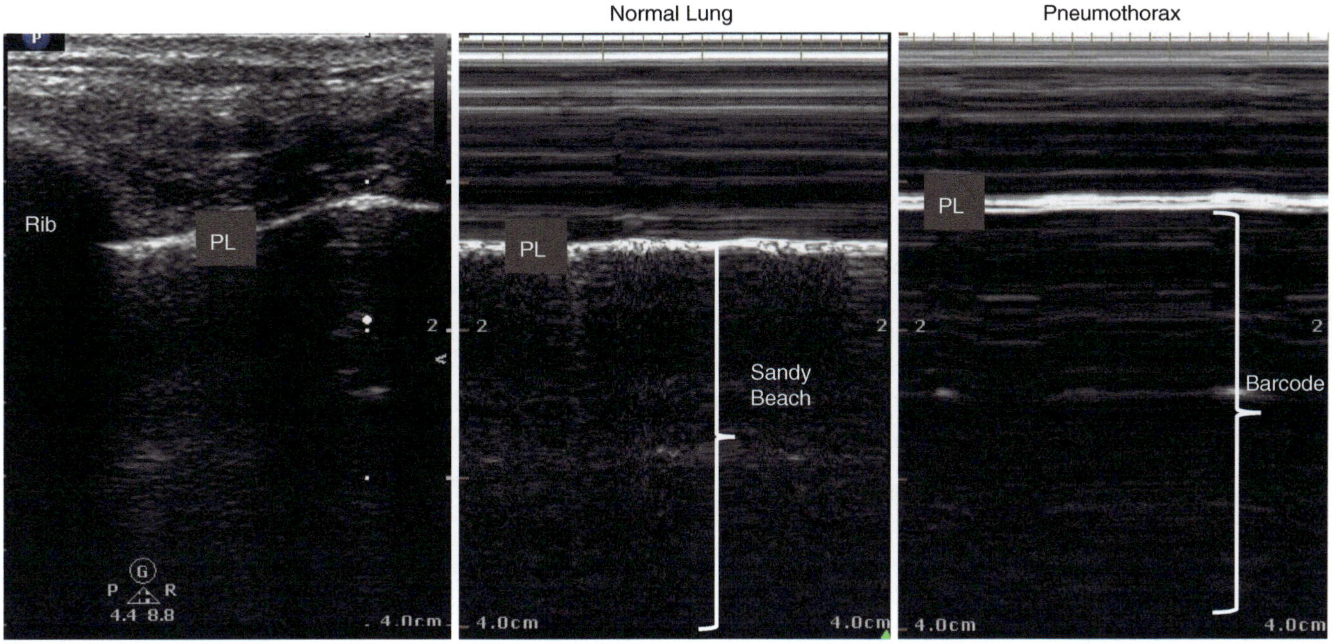

Fig. 6 Normal and abnormal M-mode. PL: pleural line. These are images obtained with M-mode in a patient at the lung point of his pneumothorax. The lung point is the transition between normal open lung and a pneumothorax. Left panel is the 2D image. Middle panel shows normal M-mode with the sandy beach sign below the pleural line. Right panel shows pneumothorax with barcode sign below the pleural line

9 Tips and Pointers

- When using M-Mode to identify for pneumothorax, it is important to match the depth of the pleural line from the 2D image and M-Mode tracing.
  - Allows correct identification of the pleural line
- This is especially important for patients with large amounts of subcutaneous tissue.

Suggested Reading

Dietrich CF, Mathis G, Blaivas M, et al. Lung B-line artefacts and their use. J Thorac Dis. 2016;8(6):1356–65.

Mayo PH, Copetti R, Feller-Kopman D, Mathis G, Maury E, Mongodi S, Mojoli F, Volpicelli G, Zanobetti M. Thoracic ultrasonography: a narrative review. Intensive Care Med. 2019;45(9):1200–11. https://doi.org/10.1007/s00134-019-05725-8. Epub 2019 Aug 15

Mojoli F, Bouhemad B, Mongodi S, Lichtenstein D. Lung ultrasound for critically ill patients. Am J Respir Crit Care Med. 2019;199(6):701–14. https://doi.org/10.1164/rccm.201802-0236CI. Erratum in: Am J Respir Crit Care Med. 2020;201(8):1015. Erratum in: Am J Respir Crit Care Med. 2020;201(11):1454. PMID: 30372119.

Right Atrial Pressure Assessment

Sagar B. Dave and Sarah B. Murthi

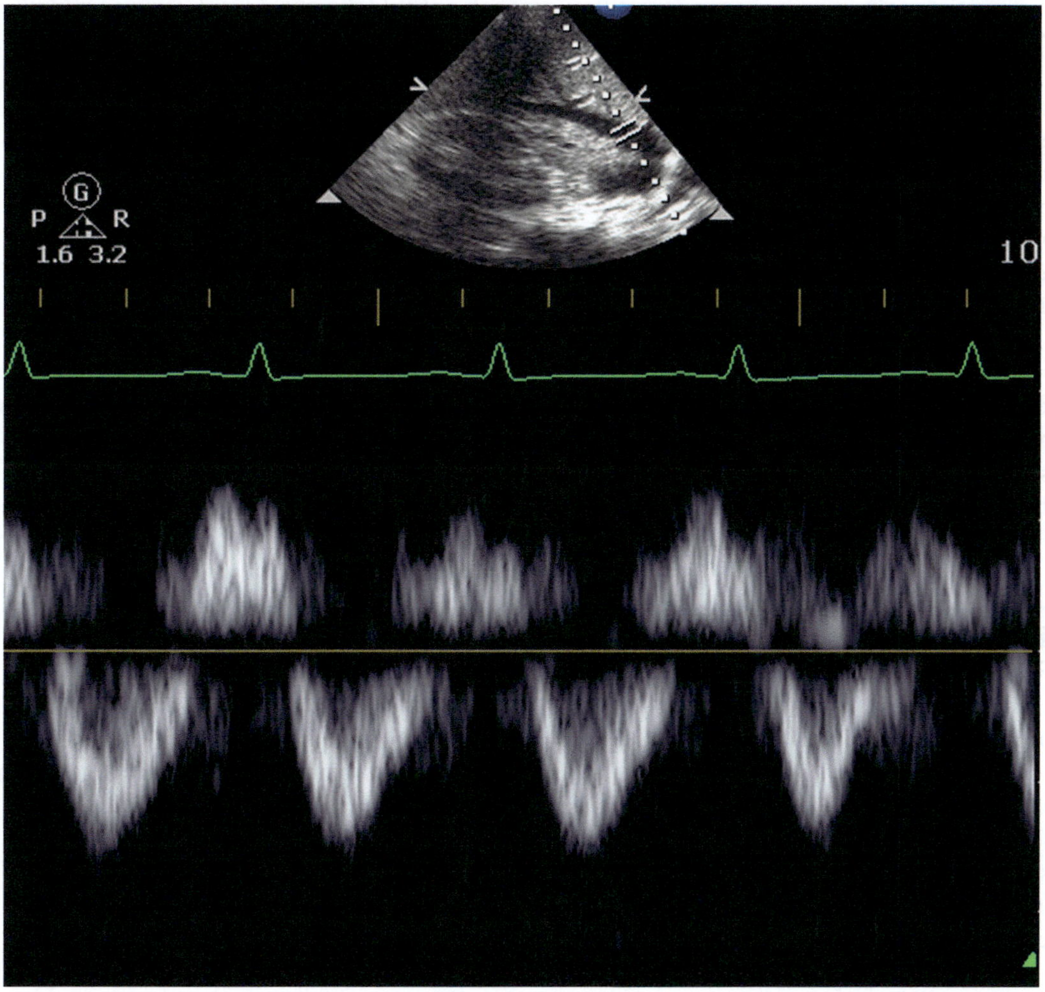

S. B. Dave
R. Adams Cowley Shock Trauma Center, University of Maryland,
Baltimore, MD, USA

S. B. Murthi (✉)
Department of Surgery, Program in Trauma and Critical Care,
R Adams Cowley Shock Trauma Center, University of Maryland
School of Medicine, University of Maryland Medical Center,
Baltimore, MD, USA
e-mail: smurthi@som.umaryland.edu

A. Salerno et al. (eds.), *Atlas of Critical Care Echocardiography*, https://doi.org/10.1007/978-3-030-74687-2_17

Abbreviations

CO	Cardiac output
CVP	Central venous pressure
D	Diastole
ECG	Electrocardiogram
IVC	Inferior vena cava
MAP	Mean arterial blood pressure
PASP	Pulmonary artery systolic pressure
RA	Right atrial pressure
RAP	Right atrial pressure
S	Systolic
SVR	Systemic vascular resistance

1 Introduction

Elevations in right atrial pressure (RAP) can cause venous congestion resulting in tissue edema. Ongoing fluid boluses will further elevate RAP leading to organ dysfunction impacting hepatic, bowel, and renal perfusion by inhibiting venous drainage. Increased RAP is difficult to detect clinically, especially in mechanically ventilated patients. Central venous pressure (CVP) and pulmonary artery catheters are affected by mean airway pressure rendering them unreliable. Echo is an exciting alternative. We use evidence of elevated RAP and venous congestion as an indication that fluid is becoming harmful and often limit administration when it is present. How to obtain these measurements is discussed in their respective chapters. In this section, we discuss how to use them together to assess RAP and determine if venous congestion is present.

2 Estimation of RAP for Calculations of SVR and PA Systolic Pressure

Estimation of RAP and CVP in Calculation of Other Metrics

Right atrial pressure and CVP are used in the calculations of systemic vascular resistance (SVR) and pulmonary artery systolic pressure (PASP).

- Estimate of RAP and CVP
  - Not the same measurement, but usually very close in value
  - On mechanical ventilation, the IVC may be dilated, in that case just use visual assessment of the right ventricle (RV) and right atria (RA). The American Society of Echocardiography suggests using similar parameters to estimate 3, 8 and 15 mmHg. We feel 5, 10, and 15 is easier and more accurately reflects that it is just an estimation.
  - Small underfilled heart, IVC < 2 cm
    - 5 mmHg
  - Euvolemic heart, IVC 1–2 cm
    - 10 mmHg
  - Full heart, large RA, IVC > 2 cm
    - 15 mmHg
  - Most of the time we use 10 mmHg
    - It simplifies assessment
    - All that is needed is a rough estimate
- Systemic vascular resistance (SVR), see Chap. 10
  - SVR = ((MAP-RAP)/CO) × 80
    - MAP = mean arterial blood pressure
    - CO = cardiac output
- Pulmonary artery systolic pressure (PASP), see Chap. 13
  - PASP = $4(\text{TRjetvmax})^2$ + RAP
    - TVjetvmax = peak velocity flow of the tricuspid jet
- Using the measurements
  - A number is generated, but *all ultrasound assessments should be considered semi-quantitative rather than exact*
  - For SVR, better to think of it as
    - Likely vasodilated
    - Likely normal
    - Likely vasoconstricted
  - For PASP, better to think of it as
    - Likely normal
    - Likely elevated
    - Likely high

3 Detection of Venous Congestion from Elevated RAP

Venous Changes (Fig. 1)

- The hepatic vein is closest to the RA and the most direct measurement of RAP
- The portal vein is after the liver and assess visceral venous pressure
  - End stage liver disease or any pathology that causes portal hypertension may cause portal pulsatility
    - Not an indication of elevated RAP
- The renal vein assesses venous congestion at the kidney
  - Once renal injury or failure is present it may not reflect RAP

Hepatic Vein (Fig. 2)

- Normal pressure
  - Systolic (S) > Diastolic (D) both below the baseline
  - Atrial (a) contraction flow is above the baseline
    - Retrograde, back into the hepatic vein
    - Not always visualized
  - Use ECG rhythm strip (Fig. 1, panel B) to identify the waves
    - S is just after the QRS
    - D is after the S
      - Falls after the T
  - Alternative method
    - Find the a wave above the baseline
      - S is just after the a

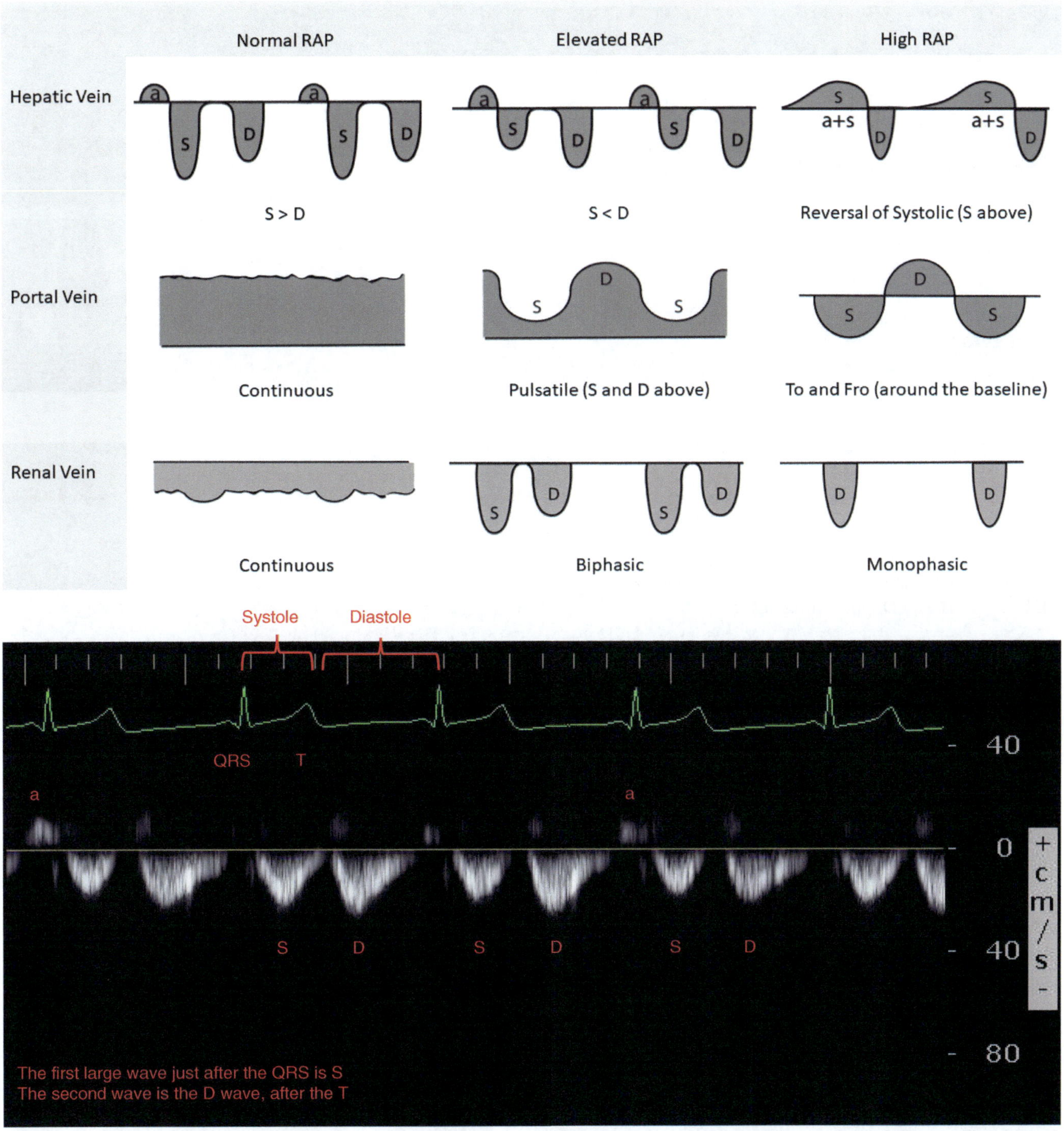

Fig. 1 Venous flow changes with right atrial pressure elevation. Upper panel: Pattern of flow changes as right atrial pressure increases. Lower panel: Identifying the S and D wave in a hepatic venous pulsed wave Doppler tracing. Find the S wave below the baseline immediately after the QRS on the ECG tracing. The D wave follows the S, after the T. This is an example of high normal RAP; S = D below the baseline. The a wave is above the baseline and can be seen intermittently

- D is after the S
- Disadvantages
  - Not possible in atrial fibrillation
  - Often difficult to distinguish from noise
- As atrial pressure increases
  - S = D
- Elevated RAP
  - S < D

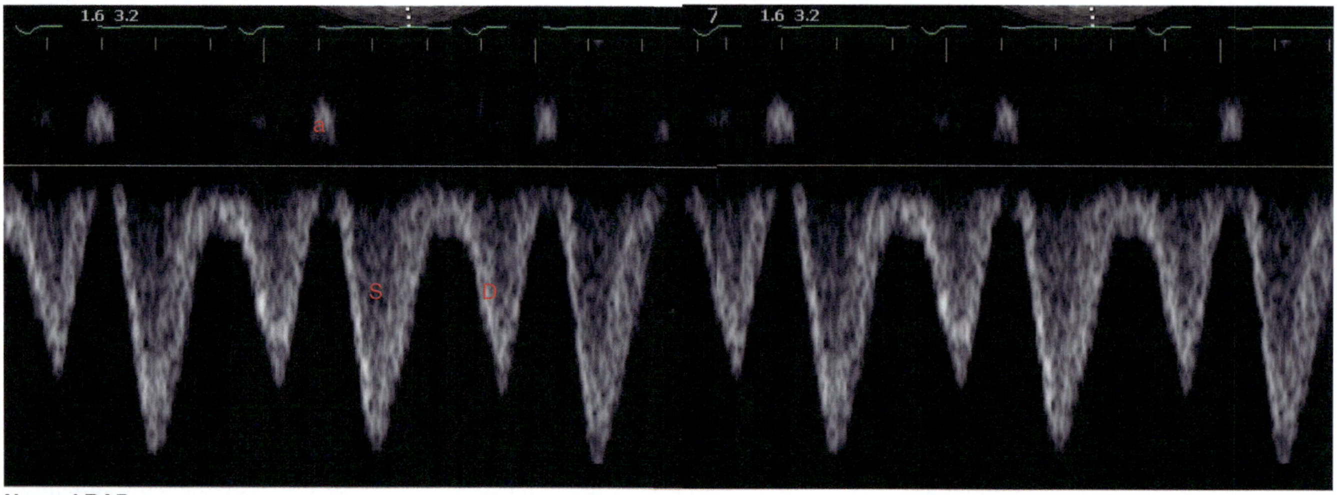

Normal RAP
S > D

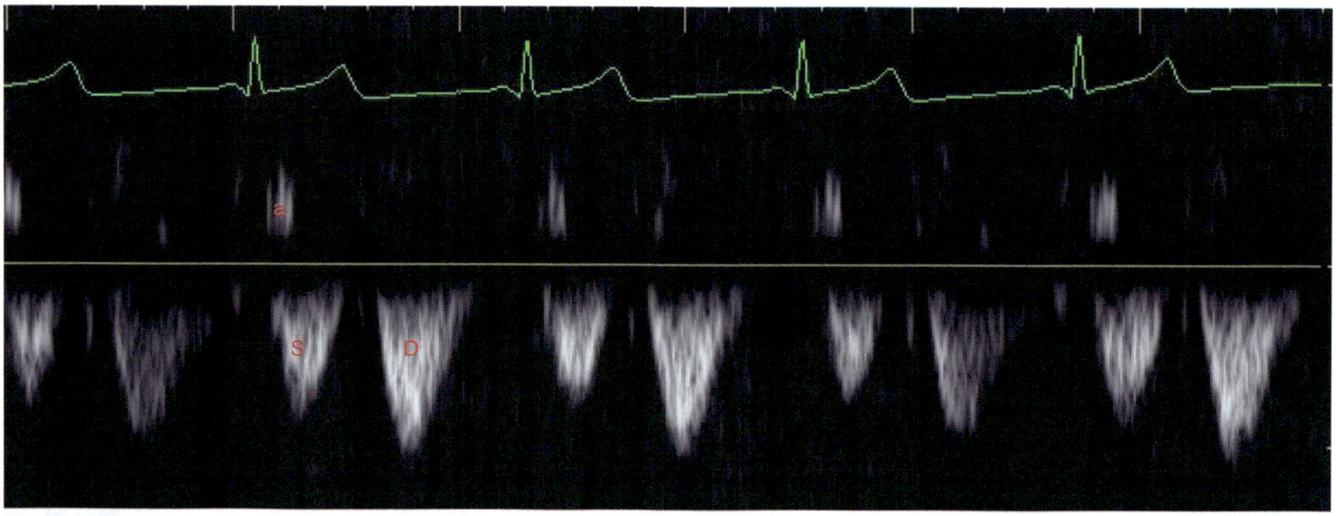

Elevated RAP
S < D

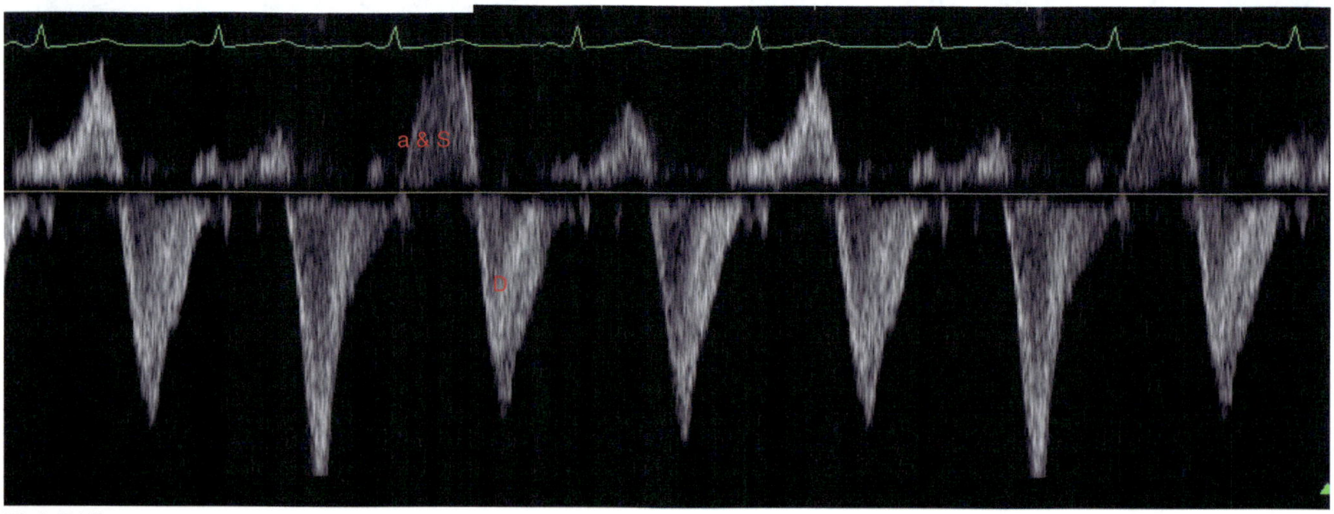

High RAP
a & S above the baseline

Fig. 2 Hepatic venous flow changes with right atrial pressure elevation. Upper panel: Normal RAP, S > D, and both are above the baseline. On this tracing, the QRS cannot be seen, but the a wave is easily identified. Middle panel: Elevated RAP. The QRS can be seen. S is immediately after the QRS. The D is after the S and falls after the T. Bottom panel: High RAP with retrograde flow in systole. Both the a and S are above the baseline. The D wave is below the baseline

- High RAP
  - Retrograde flow back into the hepatic vein
  - S flips above the baseline and often fuses with a

Portal Vein (Fig. 3)

- Normal
  - Continuous flow
  - Above the baseline
- Elevated portal pressure
  - Pulsatile flow
  - > 30% change, visual assessment or measured
    - Diminished in systole
  - Above the baseline
- High portal pressure
  - Systolic retrograde flow
  - Wraps around the baseline
  - Also called to-and-fro flow

Renal Vein (Fig. 4)

- Normal

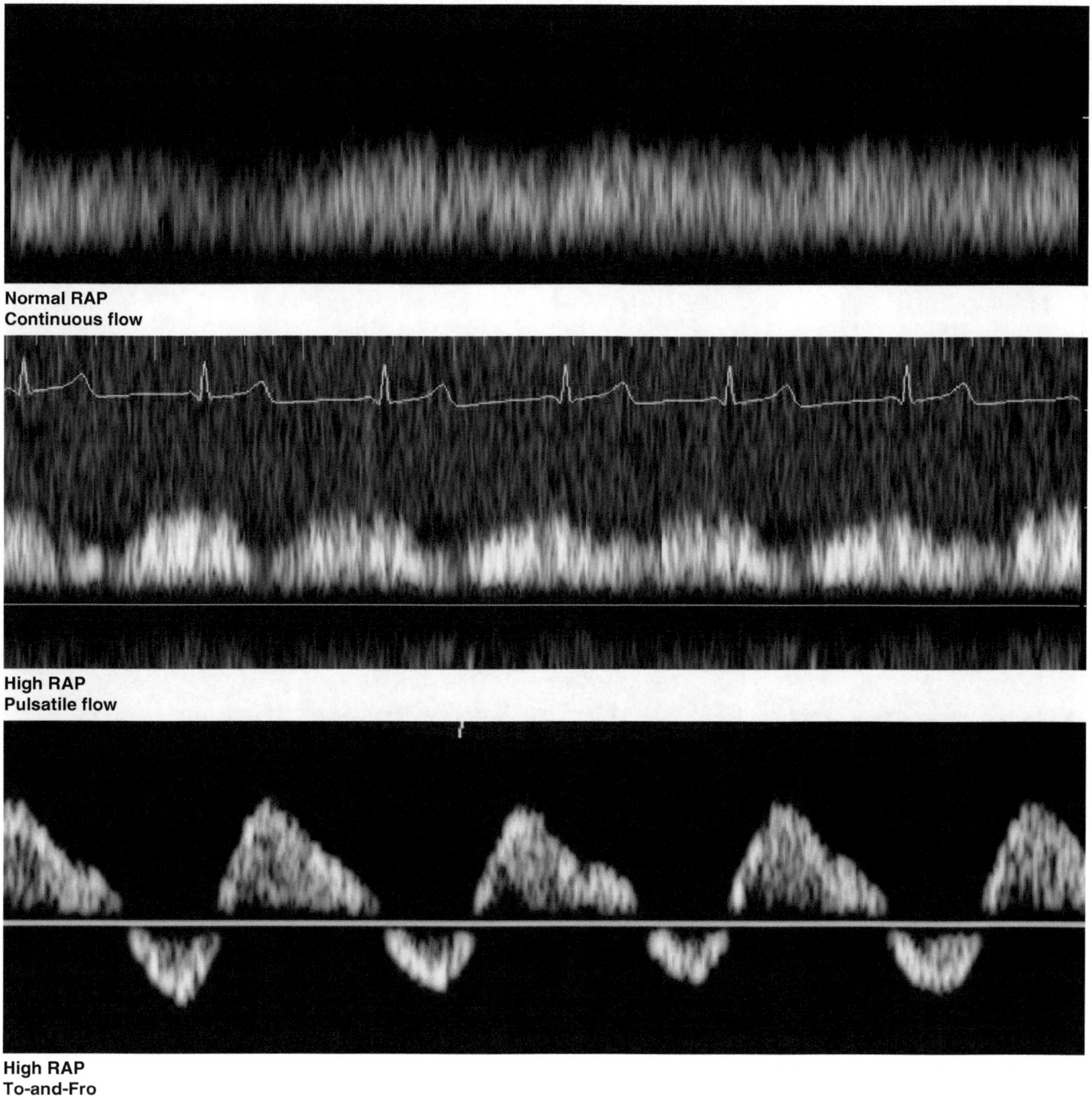

Fig. 3 Portal venous flow changes with elevations in right atrial pressure. Upper panel: Normal RAP, continuous flow in systole and diastole. Middle panel: Elevated RAP, pulsatile flow. Bottom panel: High RAP, retrograde flow in systole. The wave wraps around the baseline

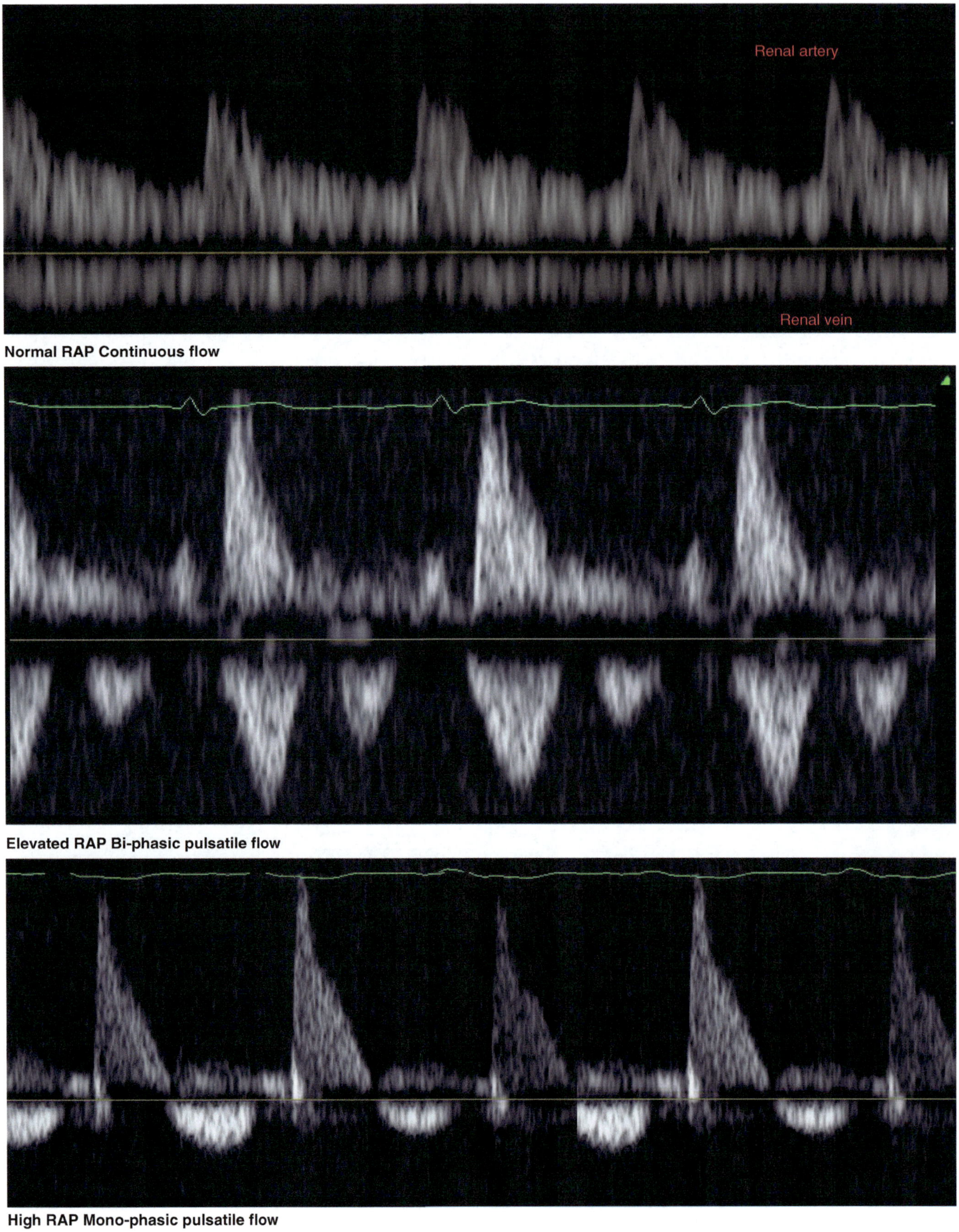

Fig. 4 Renal venous flow changes with elevations in right atrial pressure. The renal artery is above the pulsed wave Doppler baseline in all three panels. Upper panel: Normal venous flow; continuous throughout systole and diastole. Middle panel: Elevated RAP, venous flow has become pulsatile. High RAP, only monophasic diastolic flow. Systolic venous flow is absent

- Continuous flow
- As atrial pressure increases
  - Becomes pulsatile
- Elevated
  - Biphasic flow, S > D
  - As further increases S < D
- High
  - Monophasic flow
    - No venous flow in systole

We have recently finished a study (Spiegel et al.) and found that hepatic flow changes predicted major adverse kidney events to a greater extent than portal. While renal trended toward prediction, it did not reach clinical significance in a general ICU population. Others have found portal flow and renal to be predicative in a cardiac surgical population (Beaubien-Souligny et al.). We have a high acuity ICUs with high rates of pre-existing liver and renal dysfunction which may complicate those assessments.

We routinely measure both hepatic and portal flow to assess for congestion. In general, we limit fluid and consider diuresis when findings of congestion are present even if hypotension is present. We have recently stopped assessing renal flow routinely because the rate of renal failure is high in our patients, and the measurement is difficult to obtain. But we think it is an important metric that may be useful in optimizing perfusion to prevent renal injury especially early in shock.

4 Other Assessments

4.1 Right Ventricular Diastolic Function

Right ventricular diastolic dysfunction can result in elevated RAP; see Chap. 11 for further details.

4.2 Inferior Vena Cava

The cardiology literature rests heavily on the IVC as a surrogate measure of RAP. We have found unreliable in a critical care population. Positive pressure ventilation and abdominal and thoracic surgery all result in a dilated IVC with variable vessel collapse, even in small underfilled hearts with normal right ventricular function (Table 1). Also, most critically ill patients cannot perform the standard sniff.

- Place in M-mode, allow the patient to inhale, exhale, and rapidly inspire or sniff

Table 1 Positive pressure ventilation, abdominal and thoracic surgery, and dilated IVC

	Normal RAP 3 mmHg	Intermediate RAP 8–15 mmHg	High RAP 15 mmHg
IVC diameter	<21 mm	>21 mm	>21 mm
IVC collapse	>50%	>50%	<50%

  - Measure 2 cm from the RA, or just in from of the hepatic veins
- Not validated as a measure of RAP in patients on positive pressure ventilation.
- Unable to perform as described in most critically ill patients

4.3 Special Considerations

- Measurements lose accuracy with arrhythmias, valvulopathies, and mechanical ventilation
- IVC can be falsely dilated in athletes and mechanically ventilated patients
- Elevated portal pressure from end stage liver disease can cause portal pulsatility
- Renal evaluations can be attributed to ureteral obstructions
- No one evaluation in all clinical scenarios has been validated or strongly reproducible. It is important to use multiple measurements tailored to the specific clinical scenario

Suggested Reading

Beaubien-Souligny W, Benkreira A, Robillard P, Bouabdallaoui N, Chassé M, Desjardins G, Lamarche Y, White M, Bouchard J, Denault A. Alterations in portal vein flow and intrarenal venous flow are associated with acute kidney injury after cardiac surgery: a prospective observational cohort study. J Am Heart Assoc. 2018;7(19):e009961. https://doi.org/10.1161/JAHA.118.009961. PMID: 30371304; PMCID: PMC6404886

Lang RM, Badano LP, Mor-Avi V, Afilalo J, Armstrong A, Ernande L, Flachskampf FA, Foster E, Goldstein SA, Kuznetsova T, Lancellotti P, Muraru D, Picard MH, Rietzschel ER, Rudski L, Spencer KT, Tsang W, Voigt JU. Recommendations for cardiac chamber quantification by echocardiography in adults: an update from the American Society of Echocardiography and the European Association of Cardiovascular Imaging. J Am Soc Echocardiogr. 2015;28(1):1–39. e14. https://doi.org/10.1016/j.echo.2014.10.003.

Spiegel R, Teeter W, Sullivan S, Tupchong K, Mohammed N, Sutherland M, Leibner E, Rola P, Galvagno SM Jr, Murthi SB. The use of venous Doppler to predict adverse kidney events in a general ICU cohort. Crit Care. 2020;24(1):615. https://doi.org/10.1186/s13054-020-03330-6. PMID: 33076961; PMCID: PMC7574322

Potpourri of Pathology

Alexis Salerno, Daniel J. Haase, and Sarah B. Murthi

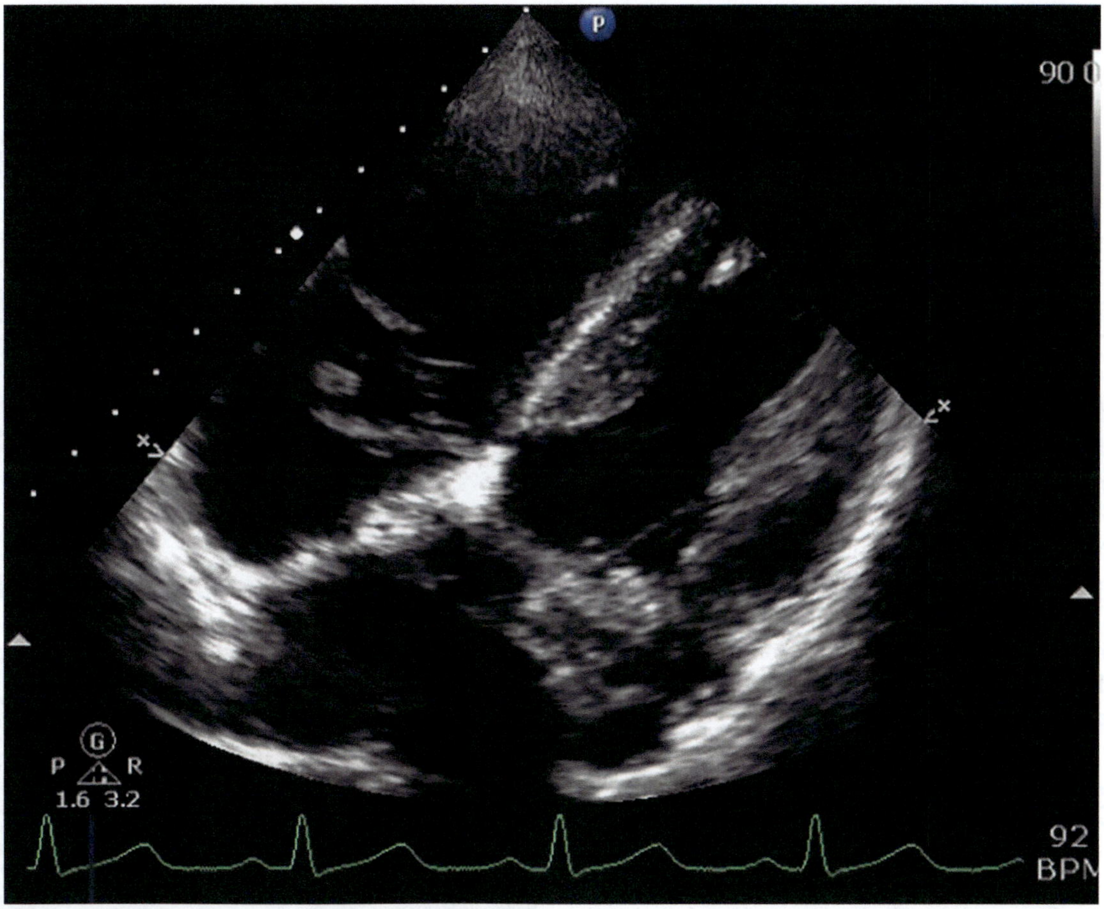

Supplementary Information The online version of this chapter (https://doi.org/10.1007/978-3-030-74687-2_18) contains supplementary material, which is available to authorized users.

A. Salerno
Department of Emergency Medicine, University of Maryland School of Medicine, Baltimore, MD, USA

D. J. Haase · S. B. Murthi (✉)
Department of Surgery, Program in Trauma and Critical Care, R Adams Cowley Shock Trauma Center, University of Maryland School of Medicine, University of Maryland Medical Center, Baltimore, MD, USA
e-mail: smurthi@som.umaryland.edu

A. Salerno et al. (eds.), *Atlas of Critical Care Echocardiography*, https://doi.org/10.1007/978-3-030-74687-2_18

Abbreviations

AP 4	Apical four chamber
AP 5	Apical five chamber
AS	Aortic stenosis
AVA	Aortic valve area
CT	Computerized tomography
CWD	Continuous wave Doppler
E	Early diastolic flow
EF	Ejection fraction
ICU	Intensive Care Unit
IVC	Inferior vena cava
LV	Left ventricle
LVOT	Left ventricular outflow tract
MV	Mitral valve
PE	Pulmonary embolus
PLA	Parasternal long axis
PSA	Parasternal short axis
PWD	Pulsed wave Doppler
RV	Right Ventricle
SVR	Systemic vascular resistance
TAPSE	Transannular systolic excursion
TEE	Transesophageal echocardiography
TR	Tricuspid regurgitant jet
TV	Tricuspid regurgitant jet
V_{max}	Maximum velocity
VTI	Velocity time integral

1 Introduction

In addition to providing information about cardiac function, volume status, and vascular resistance, point-of-care echo can detect life-threating anatomic pathology. In this chapter, we present several examples adapted from real patients in which pathologic findings are essential in determining the course of care.

2 Case 1: Cardiac Tamponade

A 50-year-old female with breast cancer on chemotherapy is admitted for a fever work-up. Twelve hours after admission she develops tachypnea and tachycardia on the cancer ward and is upgraded to the intensive care unit (ICU). On evaluation she is uncomfortable with diaphoresis and respiratory distress. Lung auscultation reveals only mild rales at the bases. An ultrasound is performed to evaluate the cause of the patient's respiratory distress. A subxiphoid view revealed a large pericardial effusion with swaying of the heart and diastolic collapse of the right ventricle. Based on the clinical picture and cardiac ultrasound findings the patient is diagnosed with cardiac tamponade.

Case Conclusion The patient remained hemodynamically unchanged. The ICU team prepared to place a pericardial drain emergently if needed and consulted a cardiologist. The patient is taken to cardiac catherization for pericardial drain placement after which her symptoms resolved.

Teaching Points The heart may move because of the effusion, and you will need to adjust where you obtain your images. Locate the heart, and reorient yourself, and then adjust the transducer to see the areas of interest.

Five Echogenic Signs of Cardiac Tamponade No one finding is highly sensitive and specific. The diagnosis is made based on a combination of findings, the clinical scenario, and changes overtime. An unstable patient with one finding may warrant drainage, whereas a stable patient with the same finding could be monitored and serially imaged.

1. Pericardial Effusion (Fig. 1)

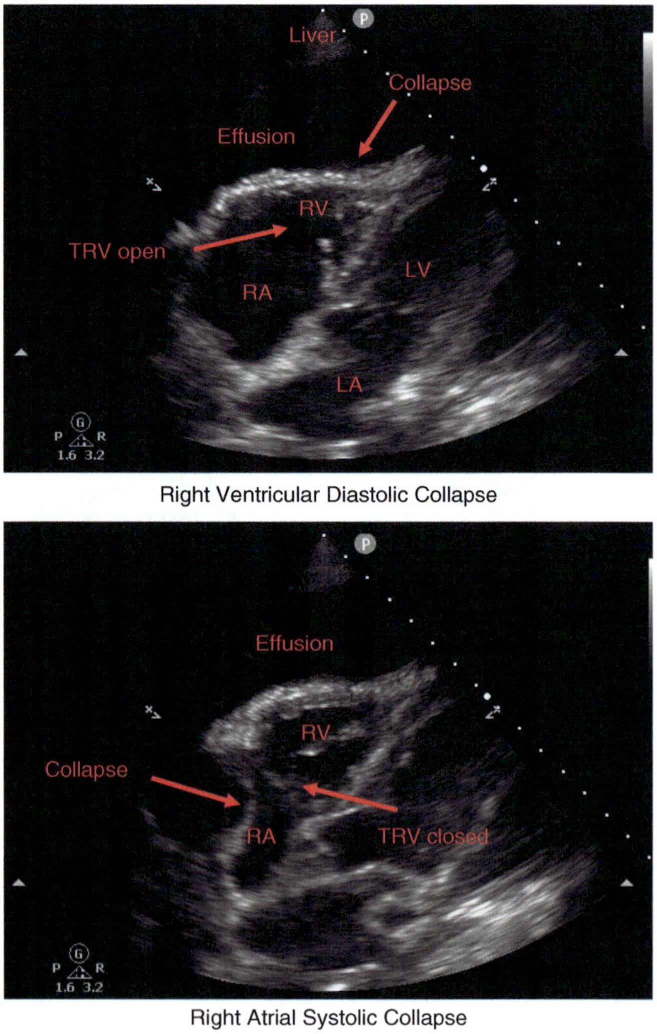

Fig. 1 Echocardiographic findings in cardiac tamponade. Upper Panel: Right ventricular diastolic collapse. RA right atria, RV right ventricle, LA left atria, LV left ventricle, TRV tricuspid valve. Note the TRV is open in diastole to allow ventricular filling. The effusion is causing collapse of the RV. Lower Panel: The TRV is closed so the heart is in systole, the effusion is causing RA collapse. Both ventricular and atrial collapse are evidence of tamponade

- A pericardial effusion can be caused by trauma, infection, and malignancy. On echo a pericardial effusion appears as an anechoic space between the heart and pericardial sac.
- The acuity of the pericardial effusion is more important than the size of the effusion.
- With larger pericardial effusions swaying of the heart is often present.

2. Right Ventricular (RV) *Diastolic* Collapse
   - RV collapse during diastole is specific for cardiac tamponade
   - 2D assessment (Fig. 1 upper panel and Video 1)
     (i) Save a video clip and carefully scroll back and forth. Look for RV free wall collapse while the tricuspid valve is open. Watch as the ventricle is filling. Look for an indent anywhere in the free wall caused by the effusion.
     (ii) In systole, the RV wall will contract, and the effusion will look bigger. This is *not* tamponade.
   - M-Mode assessment (Fig. 2)
     (i) Place the cursor over the RV and mitral valve in the parasternal long axis (PLA). Evaluate the M-Mode tracing to see if the RV collapse occurs as the mitral valve is open.
       1. Use the 2D assessment to guide where you place the cursor
     (ii) Alternative method: apply ECG leads and look for collapse in diastole: between the T and QRS waves. Early collapse will appear just before or right on the QRS.
3. Right Atrial (RA) Collapse in Systole (Fig. 1 lower panel)
   - RA collapse during systole is an early sign of cardiac tamponade.
   - Scroll carefully through the 2D clip, and look for right atrial collapse while the tricuspid valve is closed.
4. Distended Inferior Vena Cava (IVC)
   - Due to elevated right atrial pressure, the IVC becomes plethoric with minimal respiratory variation.
     (i) However, this is a common finding in mechanically ventilated patients and needs to be taken in clinical context.
5. Respiratory Variation of the Mitral Valve (MV) and Tricuspid Valve (TV) Inflow Patterns (Fig. 3)
   - Least sensitive sign for tamponade
   - Ideally a respiratory lead and ECG leads are applied.
   - In the apical 4 chamber (AP 4), place the pulse wave Doppler marker just distal to the mitral valve or tricuspid valve.
   - Decrease the sweep speed to around 25 mm/sec to see more beats on one screen.
   - Measure velocity max and velocity min with respiration (change/max).
   - A 25% decrease in the MV inflow velocities correlates with tamponade.
   - A 40% decrease in TV inflow velocities correlates with tamponade.
   - It is not valid in atrial fibrillation and other arrhythmias.

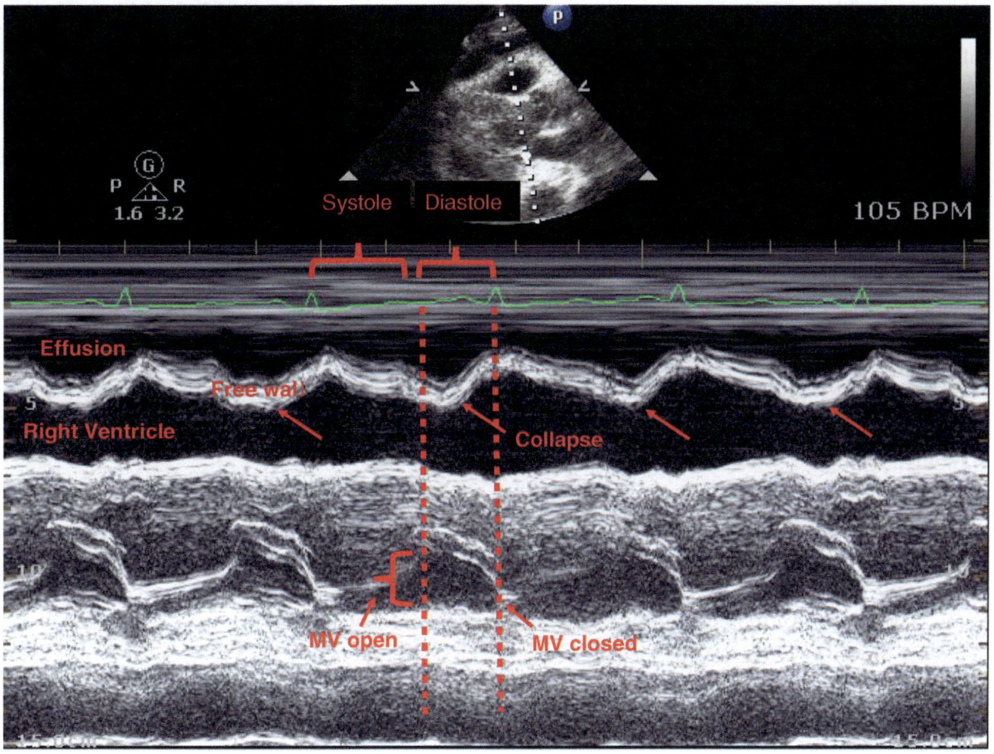

Fig. 2 M-mode of right ventricular diastolic collapse. MV mitral valve. Diastole can be identified either by the opening and closing of the mitral valve, or the EGC. Using the ECG, diastole is after the T to the middle of the QRS. In this image, RV free wall is collapsing (pushing back into the ventricle) during diastole, signifying tamponade

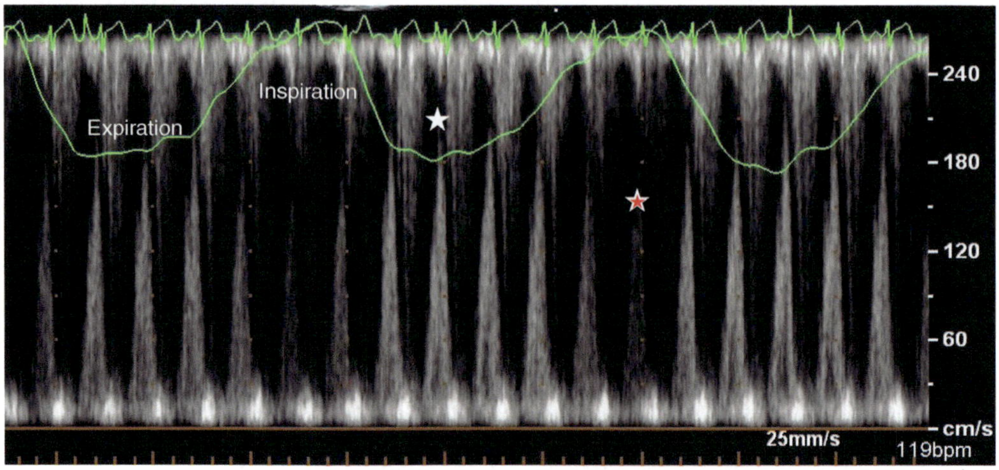

Fig. 3 Respiratory variation in mitral inflow from cardiac tamponade. White star; maximum velocity, Red star; minimum velocity. In a patient with positive pressure ventilation, there is a decrease in flow with inspiration. The maximum velocity is 210 cm/s, and the minimum is 150 or a 29% decrease; >25% is consistent with tamponade

Important Caveat If the pericardium is disrupted by trauma or cardiac surgery, blood can collect in unusual areas and be hard to visualize. Also, clotted blood has the same density as the heart and liver so it can be difficult to differentiate on ultrasound. Transesophageal echocardiography (TEE) and computerized tomography (CT) may be useful in this population. Clinical context is essential.

3 Case 2: Pulmonary Embolism

A 60-year-old male with a history of hypertension develops shortness of breath while on the trauma wards after a tibial plateau surgical repair. On exam he is tachycardic, tachypneic, and hypoxic. A beside ultrasound is performed. The AP4 view shows a dilated RV with a transannular plane systolic excursion (TAPSE) of 14 mm. There is also RV free wall akinesis with sparing of the apical portion of the RV consistent with McConnell's sign (Video 2).

Case Conclusion The echo found a large RV with signs consistent with acute failure. Based on the clinical scenario and ultrasound, systemic anticoagulation is started for suspected pulmonary embolus (PE) subsequently confirmed with CT angiogram.

Teaching Points Ultrasound is not sensitive or specific for small PEs. However, it can be very useful in detecting massive and sub-massive PEs causing hemodynamic instability.

Five Signs of Pulmonary Embolism

1. Dilated Right Ventricle (Fig. 4 upper panel)
   - The mortality in acute pulmonary embolism increases as the ratio of the RV to the left ventricle (LV) diameter approaches 1.
   - Measure the diameter of the ventricles just above the mitral and tricuspid valve on the AP 4 view.

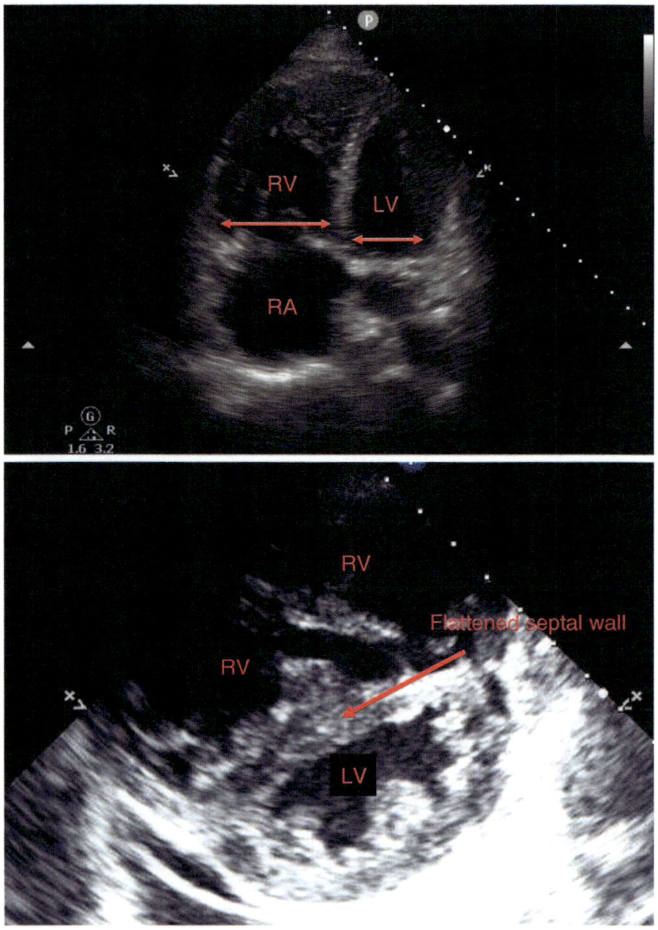

Fig. 4 Echocardiographic findings in pulmonary embolus. Upper Panel; Enlarged RV.RV right ventricle, LV left ventricle. The ratio of the diameter of the RV and LV is >1. Lower Panel; Enlarged RV and septal flattening. Note the enlarged RV. Septal flattening from RV pressure overload is causing a D-shaped LV

2. D-Sign (Fig. 4 lower panel)
   - On the parasternal short axis (PSA) view at the level of the papillary muscles, look at the intraventricular septum.

- In acute PE, there is flattening of the septum due to bowing of the RV which makes the LV appear as the letter D.

3. McConnell's Sign
   - Very sensitive for an acute PE
   - RV free wall akinesis with sparing of the apex (Video 2)
4. Low TAPSE
   - In acute pulmonary embolism, TAPSE <17 mm is concerning for a massive or sub-massive pulmonary embolism causing cardiopulmonary failure. TAPSE measurement is described in Chap. 12.
5. 60/60 Sign (Fig. 5)
   - Tricuspid regurgitant (TR) maximum pressure gradient (maxPG) >60 mmHg *and* a pulmonary acceleration time <60 msec with a mid-systolic deceleration notch are concerning for an acute PE.

- The TR maxPG = 4(TR velocity maximum)^2
  (i) Most ultrasound systems have a calculation package that includes automatic display of TR maxPG when the velocity max is measured.
  (ii) The gradient + the right atrial pressure is used to calculate the systolic artery pressure, described in Chap. 13.
    1. For the 60/60 finding in PE, the TR maxPG is used, not the estimated systolic pulmonary artery pressure.
- To measure the pulmonary acceleration time, obtain the PSA at the aortic valve, and place the pulse wave Doppler through the pulmonic valve (Fig. 5, lower panels). Measure the interval between the start of the pulmonary flow to the peak velocity; see Chap. 13 for details.

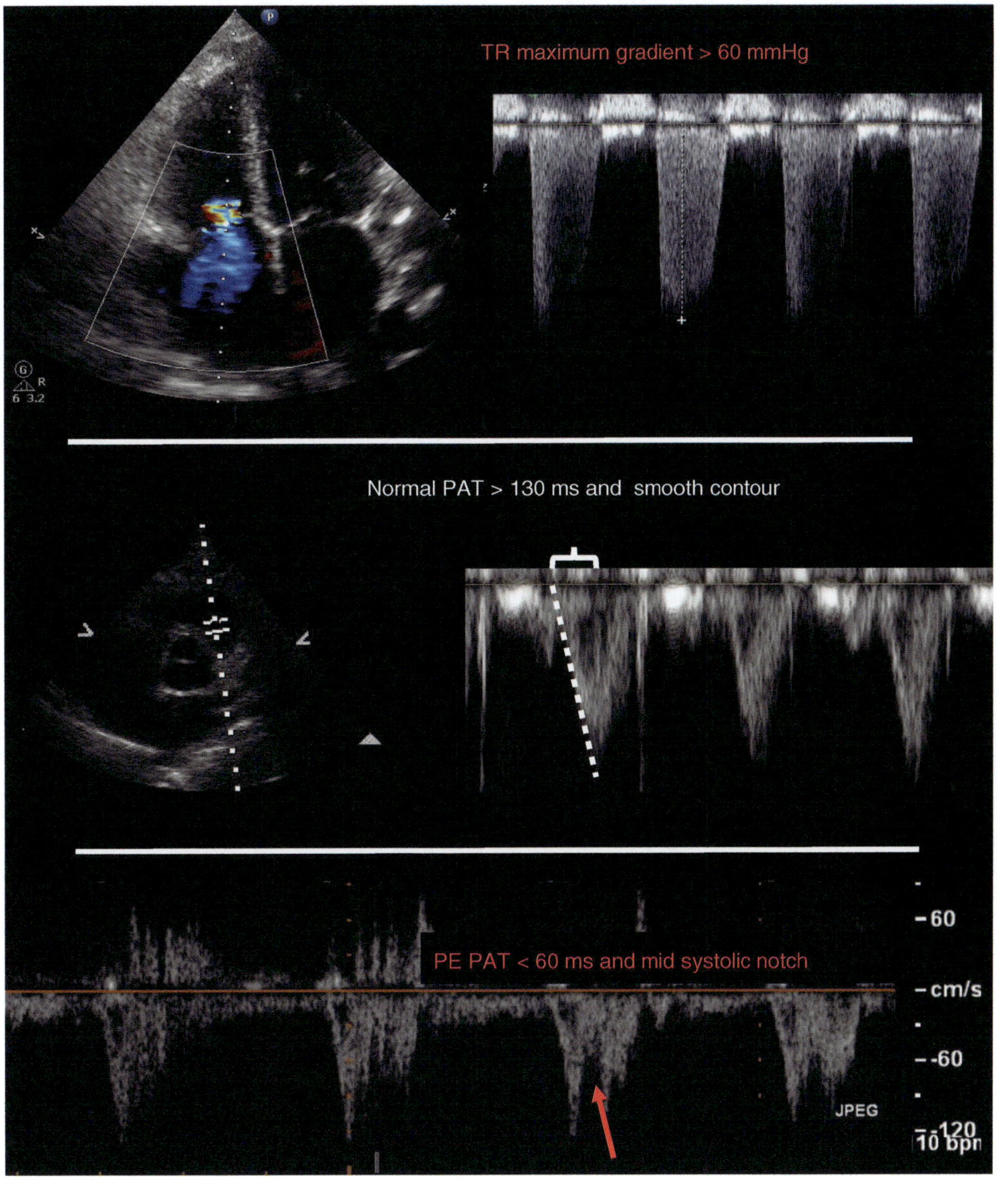

Fig. 5 Assessing 60-60 sign in pulmonary embolus. Upper Panel: The tricuspid regurgitant (TR) maximum pressure gradient (max PG). Use color flow Doppler to identify the TR jet and continuous wave Doppler to measure the peak, and the gradient is then calculated; >60 mmHg is consistent with PE. Middle Panel: Measuring pulmonic acceleration time (PAT). From the PSA at the aortic valve, use pulsed wave Doppler to measure pulmonic flow. Acceleration time is from the start of flow to the peak; >130 msec is normal. Lower Panel: PAT in PE; PAT < 60 ms, and there is often a mid-systolic notch (red arrow)

4 Case 3: COVID-19 Pneumonia

A 57-year-old female with chronic obstructive pulmonary disease and congestive heart failure presents to the emergency department by ambulance with fever and shortness of breath. The patient is hypoxic with a room air saturation of 80%. She states that she has also been vomiting and had diarrhea for the last 3 days. An ultrasound is performed to evaluate the patient's pulmonary and cardiac function.

Case Conclusion The patient is placed on high flow nasal cannula with improvement in her oxygen saturation. She is started on dexamethasone and admitted to the hospital. Her respiratory swab is positive for COVID-19.

Teaching Points Many of the specific ultrasound findings in COVID-19 are present in other viral and bacterial pneumonias; however, the constellation density is different. While ultrasound cannot be used to diagnose COVID it can identify a high-risk group. Also it can help determine the burden of lung involvement and predict those more likely to develop severe disease.

Three ultrasound signs of COVID-19 pneumonia

1. Confluent B-Lines (Fig. 6, upper left)
   - B-Lines are an indicator of interstitial fluid.
   - The B-Lines in COVID-19 pneumonia are broad compared to normal B-lines.
   - B-lines are found in multiple lobes of the lungs but more common in the posterior lateral lobes.
2. Irregular Pleural Line (Fig. 6, upper right)
   - As with bacterial pneumonia, COVID-19 will show an irregular coursed pleural line, best seen using a linear probe.
   - Small round subpleural abscesses are often seen.
3. Subpleural Collections (Fig. 6 lower panel)
   - Subpleural collections will appear as focal hyperechoic artifacts deep to the pleural line.
   - These can be seen using a linear or curvilinear probe, but the curvilinear probe allows seeing more of the lung.

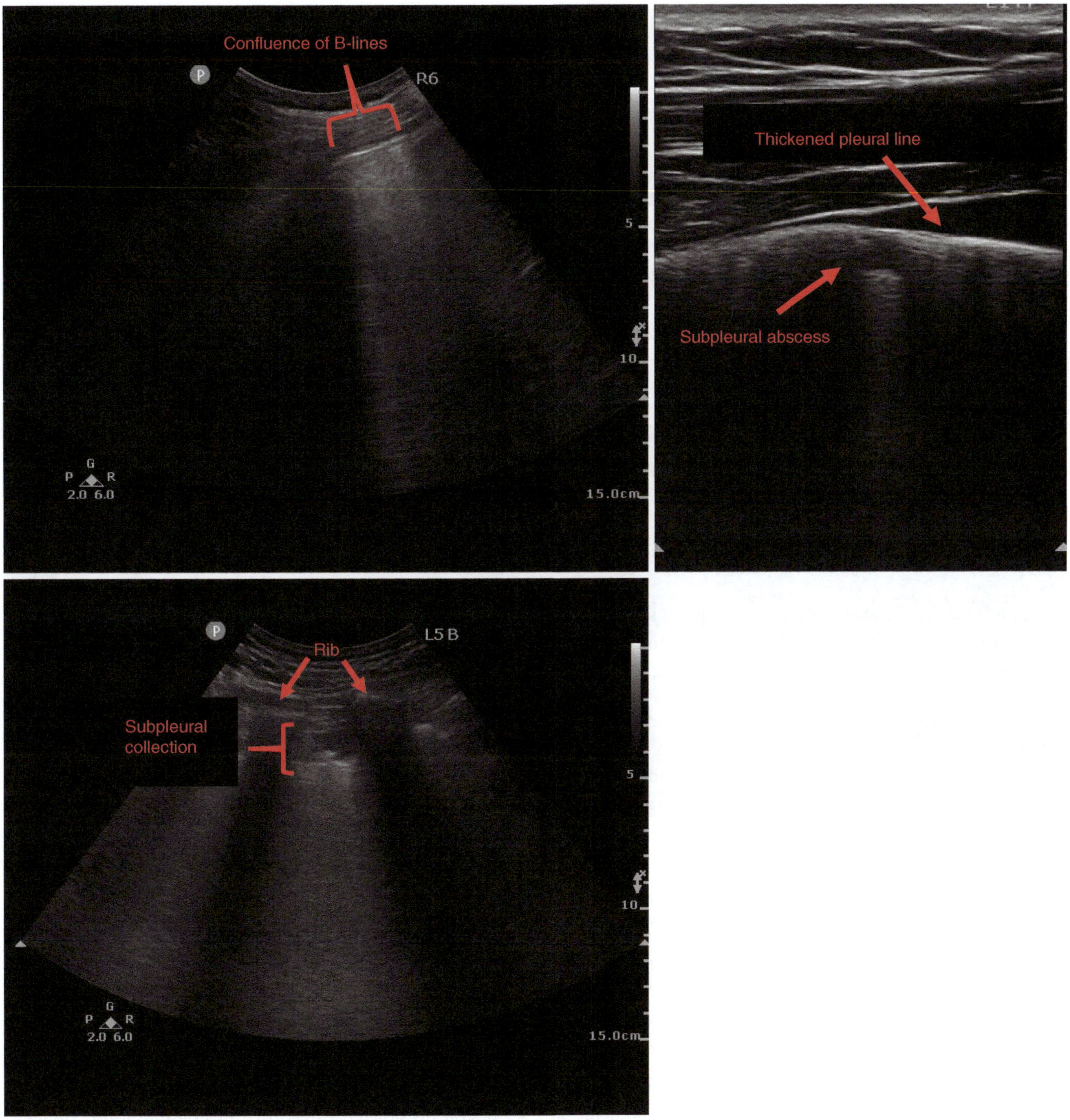

Fig. 6 Lung ultrasound findings in COVID-19. Upper left: Confluence of B-lines. Upper right: Thickened pleural and small round subpleural abscess. Lower panel complex sub-pleural collection

5 Case 4 Severe Aortic Stenosis

A 76-year-old male post-op from a sigmoid colectomy for perforated diverticulitis is tachycardic, dyspneic, and hypotensive 24 hours after being extubated. A point-of-care echocardiogram is done to assess cardiac function and volume status. Aortic stenosis is detected. LV ejection fraction (EF) is >70%. No B-lines are seen on lung imaging (Fig. 7 and Video 3).

Pulsed wave Doppler (PWD) and continuous wave Doppler (CWD) are performed. Severe aortic stenosis (AS) is confirmed (Fig. 8).

Case Conclusion The patient's respiratory status continues to decline, and intubation is planned. An arterial line is placed, a fluid bolus is given, and phenylephrine started. Etomidate is used as the induction agent and he is safely

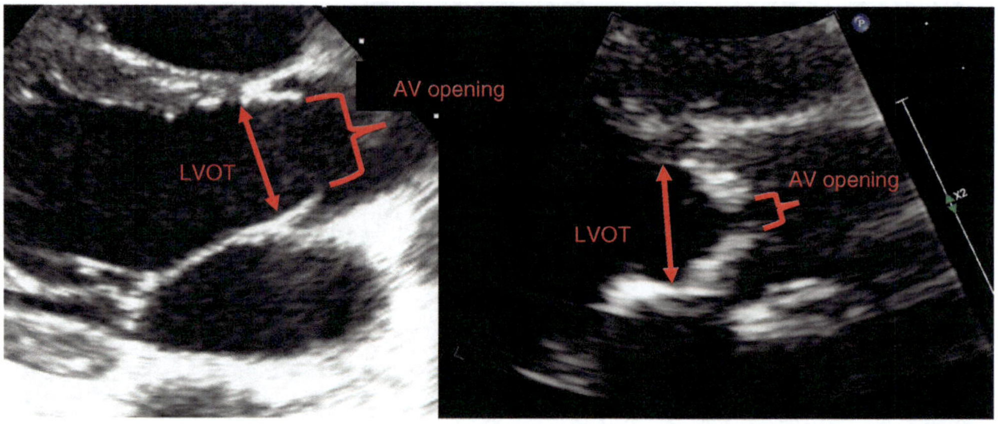

Fig. 7 Severe aortic stenosis. Left panel: Normal aortic valve. LVOT; left ventricular outflow tract, AV; aortic valve. Right panel: Severely stenotic aortic valve. Note how in the normal image the LVOT and the AV valve opening are about the same diameter, but in stenosis, the AV valve opening is decreased and much narrower than the LVOT

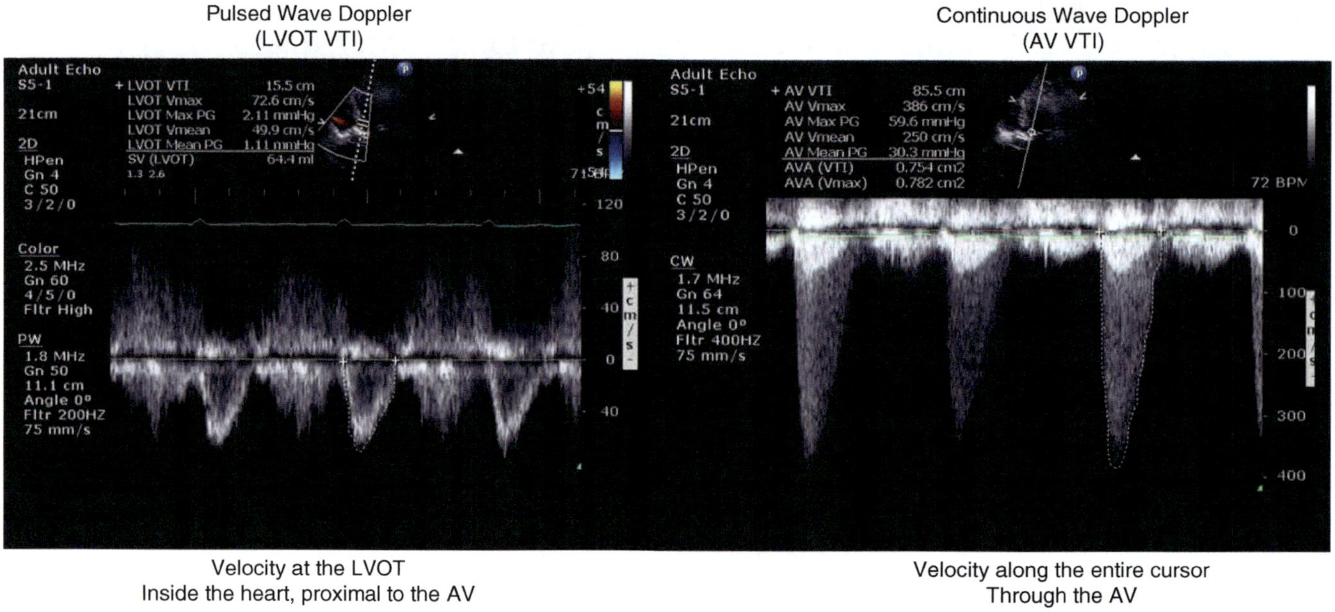

Fig. 8 Pulsed and continuous wave Doppler in aortic stenosis. Left Panel: Pulsed wave Doppler. LVOT left ventricular outflow tract, VTI velocity time integral, AV aortic valve. Right Panel: Continuous wave Doppler

intubated. Cardiology is consulted, and a transcatheter aortic valve replacement is planned.

Teaching Points Detection and grading of AS

- Close examination of the aortic valve in the PLA and the Apical 5 chamber (AP 5) views are crucial elements in detecting AS.
  - In the PLA, use active zoom to magnify the valve and closely examine the opening and closing of the valve.
    - Moderate to severe AS is not a subtle finding; the valve appears stenotic and the leaflets barely open.
  - Apply color flow Doppler over the valve in both windows.
    - Look for a narrowing in the column of flow at the valve.
  - If AS is present, then the stroke volume cannot be assessed with echo.
    - The stenotic aortic valve is the narrowest area in the column of blood flow not the left ventricular outflow tract (LVOT).
- If you do not have expertise in grading aortic stenosis, obtain a full-service cardiology transthoracic echocardiogram**.**
  - It is easy to underestimate the AS; measurement of the gradient is operator dependent.
  - In severe AS or AS with low left ventricular ejection the gradient may be low due to low flow through the valve.
- Pulsed wave Doppler (PWD) measures velocity at the LVOT before the valve.

- LVOT velocity time integral (LVOT VTI) and LVOT velocity peak (LVOT V_{max})
- Pulsed wave is pulsed and therefore has a pause period to listen for the return signal
- Allows for listening at a specific point along the cursor, set by the marker
- But with high velocity flow PWD will alias

- Continuous wave Doppler (CWD) measures velocity along the entire cursor, so measures flow through the valve
  - AV VTI and AV V_{max}
  - Continuous wave uses two crystals to continuously send and receive the signals
  - Cannot listen at various depths, listens along the entire cursor
  - Does not alias
- Normally when the AV leaflets are open the narrowest part of flow and thus highest velocity flow is at the LVOT
  - So LVOT and AV velocities are similar.
    - AV flow is always a little bit faster.
- In aortic stenosis, the stenotic leaflets become the narrowest region of flow
  - So CWD velocities will be much higher than PWD velocities.
    - AV VTI and AV V_{max}>>> LVOT VTI and LVOT V_{max}
- CWD and PWD are used together to estimate the aortic valve area (AVA) measure the velocity ratio. CWD is used to measure the peak and mean gradient.
  - AVA = πr^2PWD Velocity/CWD Velocity
  - r (radius) = LVOTDiameter/2
  - Velocity can be VTI or V_{max}.
- Velocity is dependent on flow so low LV EF and severe aortic stenosis can decrease the peak and mean gradient changes causing inaccurate grading (Table 1).

Teaching Points Medical management of respiratory failure and hypotension in severe aortic stenosis.

- The pressure gradient across the AV causes high pressure in the LV and low pressure in the aortic root where the coronary arteries take off.
  - Decreases coronary artery perfusion pressure
- Increases in heart rate and contractility, or decreases in systemic vascular resistance (SVR) increase the gradient across the valve and risks cardiovascular collapse.

Table 1 This table describes the changes to the aortic valve area and flow gradients across the aortic valve as severity of aortic stenosis increases

	No stenosis	Mild	Moderate	Severe
Max jet velocity (m/s)	< 2.6	2.6–3	3–4	>4
Mean gradient (mmHg)	–	<30	30–50	>50
AVA (cm^2)	–	>1.5	1–1.5	<1
Indexed AVA (cm^2/m^2)	–	>0.9	0.6–0.9	<0.6
Velocity ratio	–	>0.5	0.25–0.50	<0.25

- Beta-agonists like norepinephrine and epinephrine increase contractility and heart rate risking myocardial ischemia.
  - Pure alpha agonists, like phenylephrine, which increase the SVR without increasing heart rate or contractility are safer agents in treating hypotension with severe AS.
- Intubation WILL increase the gradient across the aortic valve and can precipitate decompensation.
  - Prepare prior to intubation
    - Place an arterial line.
    - Give fluid if no evidence of pulmonary edema.
    - Etomidate is the ideal induction agent.
      - Minimal hemodynamic effects

6 Case 5 Endocarditis

A 28-year-old women who abuses intravenous drugs presents to the emergency room with a 3-day history of worsening left lower extremity cellulitis, fatigue, and fever. She is febrile to 39 °C and is in respiratory distress. After intubation, she becomes hypotensive; an echo is preformed to assess cardiac function and volume status. She is found to have a thickened mitral leaflet with a mass and a mobile lesion on the tricuspid valve (Fig. 9 and Video 4). She has wide-open tricuspid regurgitation with reversal of flow during systole in her hepatic veins and portal pulsatility, indicating elevated right atrial pressure (Fig. 10 and Video 5). She also has diffuse B-lines lung imaging (Fig. 10).

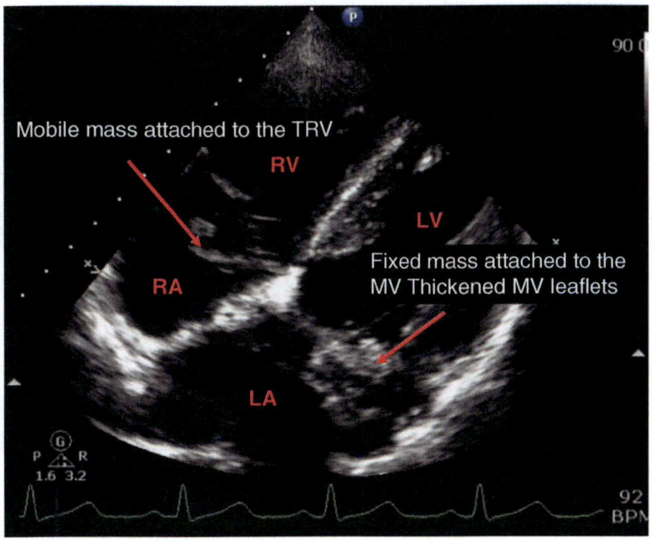

Fig. 9 Echocardiographic findings in endocarditis. RA right atria, RV right ventricle, LA left atria, LV left ventricle, TRV tricuspid valve, MV mitral valve. This patient has both tricuspid and mitral valve endocarditis. The TRV lesion is attached to the valve and mobile. It flaps freely in the video clip. The MV lesion is bigger and more fixed to the valve

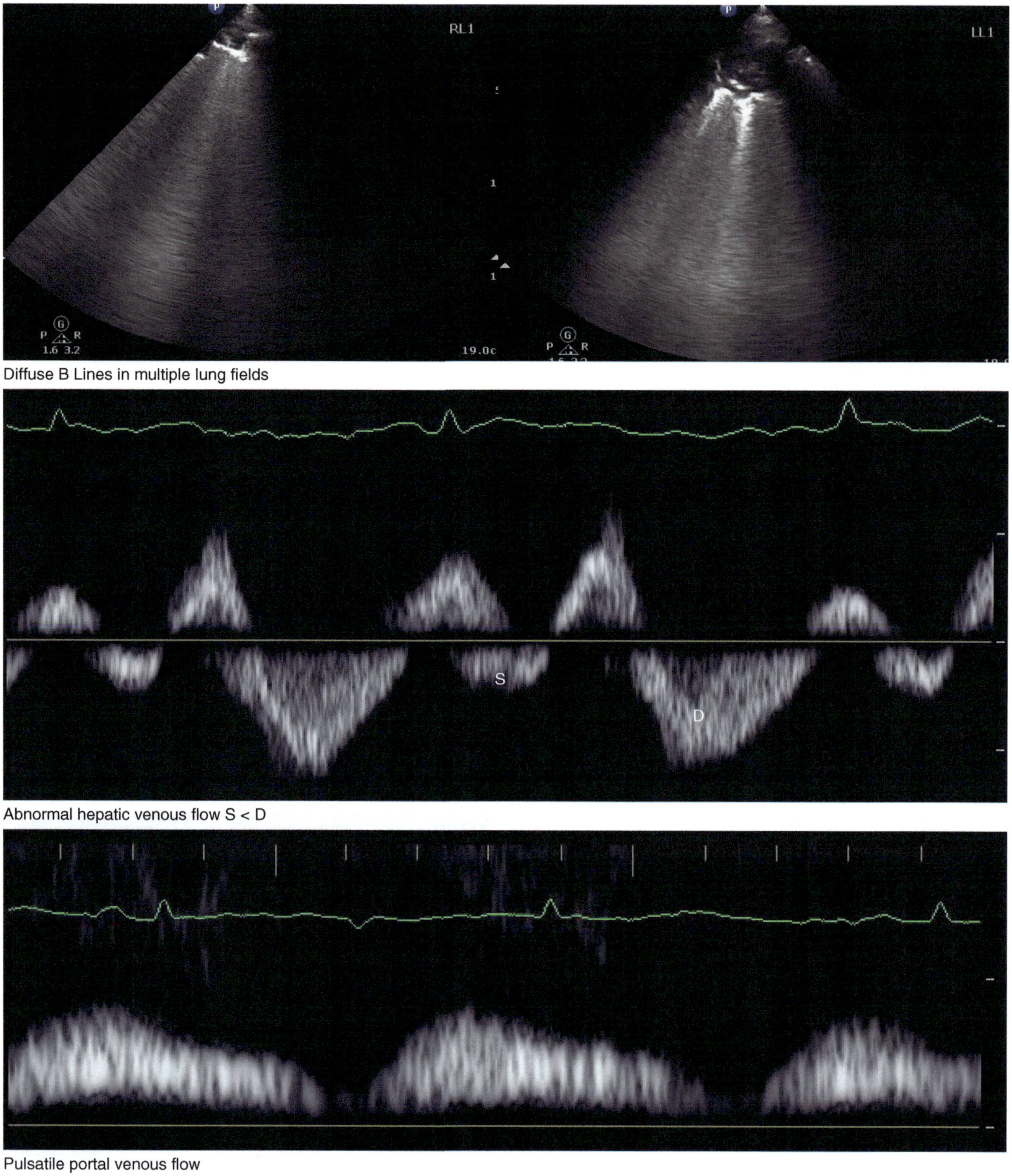

Fig. 10 Findings of volume overload in endocarditis. Upper panel: Diffuse B-lines in multiple lung fields. Middle Panel: Abnormal hepatic venous flow. S systolic, D diastolic. S < D is consistent with elevated right atrial pressure. Lower Panel: Pulsatile portal flow. Portal pusatility is consistent with elevated right atrial pressure

Case conclusion She is diuresed. Broad spectrum antibiotics are started. Her blood cultures are positive for gram (-) rods. She is transferred to the ICU with a diagnosis of mitral and tricuspid endocarditis. Cardiac surgery and cardiology are consulted. Her lower extremity cellulitis is closely monitored and does not require surgical debridement.

Teaching Points

- Endocarditis can be an important incidental finding in an echo preformed for other indications.
- The mitral, aortic, and tricuspid valves should be carefully examined with every point-of-care echo, especially in high-risk populations. The pulmonic valve is not well visualized.
  - Look for mobile mass attached to the valve leaflets (flibbertigibbets).
    - If endocarditis is present, it should be seen in more than one window.
  - Look carefully to see if the valve leaflets are co-opting normally.
  - Activate Zoom when appropriate to more fully understand the mass and assess valvular function.
  - Use color flow Doppler to look for abnormal flow across the valve.
- A dedicated exam to rule out endocarditis should be performed by a service with expertise in both TTE and transesophageal echocardiography.

Suggested Reading

Alerhand S, Carter JM. What echocardiographic findings suggest a pericardial effusion is causing tamponade? Am J Emerg Med. 2019;37(2):321–6. https://doi.org/10.1016/j.ajem.2018.11.004. Epub 2018 Nov 17

Fields JM, Davis J, Girson L, Au A, Potts J, Morgan CJ, Vetter I, Riesenberg LA. Transthoracic echocardiography for diagnosing pulmonary embolism: a systematic review and meta-analysis. J Am Soc Echocardiogr. 2017;30(7):714–723.e4. https://doi.org/10.1016/j.echo.2017.03.004. Epub 2017 May 9

Allinovi M, Parise A, Giacalone M, et al. Lung ultrasound may support diagnosis and monitoring of COVID-19 pneumonia. Ultrasound Med Biol. 2020;46(11):2908–17. https://doi.org/10.1016/j.ultrasmedbio.2020.07.018.

Alzahrani H, Woo MY, Johnson C, Pageau P, Millington S, Thiruganasambandamoorthy V. Can severe aortic stenosis be identified by emergency physicians when interpreting a simplified two-view echocardiogram obtained by trained echocardiographers? Crit Ultrasound J. 2015;7(1):5.

Baddour LM, Wilson WR, Bayer AS, Fowler VG Jr, Tleyjeh IM, Rybak MJ, Barsic B, Lockhart PB, Gewitz MH, Levison ME, Bolger AF, Steckelberg JM, Baltimore RS, Fink AM, O'Gara P, Taubert KA. Infective endocarditis in adults: diagnosis, antimicrobial therapy, and management of complications: a scientific statement for healthcare professionals from the American Heart Association. Circulation. 2015;132(15):1435–86. https://doi.org/10.1161/CIR.0000000000000296.

Part III

Shock Protocols

The Focused Sonogram for Trauma (FAST)

Kevin Flanagan and Sarah B. Murthi

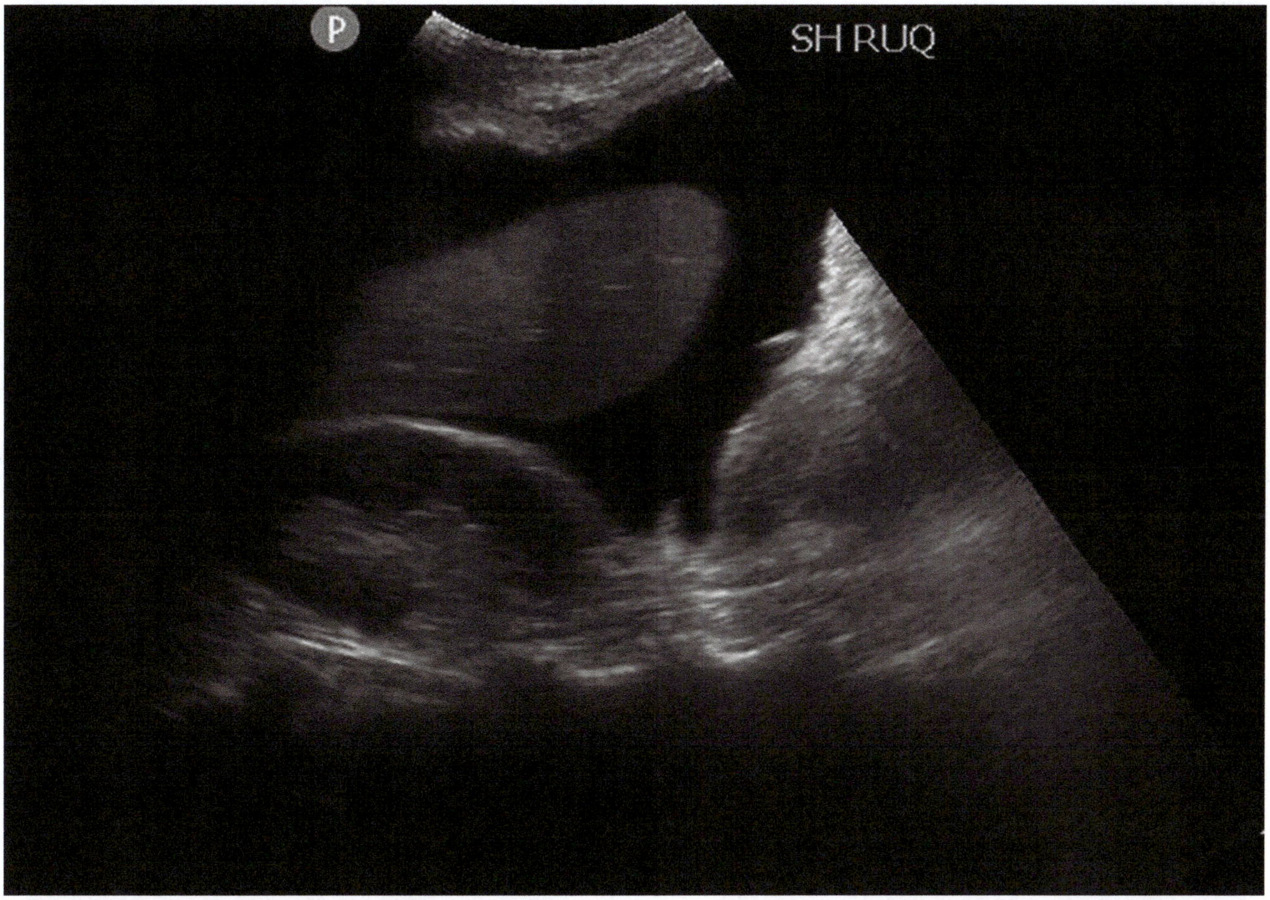

Supplementary Information The online version of this chapter (https://doi.org/10.1007/978-3-030-74687-2_19) contains supplementary material, which is available to authorized users.

K. Flanagan
Department of Emergency Medicine, University of Maryland School of Medicine, Baltimore, MD, USA

S. B. Murthi (✉)
Department of Surgery, Program in Trauma and Critical Care, R Adams Cowley Shock Trauma Center, University of Maryland School of Medicine, University of Maryland Medical Center, Baltimore, MD, USA
e-mail: smurthi@som.umaryland.edu

A. Salerno et al. (eds.), *Atlas of Critical Care Echocardiography*, https://doi.org/10.1007/978-3-030-74687-2_19

Abbreviations

FAST	Focused assessment with sonography in trauma
IVC	Inferior vena cava
LUQ	Left upper quadrant
PSL	Parasternal long axis view
RUQ	Right upper quadrant
SX	Subxiphoid
TTE	Transthoracic echocardiography

1 Introduction

The focused assessment with sonography in trauma (FAST) is commonly used to rapidly detect abdominal hemorrhage causing hypotension in trauma patients. Many centers are now performing the extended FAST (eFAST) which includes evaluating the chest for hemothorax and pneumothorax. In hypotensive trauma patients, fluid is assumed to be blood from traumatic hemorrhage and is an indication for intervention depending on the clinical scenario.

2 Uses

- Identification of abdominal free fluid
- Identification of thoracic free fluid
- Identification of pneumothorax
- Identification of pericardial fluid

3 The FAST Protocol

The FAST protocol (Figs. 1 and 2) is performed with a phased array or a curvilinear transducer in abdominal presets. The provider examines Morrison's pouch in the right upper quadrant (RUQ), the splenorenal space in the left upper quadrant (LUQ), the pelvis, and the pericardium in subxiphoid (SX) widow and for free fluid. In the typical eFAST, the transducer is fanned into the chest in RUQ and LUQ windows to look for hemothorax, and parasternal thoracic windows are added to evaluate for pneumothorax. The order of windows varies, with some centers starting with the SX and finishing with the pelvis, while others start with the RUQ. A FAST/eFAST is positive if free fluid is seen and negative if none is visualized. Free fluid in the context of traumatic shock is assumed to be blood from hemorrhage (Fig. 2) causing hypotension. A negative FAST does not rule out traumatic injury.

- *RUQ*: Place the transducer on the right mid axillary line with the marker toward the patient's head. Identify the potential space between the liver and the kidney called Morrison's pouch. Fully investigate this area by sweeping through the kidney and observing the liver tip. A dark anechoic area between the liver and the kidney suggests free fluid (Fig. 3). If preforming an e-FAST, fan the transducer into the chest to look for hemothorax.
- *LUQ*: Similarly place the transducer on the left mid axillary line with the probe marker toward the patient's head. The LUQ can be difficult to get; it is often posterior so the transducer may need to be moved all the way down to the bed. Identify the potential space between the spleen and

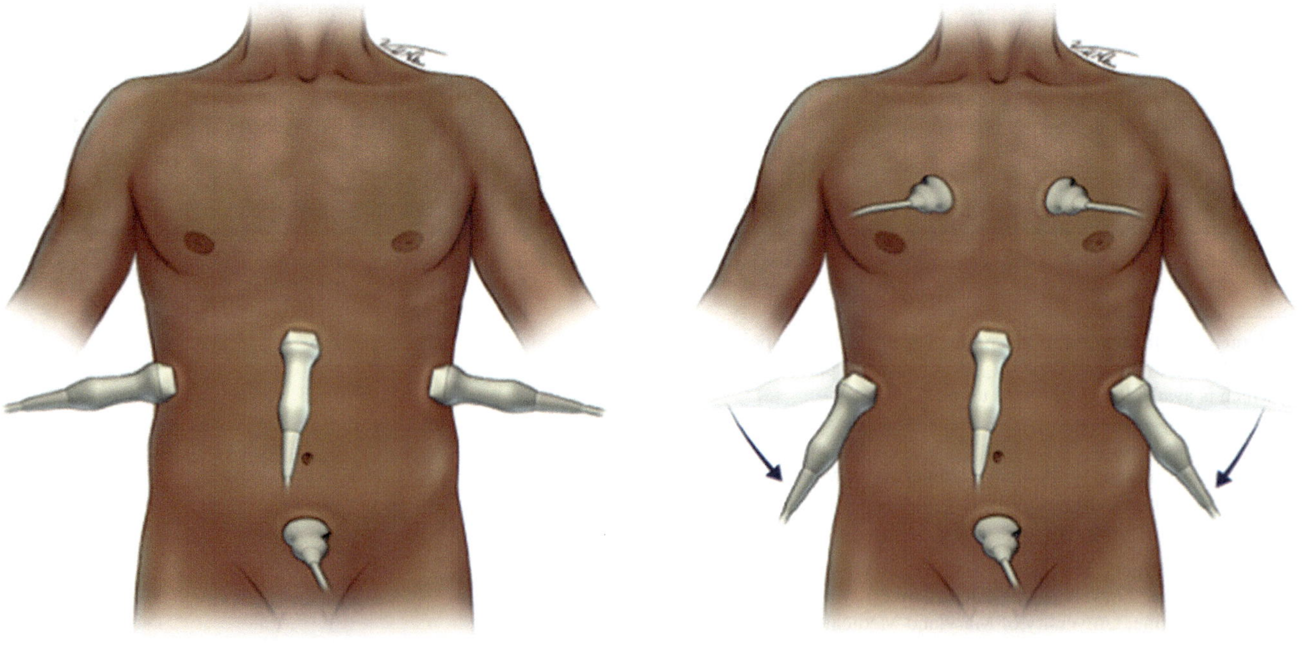

Fig. 1 Transducer placement for the FAST and the eFAST

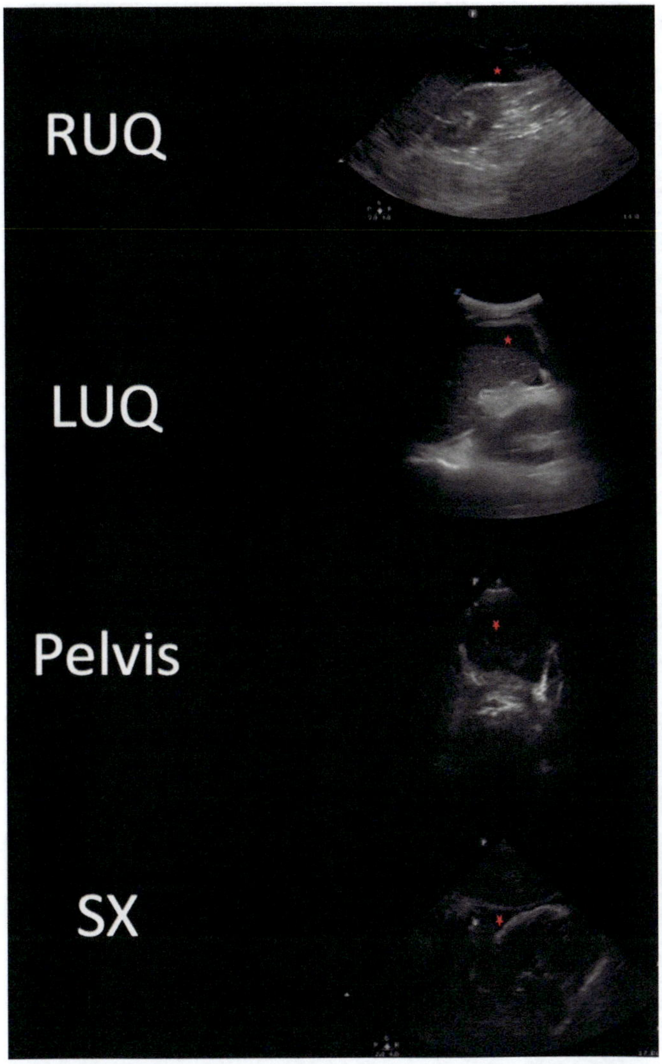

Fig. 2 Standard windows for the FAST. All of the images are positive for fluid, indicated by the red dot

the kidney. Fully investigate this area by sweeping through the kidney. A dark anechoic area between the spleen and the kidney suggests free fluid. It is important to image above the spleen as well (Video 1). Anechoic fluid above the spleen suggests injury. If preforming an e-FAST, fan the transducer into the chest to look for hemothorax (Fig. 4).

- *Pelvis*: Transducer the probe in the suprapubic region with the marker toward the patient's right. Identify the bladder and sweep through the bladder. A dark anechoic line adjacent to the bladder border is concerning for free fluid (Fig. 5 and Video 2). For a complete exam, the bladder should be imaged in cross section and long axis; this is especially important in pediatric patients.

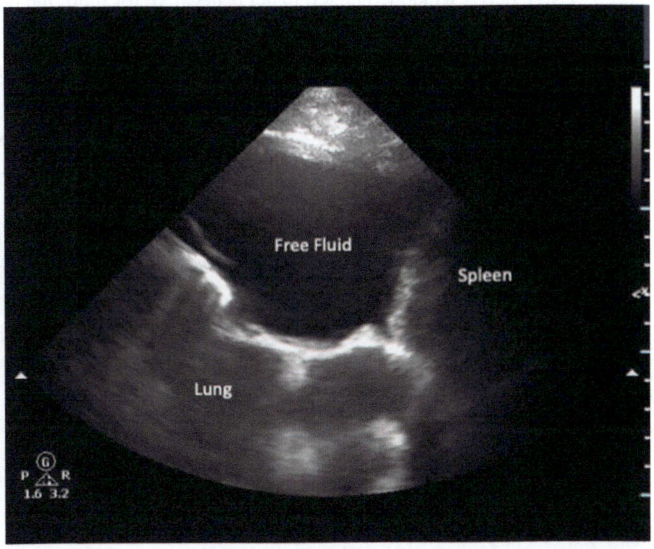

Fig. 4 eFAST left upper quadrant window positive for free fluid in the thorax

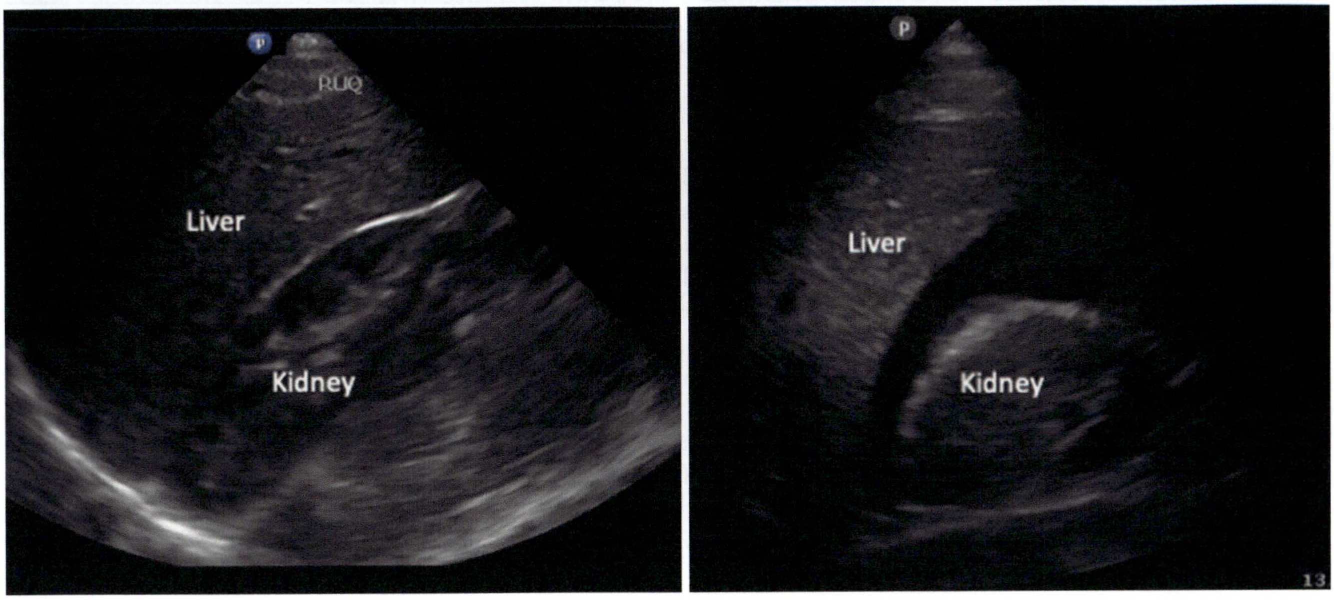

Fig. 3 FAST, right upper quadrant view. The panel on the left negative for free fluid. The panel on the right shows fluid in between the kidney and liver

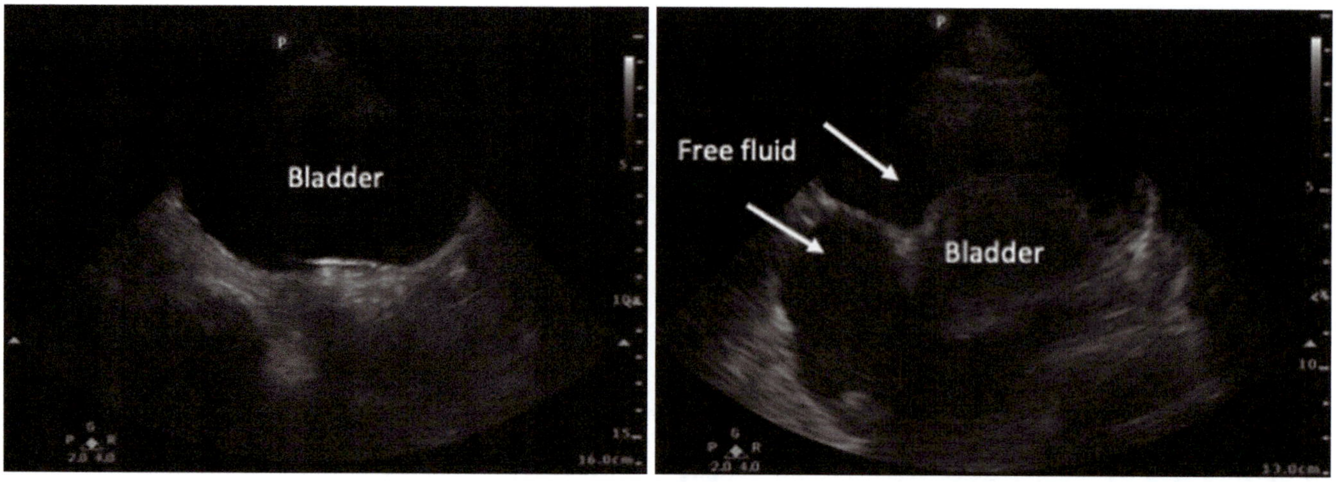

Fig. 5 FAST pelvis window. The left panel is negative for fluid; the right panel is positive for fluid

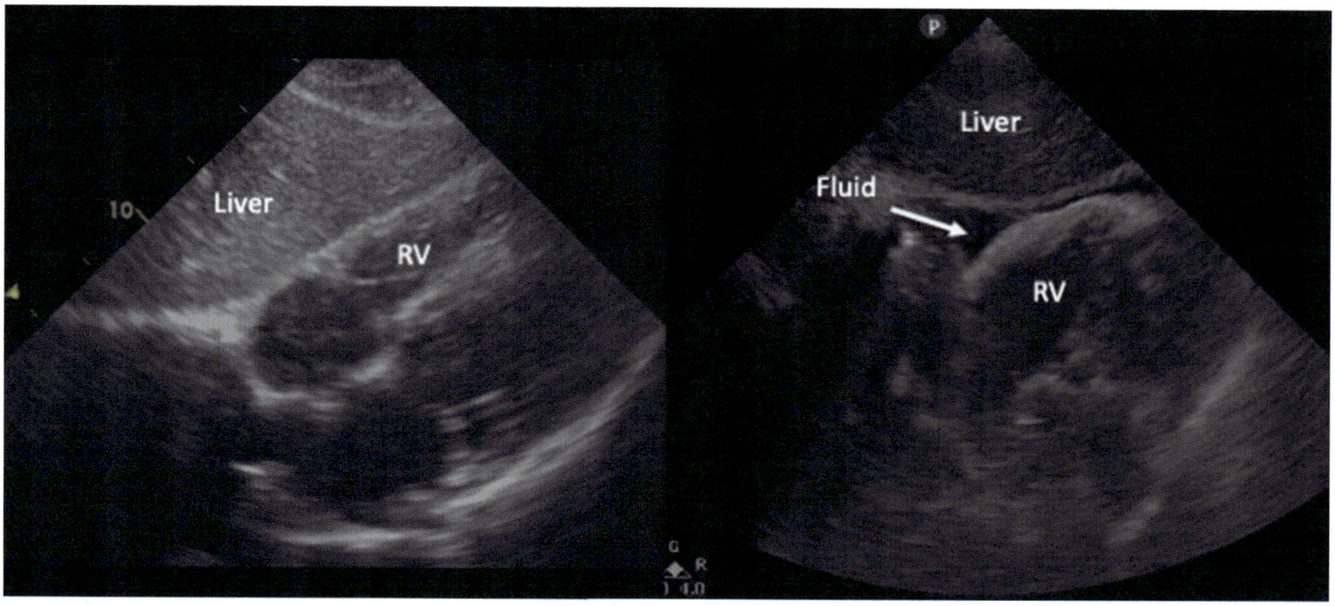

Fig. 6 FAST subxiphoid window. The left panel is negative for pericardial fluid. The right panel is positive for pericardial fluid. Right ventricle (RV)

- *Subxiphoid*: Place the transducer two centimeters below the xiphoid process. Angle the face under the xiphoid and image the RV at the liver; turn the indicator to the patient's right to see the four chambers of the heart. Pericardial fluid will appear as a dark stripe in between the RV and the liver (Fig. 6 and Video 3).
  - Penetrating chest injury, clear pericardial effusion
    - Thoracotomy/median sternotomy (depending on clinical scenario)
  - For low/moderate risk injury, patient with risk factors for preexisting effusion (cancer, renal failure), and clinical suspension the effusion is not blood
    - Monitor with serial transthoracic echocardiography (TTE)
    - Consider pericardiocentesis in the operating room with plan for rapid conversion to thoracotomy/sternotomy
  - Low risk injury, small/trace effusion
    - Monitor, serial TTE
- Lung (eFAST): Place the transducer to the left and right of the sternum with the indicator aimed toward the patient's head to rapidly rule out tension pneumothorax causing hypotension. If a more complete evaluation is indicated, consider transitioning to a linear, high-frequency transducer and performing a complete lung exam (Video 4) (see See Chap. 8).
- The FAST/eFAST are intended to be rapidly performed during the primary survey to rapidly diagnose reversible

causes of traumatic shock. Once the primary and secondary surveys are complete, the patient can be more fully evaluated.

4 Tips and Pointers

- Stabilization and care of the patient supersedes obtaining and interpreting the FAST. While the FAST is important, its performance must not interfere with patient care.
- This study is intended to be a *rapid* assessment for overt sonographic evidence of pathology. Nuanced measurements or overly comprehensive assessments are not recommended unless there is obvious pathology already identified.

5 Special Considerations

- Ulltrasound is unable to differentiate blood from ascites fluid in the abdomen. Patients with ascites will have a positive FAST but does not necessarily mean hemorrhage. Similarly, we are now able to detect small pericardial effusions which may exist prior to the traumatic event. In a case of penetrating chest injury with clear pericardial fluid, it is reasonable to assume there is a cardiac injury and proceed to the OR. But in a blunt trauma with a small effusion, monitoring with serial exams may be adequate.

Suggested Reading

Lichtenstein DA, et al. Ultrasound diagnosis of occult pneumothorax. Critical Care Medicine. 2005;33(6):1231–8.

Ma OJ, Mateer J, Blaivas M, editors. Critical care in emergency ultrasound. New York: McGraw-Hill Professional; 2007. p. 191–223.

Weingart S, Duque D, Nelson B. The RUSH exam—rapid ultrasound for shock and hypotension; 2009.

The Rapid UltraSound in Shock (RUSH)

Kevin Flanagan and Alexis Salerno

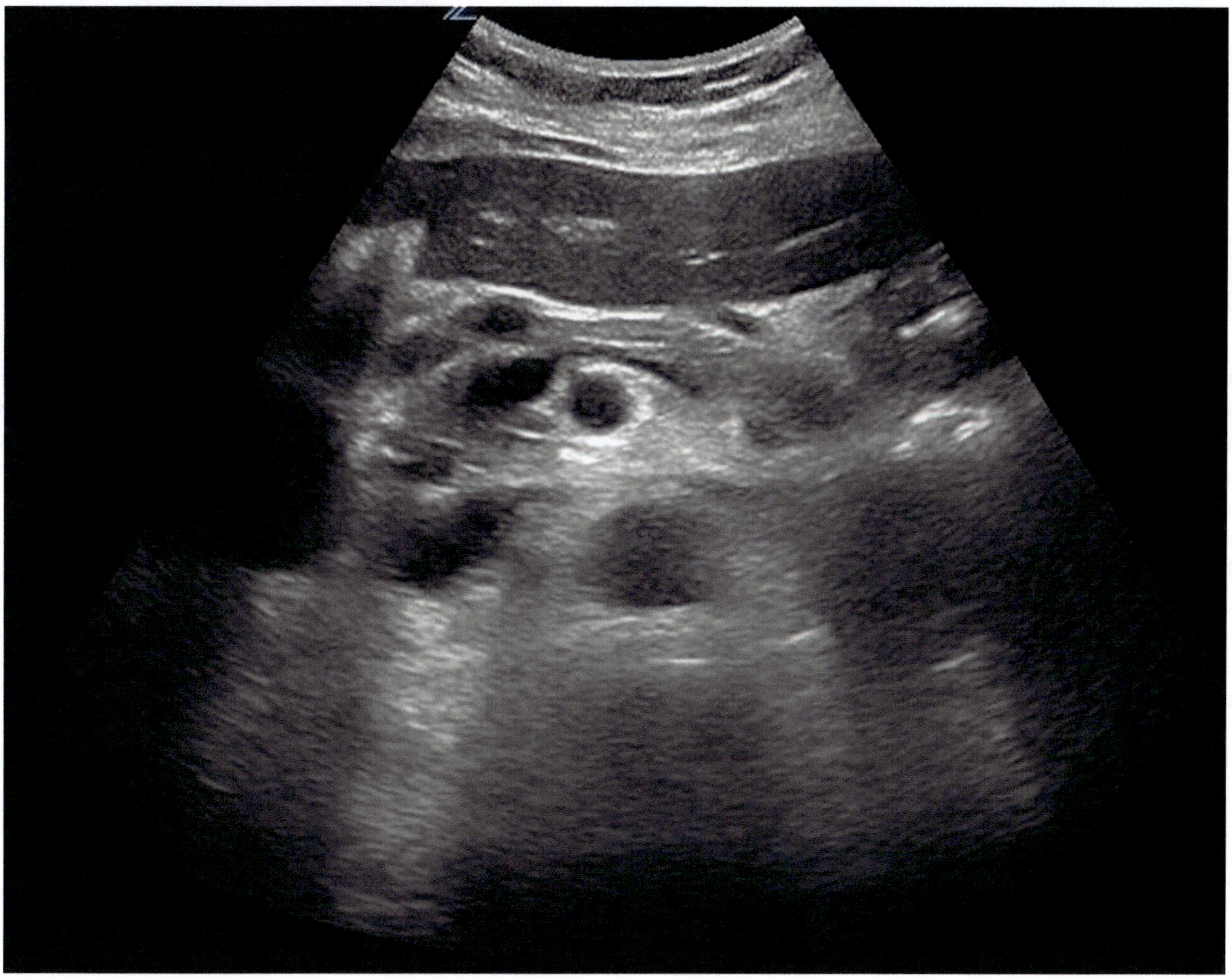

Supplementary Information The online version of this chapter (https://doi.org/10.1007/978-3-030-74687-2_20) contains supplementary material, which is available to authorized users.

K. Flanagan · A. Salerno (✉)
Department of Emergency Medicine, University of Maryland School of Medicine, Baltimore, MD, USA
e-mail: Alexis.Salerno@som.umaryland.edu

A. Salerno et al. (eds.), *Atlas of Critical Care Echocardiography*, https://doi.org/10.1007/978-3-030-74687-2_20

1 Introduction

The rapid ultrasound in shock (RUSH) is designed to rapidly diagnose the cause of undifferentiated hypotension. It was developed in the emergency department to systematically evaluate a patient with ultrasound to identify life-threatening pathologies. The RUSH includes heart, inferior vena cava (IVC), and aortic assessments for diagnosing the etiology of acute hypotension in the emergency department. The RUSH can detect pathologies causing hypotension that may not be evident on physical examination including acute MI, ruptured aortic aneurism, and tension pneumothorax.

2 Uses

- Evaluation for reversible causes of hypotension
- Identification of pericardial tamponade
- Identification of abdominal free fluid
- Identification of abdominal aortic aneurysm
- Identification of pneumothorax

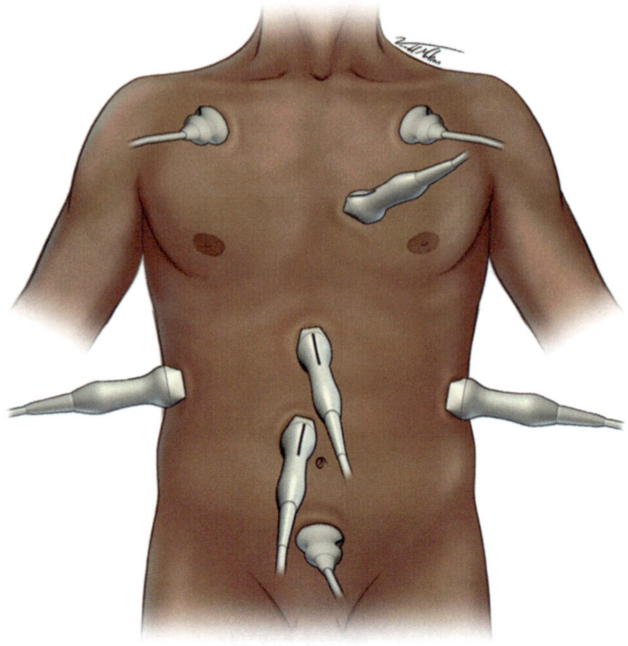

Fig. 1 This image shows the probe placement for the RUSH views

3 FAST and RUSH Protocols

The RUSH exam is performed with a curvilinear transducer in abdominal pre-sets. The provider briefly evaluates the heart for cardiogenic dysfunction, the IVC for hypovolemia, performs a FAST exam for evidence of abdominal free fluid, and evaluates the abdominal aorta for rupture and the lungs for evidence of tension pneumothoraces. The pneumonic "HI-MAP" is used to remember this series of examination: **H**eart, **I**VC – **M**orrison's pouch/FAST, **A**orta, **P**neumothorax (Figs. 1 and 2).

Heart (Cardiac)

- Parasternal long axis (PLA) or subxiphoid view of the heart. See Chaps. 2 and 5 for further description of how to obtain these views.
  - Assess for pericardial fluid and tamponade (Video 1).
  - Assess relative ventricular diameters for evidence of primary RV failure, pulmonary hypertension, or pulmonary embolism (Fig. 3).
  - Assess relative ventricular contractility for evidence of lateralizing or global systolic dysfunction.

IVC

- Obtain a long axis view of the IVC. See Chap. 5 for further description of how to obtain these views.
  - This is a rough estimation of volume status by noting overdistension or collapse of the IVC with each respiratory cycle. Also, evidence of RV failure with IVC overdistension can be seen (Fig. 4 and Video 2).

Morrison's Pouch/FAST

- Observe for abdominal free fluid within Morrison's pouch but can also extend to perform the full FAST examination (see Chap. 19).

Abdominal Aorta

- Place the probe just below the subxiphoid process with the probe marker toward the patient's right side. Identify the aorta as a circular beating structure on the right of the screen adjacent to the IVC (Fig. 5).
- Scan caudally along the aorta from the celiac branch to aortic bifurcation (Video 4).
- When measuring the aorta, look for the upper outer wall of the aorta, and measure down to just above the vertebral

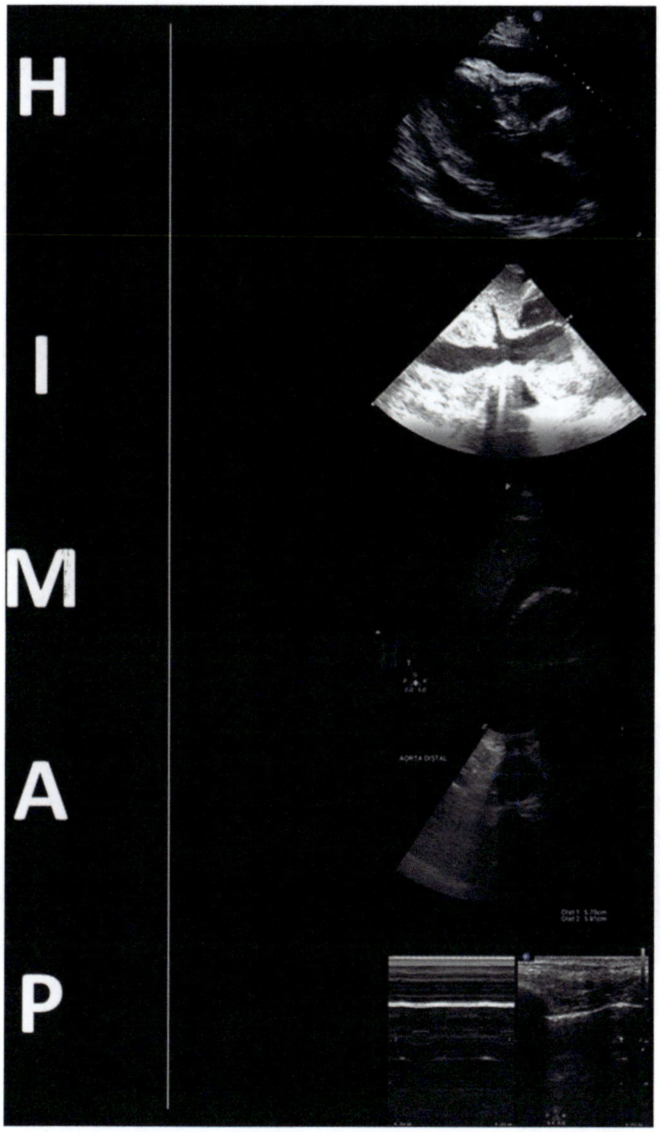

Fig. 2 This image shows examples of potential pathology found using the RUSH examination

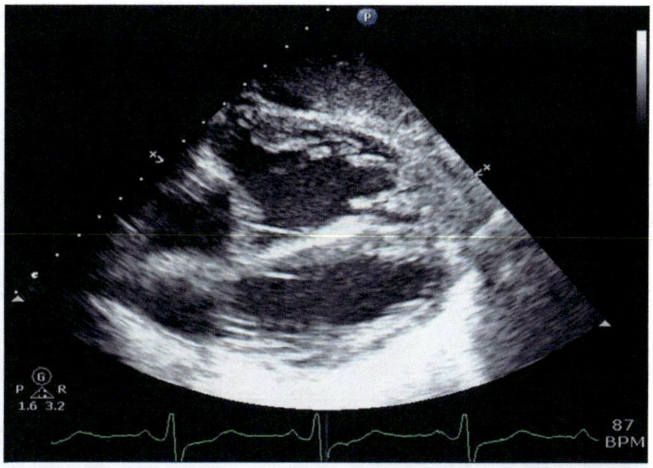

Fig. 3 This image shows an example of RV strain on subxiphoid view

line. This may be tricky when there is atherosclerosis (Fig. 6).

- Any segment with a diameter >5.0 cm should raise immediate concern for abdominal aortic aneurysmal with a potential for rupture.

Pneumothorax

- Bilateral exam 2nd and 4th intercostal spaces, midclavicular line, longitudinal axis. See Chap. 8 for further description of how to obtain views.
- Observe for loss of pleural sliding visually and using M-Mode. Also look for lung point(s) with respiration (Fig. 7 and Video 4).

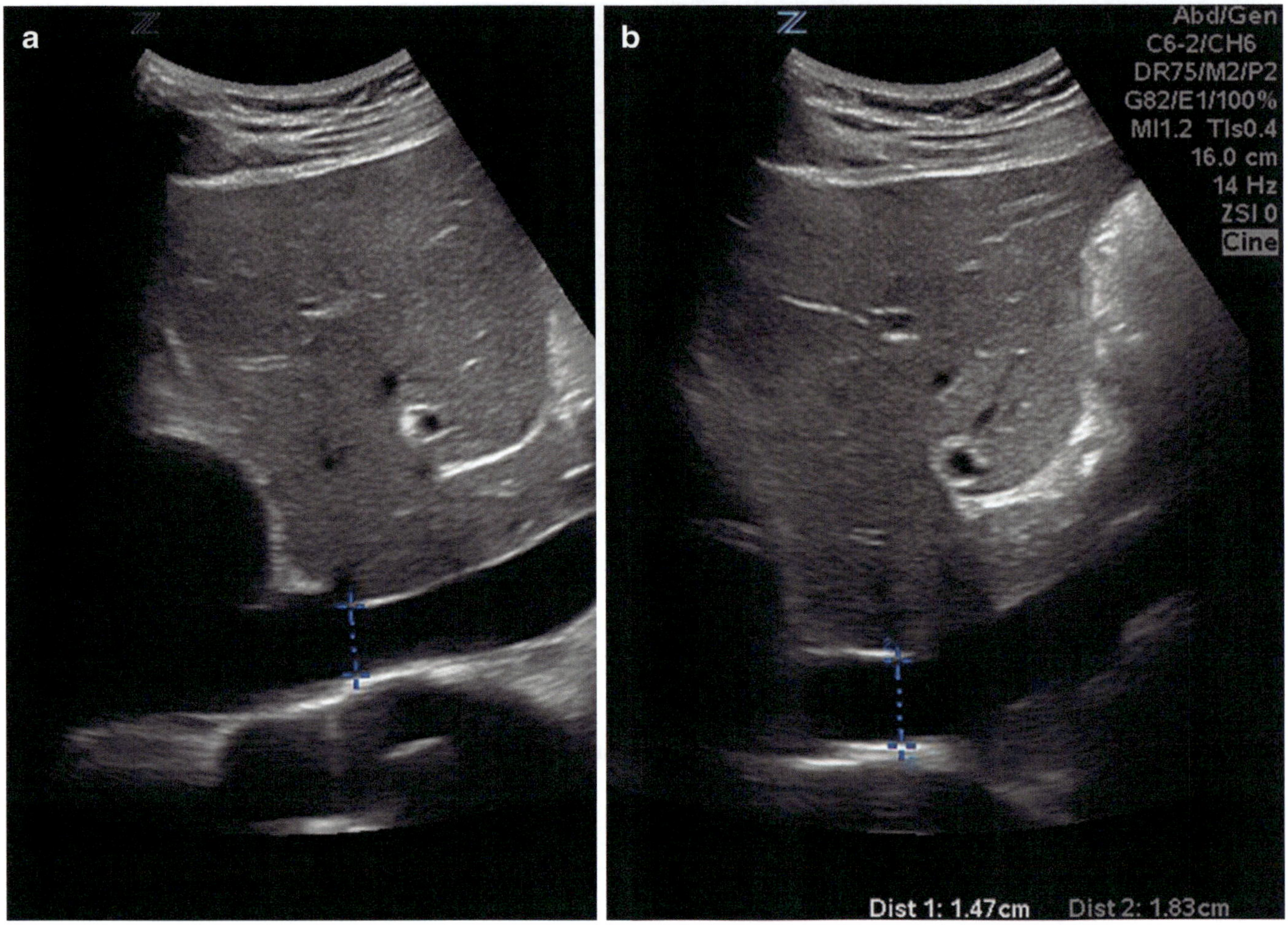

Fig. 4 IVC examination and measurement during inspiration. The patient shows signs of volume responsiveness

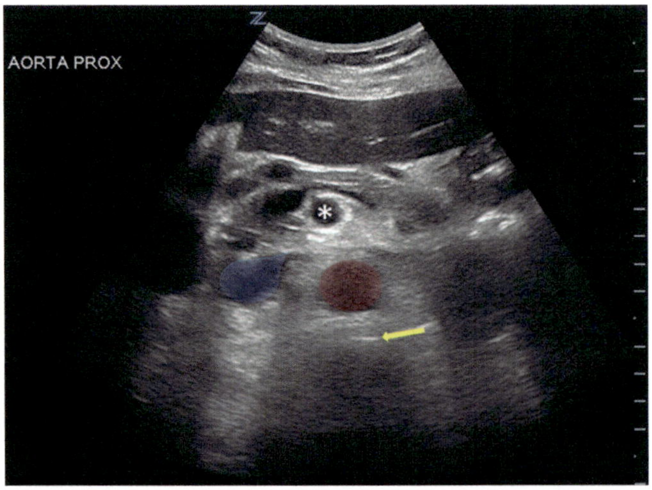

Fig. 5 This image shows an example of the abdominal aorta view. The blue is the IVC, the red is the aorta. The star is the superior mesenteric artery. The arrow points to the vertebral line

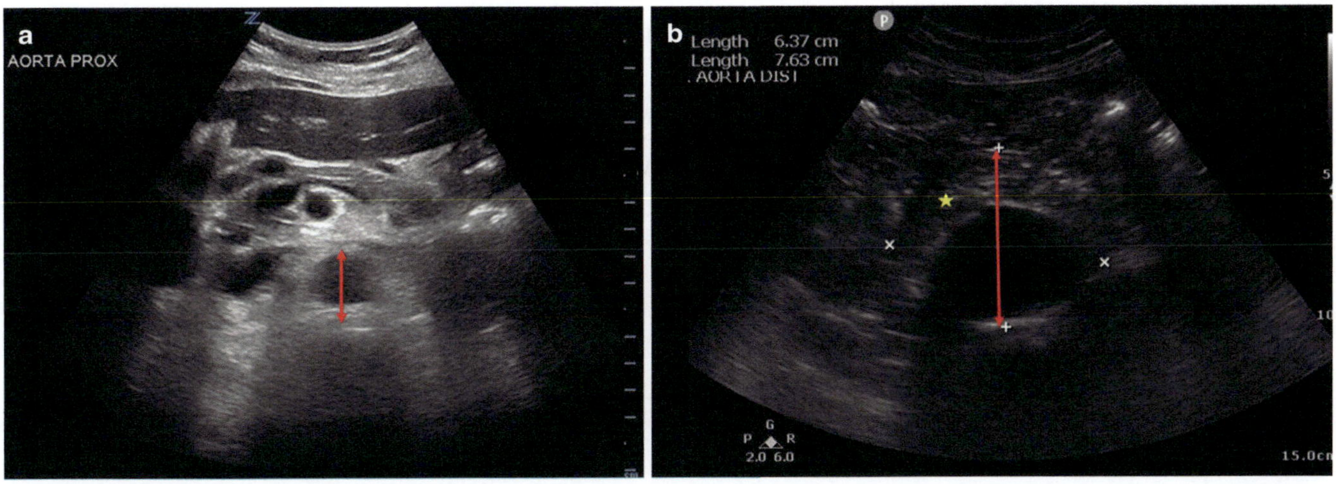

Fig. 6 This image shows an example of an abdominal aortic aneurysm (**b**) vs a normal aorta (**a**) and how to properly measure. The yellow star is atherosclerosis in the lumen of the aorta. (Image B is courtesy of University of Maryland Emergency Medicine Department)

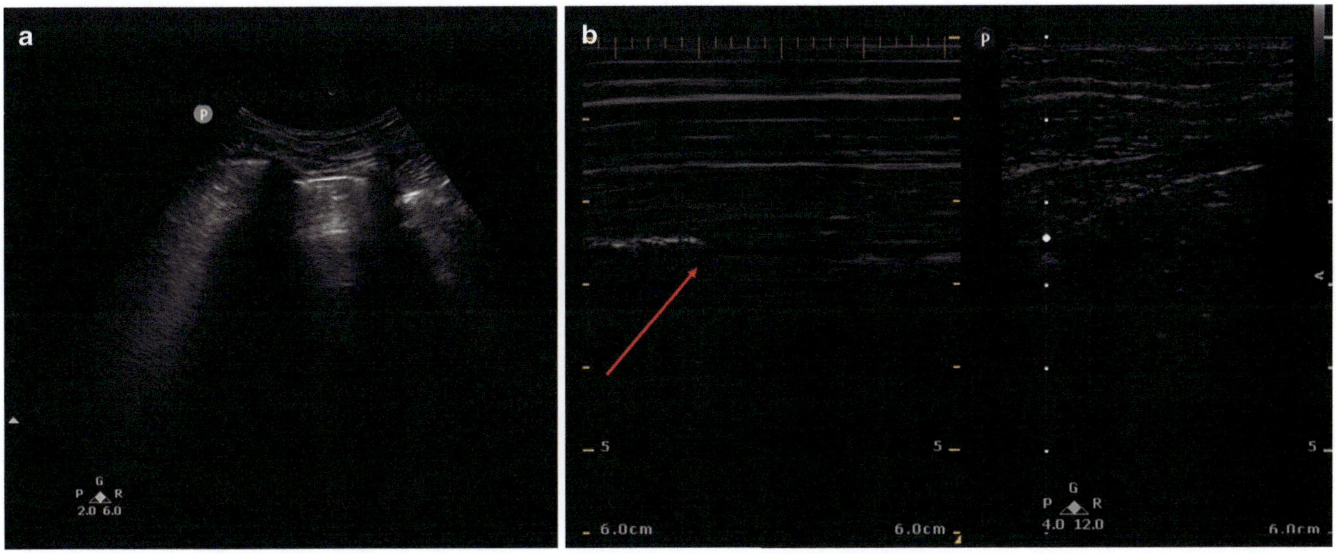

Fig. 7 This image shows an example of a lung exam during a RUSH examination. The patient had A-lines but abnormal movement along the lung line (image A). On further evaluation with M-mode, the patient was found to have a lung point (arrow in image B)

4 Tips and Pointers

- This study is intended to be a *rapid* assessment for overt sonographic evidence of pathology. Nuanced measurements or overly comprehensive assessments are not recommended unless there is obvious pathology already identified.
- Using a curvilinear transducer on the FAST or abdominal setting for this examination will help to avoid the need to allocate time to adjusting transducers and machine parameters.

5 Special Considerations

- In patients with chronic pulmonary disease or on positive pressure ventilation, the RV and IVC may demonstrate findings concerning for RV dysfunction, pulmonary hypertension, or pulmonary embolism.
- Ultrasound machine is unable to differentiate blood from ascites in the abdomen. Patients who have a history of ascites will have a positive FAST but does not necessarily mean hemorrhage.
- Always consider the epidemiology of specific pathologies within this study, for example:

- Younger patients are less likely to have an aortic aneurysm and tailor the exam as needed.
- Suspicion for ectopic pregnancy should remain high in female patients of child-bearing age.
- Consider also interrogating the lower extremities for evidence of a deep vein thrombosis in patients with bedside echocardiography findings concerning for an acute pulmonary embolism.

Suggested Reading

Lichtenstein DA, Mezière G, Lascols N, Biderman P, Courret JP, Gepner A, et al. Ultrasound diagnosis of occult pneumothorax. Crit Care Med. 2005;33(6):1231–8.

Ma OJ, Mateer J, Blaivas B. Critical care in emergency ultrasound. New York: McGraw-Hill Professional; 2007. p. 191–223.

Weingart S, Duque D, Nelson B. The RUSH exam—rapid ultrasound for shock and hypotension. EM Crit Project. 2009. https://emcrit.org/rush-exam.

Cardiac Arrest Sonographic Assessment (CASA)

Ahmed Al Hazmi

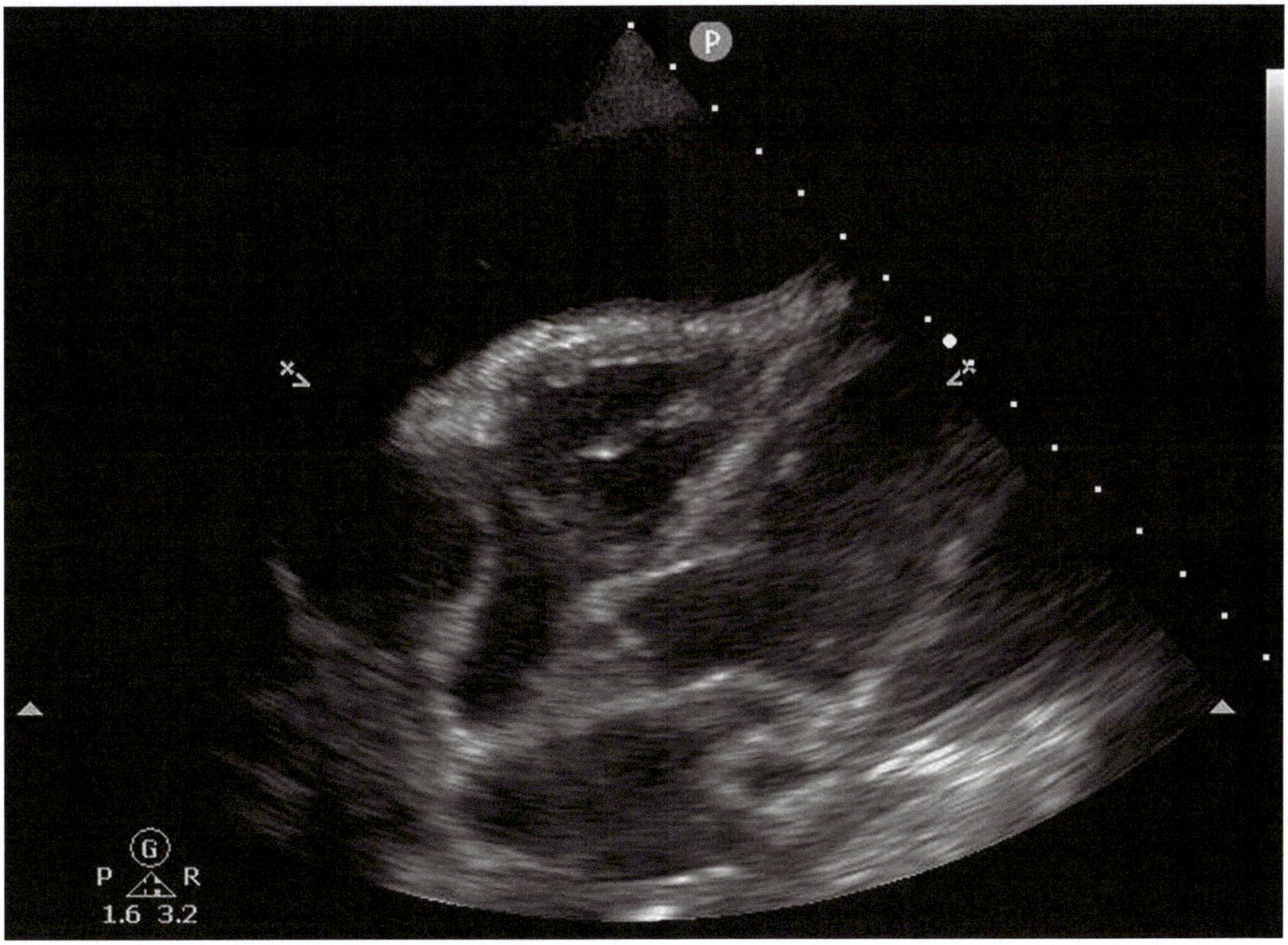

Supplementary Information The online version of this chapter (https://doi.org/10.1007/978-3-030-74687-2_21) contains supplementary material, which is available to authorized users.

A. Al Hazmi (✉)
Jeddah, Saudi Arabia

A. Salerno et al. (eds.), *Atlas of Critical Care Echocardiography*, https://doi.org/10.1007/978-3-030-74687-2_21

1 Introduction

The role of point of care ultrasound (POCUS) in cardiac arrest has evolved over the last several years. Reports have shown that POCUS performed during arrest can length pulse checks. In response, the Cardiac Arrest Sonographic Assessment (CASA) was developed. CASA identifies reversible causes of cardiac arrest while minimizing interruptions in high-quality CPR [1–3]. Additionally, CASA provides a simplified, stepwise approach to minimize provider's cognitive load during resuscitation. In the future, we may see a change in cardiac arrest protocol as transesophageal echocardiography (TEE) use more widespread.

2 Uses for CASA

1. Identify the presence of pericardial effusion.
2. Evaluate the sequelae of PE, presence of a right heart strain.
3. Assess cardiac activity.
4. Rule out pneumothorax.
5. Determine the presence or absence of peritoneal free fluid.

These last two bullet points can be done at any time during the resuscitation, taking care not to interfere with compression. The first three bullet points can be evaluated during pulse check pauses. At no time should performing the ultrasound interfere with running the code.

3 CASA Protocol

During Pulse Check Pause

1. Using the subxiphoid view record a 10 second clip or for as long as the pulse check. Do not extend the time to obtain images. If possible, image all chambers for thorough evaluation of the heart. If unable to obtain a subxiphoid view, obtain a parasternal long axis PLA view (Fig. 1).
2. Review captured clip once CPR is resumed.
   - Presence or absence of pericardial fluid (Fig. 2): Rapid identification and treatment can resolve PEA. Once pericardial effusion is identified, pericardiocentesis should be performed promptly.
   - Right ventricular strain (dilation) (Fig. 3): Look at the size of the RV as compared to the LV. A RV > LV can suggest PE as a cause of the arrest.
   - Visualization of cardiac activity (Video 1): Assess for global cardiac activity vs fibrillations. If cardiac activity is present, check for a pulse and blood pressure to guide resuscitative efforts. If no pulse, continue CPR even if cardiac activity is seen on US.
   - In the absence of cardiac activity, prognostic factors such as prolonged CPR, low end tidal CO_2, or pH should be evaluated for continuation vs termination of resuscitation.

During CPR

1. Evaluate anterior chest for lung sliding on both sides (Fig. 4).
   - Rule out tension pneumothorax as a cause.
   - If a pneumothorax is detected, a needle decompression or thoracostomy should be considered.
2. FAST exam to detect peritoneal free fluid (Fig. 5)
   - Assess for ruptured AAA.
   - Rule out ectopic pregnancy.

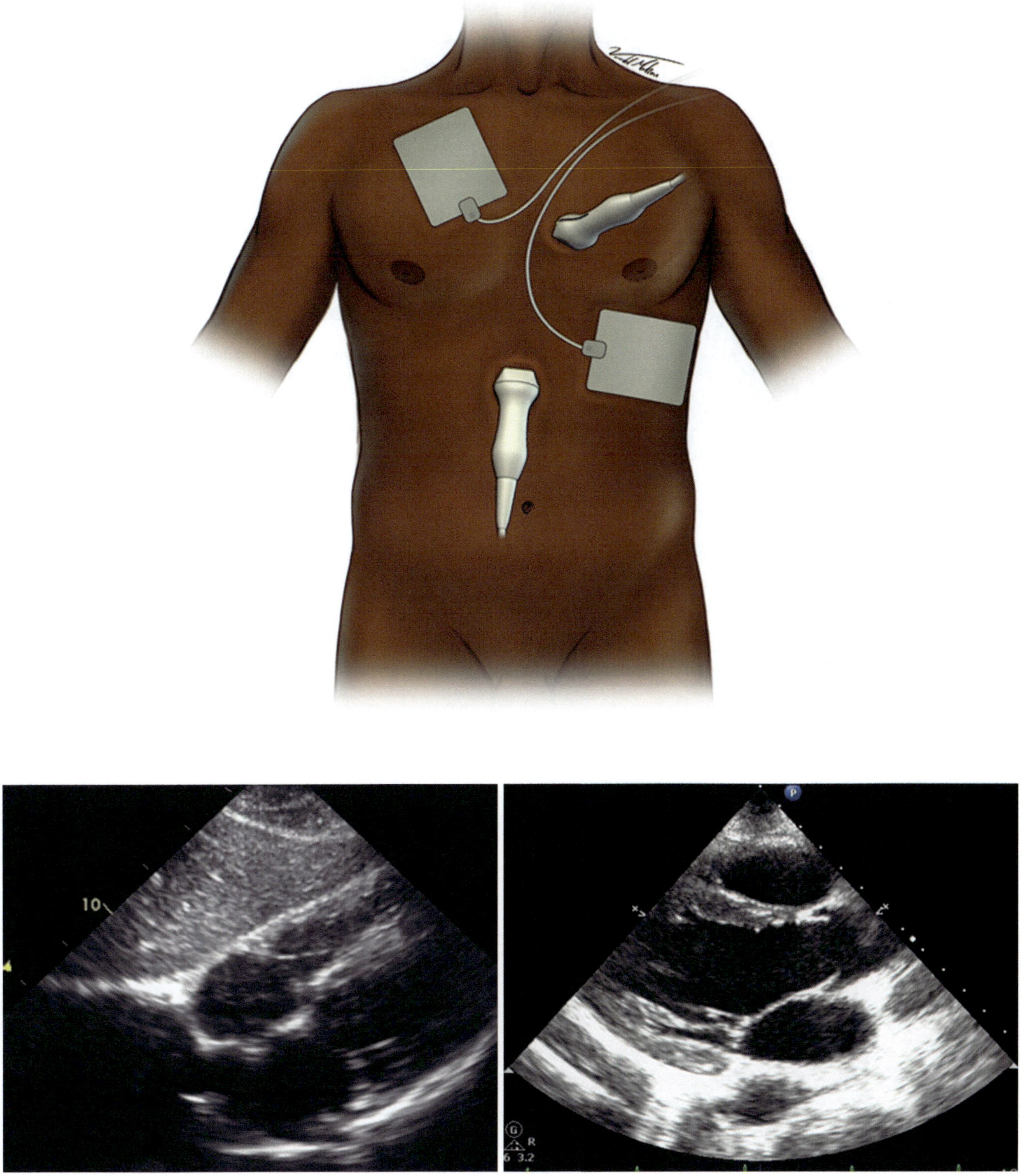

Fig. 1 Ideal transducer location for CASA. Upper panel shows the SX, the preferred location and the PLA. Lower left is a SX image, lower right is a PLA image

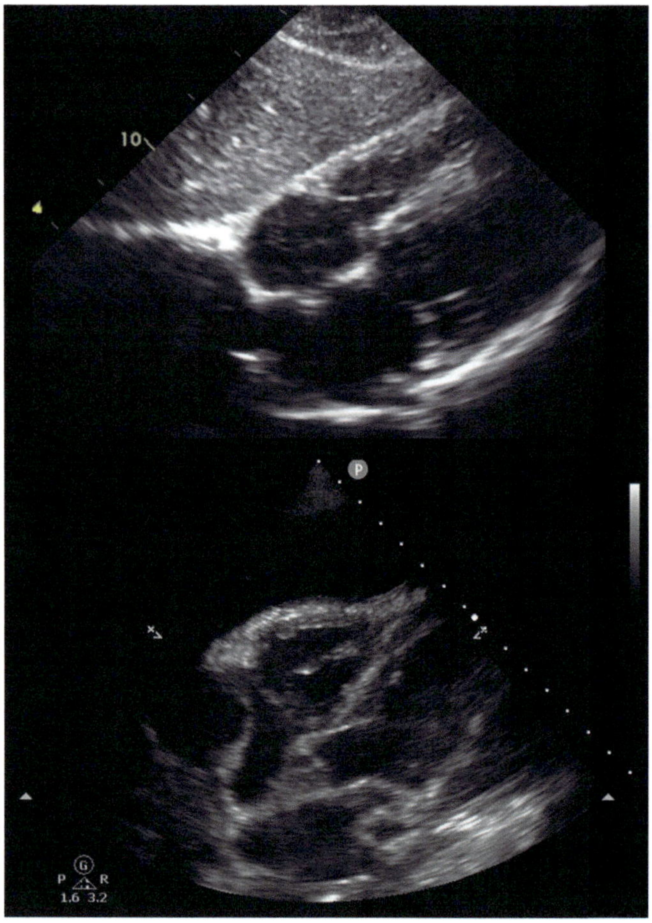

Fig. 2 Pericardial effusion with tamponade. Upper panel: A normal RV with no effusion. Lower panel: A large pericardial effusion concerning for tamponade

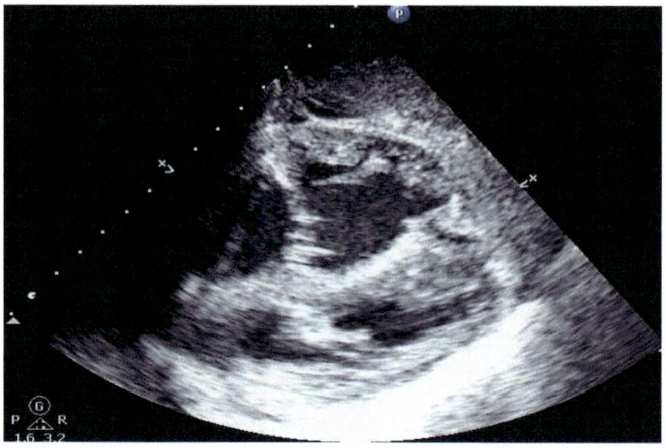

Fig. 3 RV dilation concerning for pulmonary embolus. A dilated RV which can be related to PE but can also represent changes from positive pressure ventilation, post arrest physiology, or chronic pulmonary hypertension

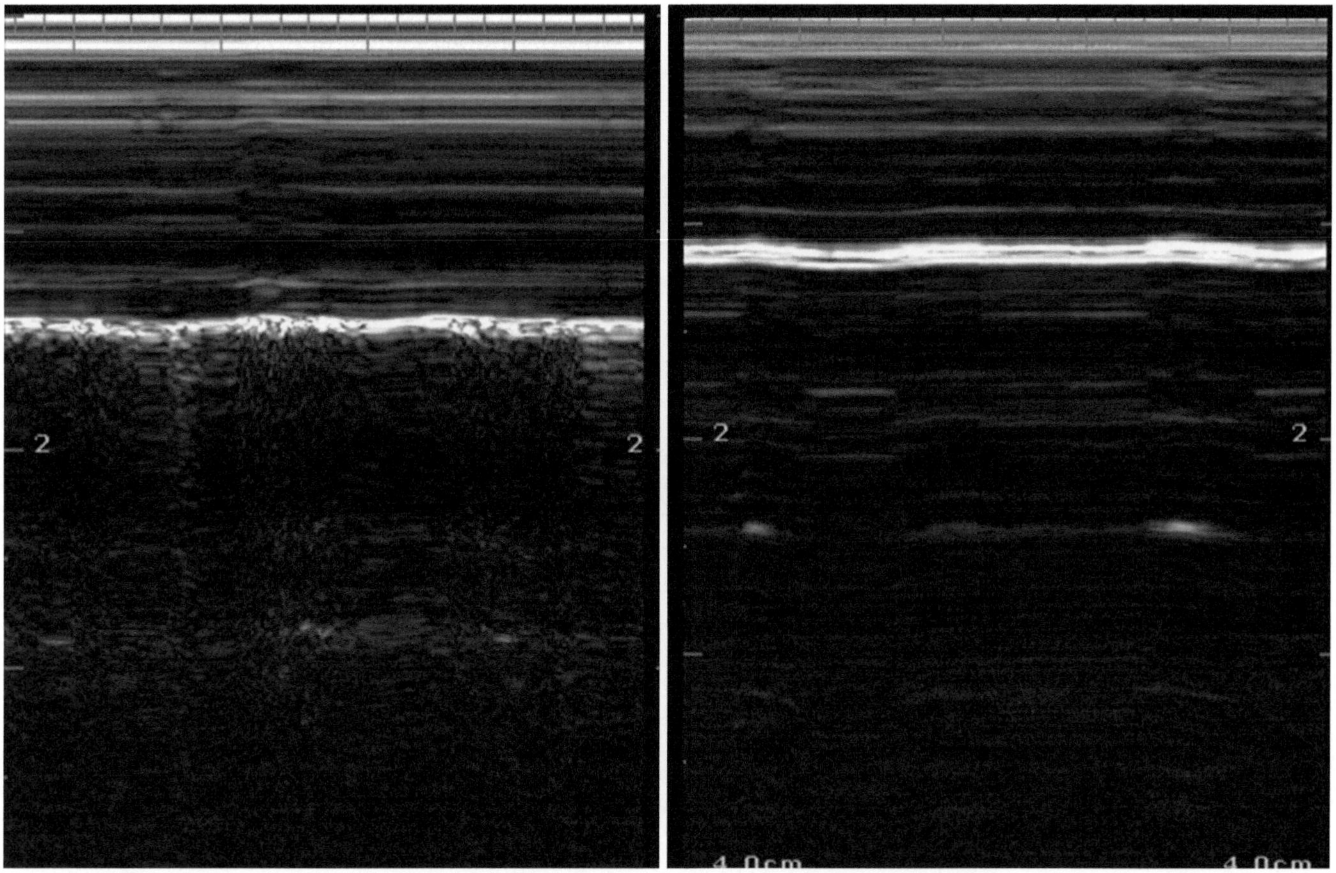

Fig. 4 Pneumothorax. Left panel: M-mode a normal lung using a linear probe. Right Panel: M-mode showing "bar-code sign" diagnostic of pneumothorax

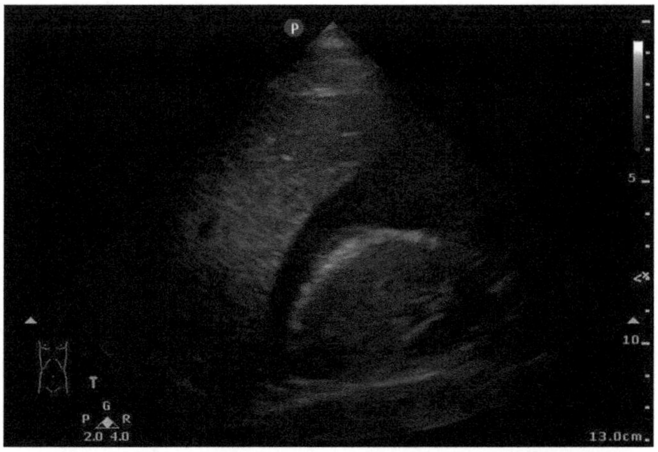

Fig. 5 Positive abdominal fluid. Abdominal ultrasound showing free fluid between the liver and kidney

4 Tips and Pointers

- Do not interrupt or delay compressions to obtain images.
- Use the phased array transducer with cardiac presets. If using abdominal or FAST preset, the image resolution will make it difficult to accurately assess for cardiac activity.
- Place ultrasound transducer on chest and find view BEFORE CPR pause.
- Rapidly obtain and save the clip.
- Review it AFTER compressions have resumed.
- Wipe the ultrasound gel once images acquired to prevent interference with compressions and defibrillation pads.
- Although RV strain can be due to PE, please consider chronic changes in patients who have a history of COPD or right heart failure.

References

1. Gardner KF, Clattenburg EJ, Wroe P, Singh A, Mantuani D, Nagdev A. The Cardiac Arrest Sonographic Assessment (CASA) exam – a standardized approach to the use of ultrasound in PEA. Am J Emerg Med. 2018;36(4):729–31.
2. Clattenburg EJ, Wroe PC, Gardner K, et al. Implementation of the Cardiac Arrest Sonographic Assessment (CASA) protocol for patients with cardiac arrest is associated with shorter CPR pulse checks. Resuscitation. 2018;131(May):69–73.
3. Gardner K, Clattenburg E, Wroe P, Nagdev A. Introducing the CASA exam: a new protocol to guide point-of-care ultrasound in cardiac arrest - ACEP Now. [online] ACEP Now. 2018. Available at: https://www.acepnow.com/article/introducing-the-casa-exam-a-new-protocol-to-guide-point-of-care-ultrasound-in-cardiac-arrest/.

Part IV

The Focused Rapid Echocardiographic Evaluation (FREE)

There Is No @#$% Tank! It is a Pump!!

Sarah B. Murthi

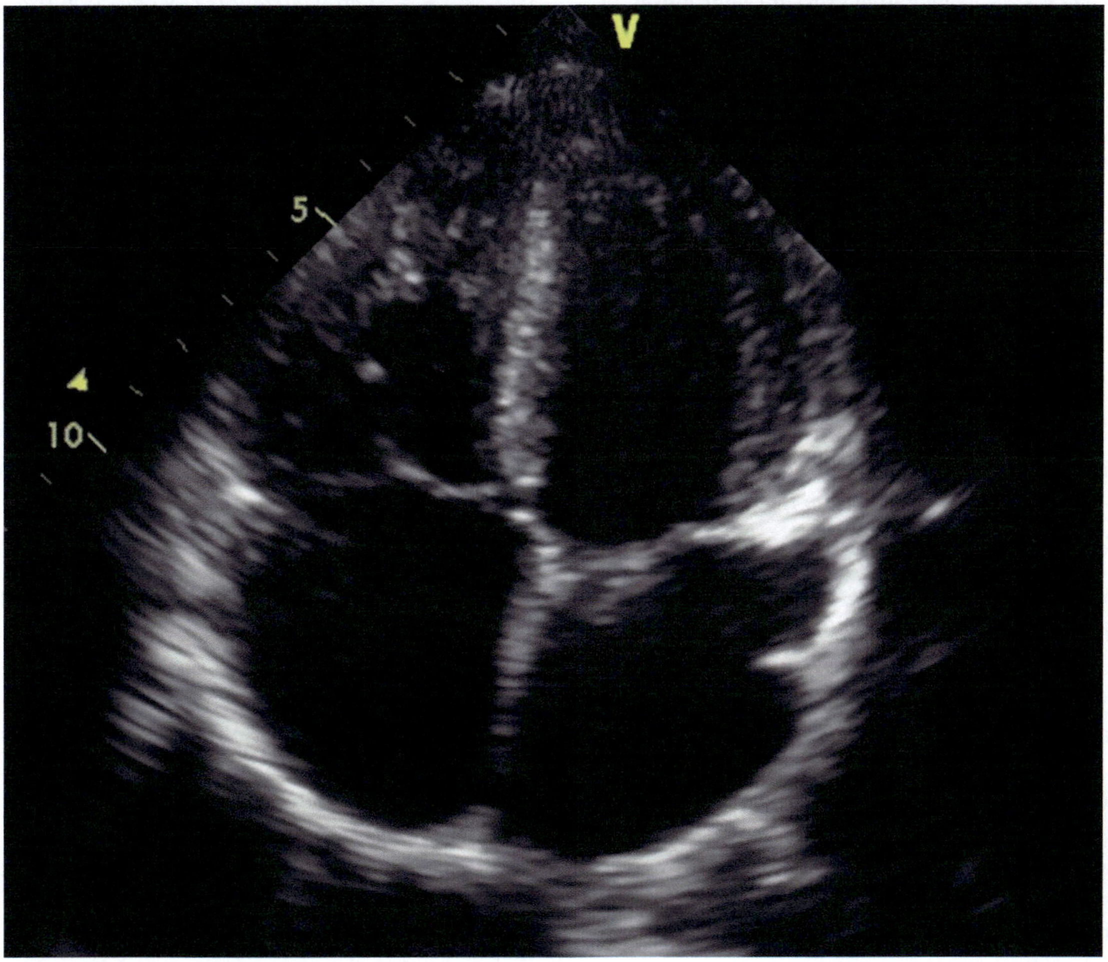

Supplementary Information The online version of this chapter (https://doi.org/10.1007/978-3-030-74687-2_22) contains supplementary material, which is available to authorized users.

S. B. Murthi (✉)
Department of Surgery, Program in Trauma and Critical Care, R Adams Cowley Shock Trauma Center, University of Maryland School of Medicine, University of Maryland Medical Center, Baltimore, MD, USA
e-mail: smurthi@som.umaryland.edu

A. Salerno et al. (eds.), *Atlas of Critical Care Echocardiography*, https://doi.org/10.1007/978-3-030-74687-2_22

Abbreviations

a	Atrial contraction flow
CO	Cardiac output
E	Early diastolic flow
E′	Early diastolic ventricular movement
ECG	Electrocardiogram
EF	Ejection fraction
IJ	Internal Jugular
ITP	Intrathoracic pressure
IVC	Inferior vena cava
LA	Left atria
LV	Left ventricle
MSFP	Mean systemic filling pressure
NPV	Negative Pressure Ventilation
O_2	Oxygen
PA	Pulmonary artery
PEEP	Positive end expiratory pressure
PG	Pressure gradient
PPV	Positive pressure ventilation
RA	Right atria
RAP	Right atrial pressure
RV	Right ventricle
SV	Stroke volume
SVC	Superior vena cava
SVR	Systemic vascular resistance
TAPSE	Transannular plane systolic excursion
TR pk	Tricuspid regurgitant peak velocity
VTI	Velocity time integral

1 Introduction

Cardiology interprets echo with a focus on the heart itself. Hemodynamic ultrasound interprets echo with a focus on end organ perfusion. Our central question is how can the cardiovascular system be optimized to perfuse capillary beds. Incorporating echo into a critical care practice leads to a richer understanding of cardiac function, blood flow, perfusion, and shock.

The ultrasound findings are discussed in detail in their respective chapters.

2 There Is No @#$% Tank! It Is a Pump!!!

A common shorthand for the cardiovascular system is a tank which needs to be filled-up prior to starting vasopressors. This leads to a heavy-handed approach to fluid which undervalues the importance of venous congestion. Instead, think of it how it is: a four-chambered pump. The heart pumps deoxygenated blood from end organ capillary beds via the lower pressure right side through the pulmonary vasculature where it is oxygenated by the lungs and into the left side of the heart. The high pressure left side pumps out oxygenated blood into the aorta, through arteries and arterioles into the capillary beds (Fig. 1 and Video 1).

Four-Chambered Pump (Fig. 1)

- Two functions: ejection and filling
  - Systolic function
    - Ejection of blood from the ventricles
      - *Ultrasound assessments*
        - *Left ventricular (LV) ejection fraction (EF)*
        - Right ventricular (RV) global assessment
        - RV transannular plane systolic excursion (TAPSE)
  - Diastolic function
    - The ventricles actively relax
      - ATP requiring process
      - The ventricles untwist and rapidly descend pulling blood in
      - *Ultrasound assessments*
        - Tissue Doppler

Two Tasks

- Pump blood out of the heart towards organs
  - Oxygenated blood from the LV through the aorta to end organs
  - Deoxygenated blood from the RV through the pulmonary artery (PA) into the lungs
    1. Failure of Task One (Fig. 2): Low cardiac output *relative* to end organ needs
       - Hypotension
       - End organ hypoperfusion
- Pump blood off organs into the heart
  - Deoxygenated blood from end organs into the right atria (RA) through the superior and inferior vena cava (SVC, IVC)
  - Oxygenated blood from the lungs into the left atria (LA) via the pulmonary veins
    1. Failure of Task 2 (Fig. 3): Venous congestion, end organ edema
       - Right side
         - Hepatic, visceral, renal edema, and dysfunction
       - Left side
         - Pulmonary edema, respiratory failure

Blood Flow (Fig. 1)

- Right atrium: Thin walled, lower pressure flow

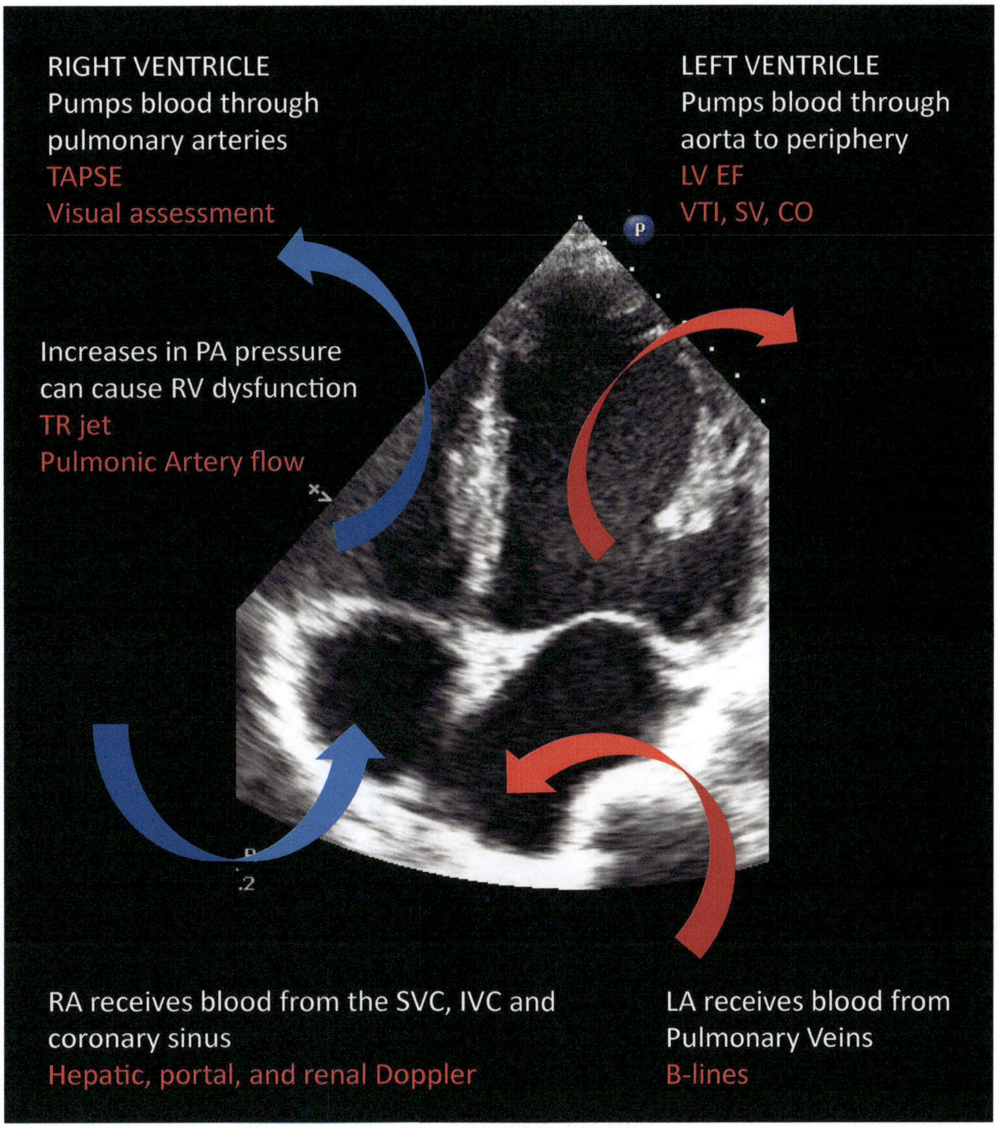

Fig. 1 The Pump. Deoxygenated blood is pumped off end organs and flows into the low-pressure right side of the heart. It pulsates through the pulmonic vasculature where it is oxygenated. Blood fills the left side and is pumped out into the high-pressure arterial circulation. Blue arrows: deoxygenated blood; red arrows: oxygenated blood; red type: relevant ultrasound findings

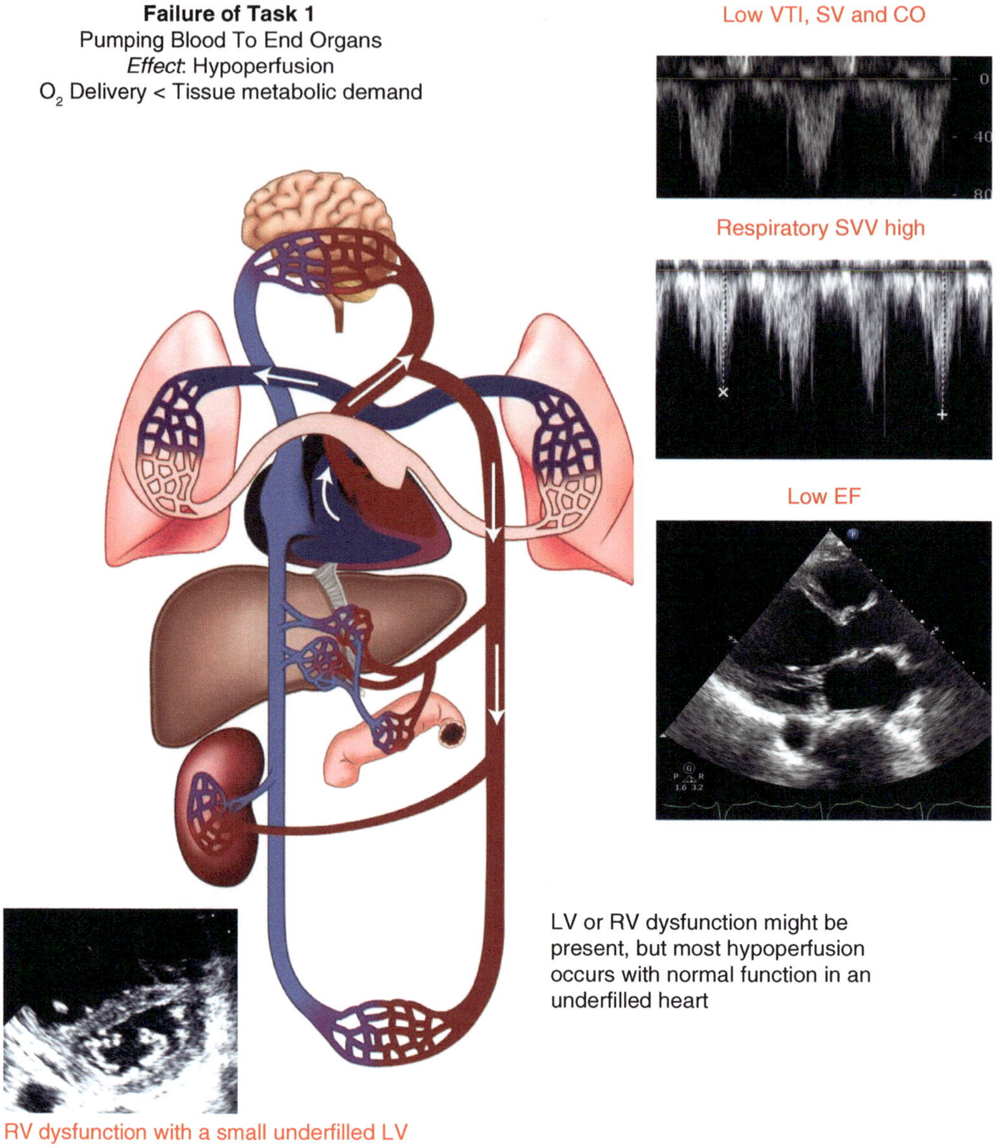

Fig. 2 Hypoperfusion, failure of Task 1. Hypoperfusion occurs when oxygen delivery is less than the metabolic needs of end organs. White arrows: blood flow out of the RV and LV. Red type relevant ultrasound findings

  - Receives deoxygenated blood from the IVC and SVC
  - Contracts in late diastole to finish filling the RV
    1. *Ultrasound assessments*
       - Hepatic vein flow
         - Assess right atrial pressure (RAP)
       - Size of the RA
       - Quality of contraction
- Right ventricle (RV): Thin walled, lower pressure flow
  - Actively relaxes in diastole to accept blood from the RA
  - Contracts in systole to pump blood into the PA and through the lungs into the pulmonary veins
    1. *Ultrasound assessments*
       - Size of the RV
       - Quality of contraction
       - TAPSE
       - Tricuspid valve regurgitant jet velocity peak flow (TRpk)
         - Assess PA systolic pressure
- Left atrium (LA): Thicker walled, accustomed to higher pressure flow
  - Receives oxygenated blood from the pulmonary veins
  - Contracts in late diastole to finish filling the left ventricle
    1. *Ultrasound assessments*
       - *Size of the LA*
       - *Quality of contraction*
       - *Characterization of B-Lines on lung imaging*

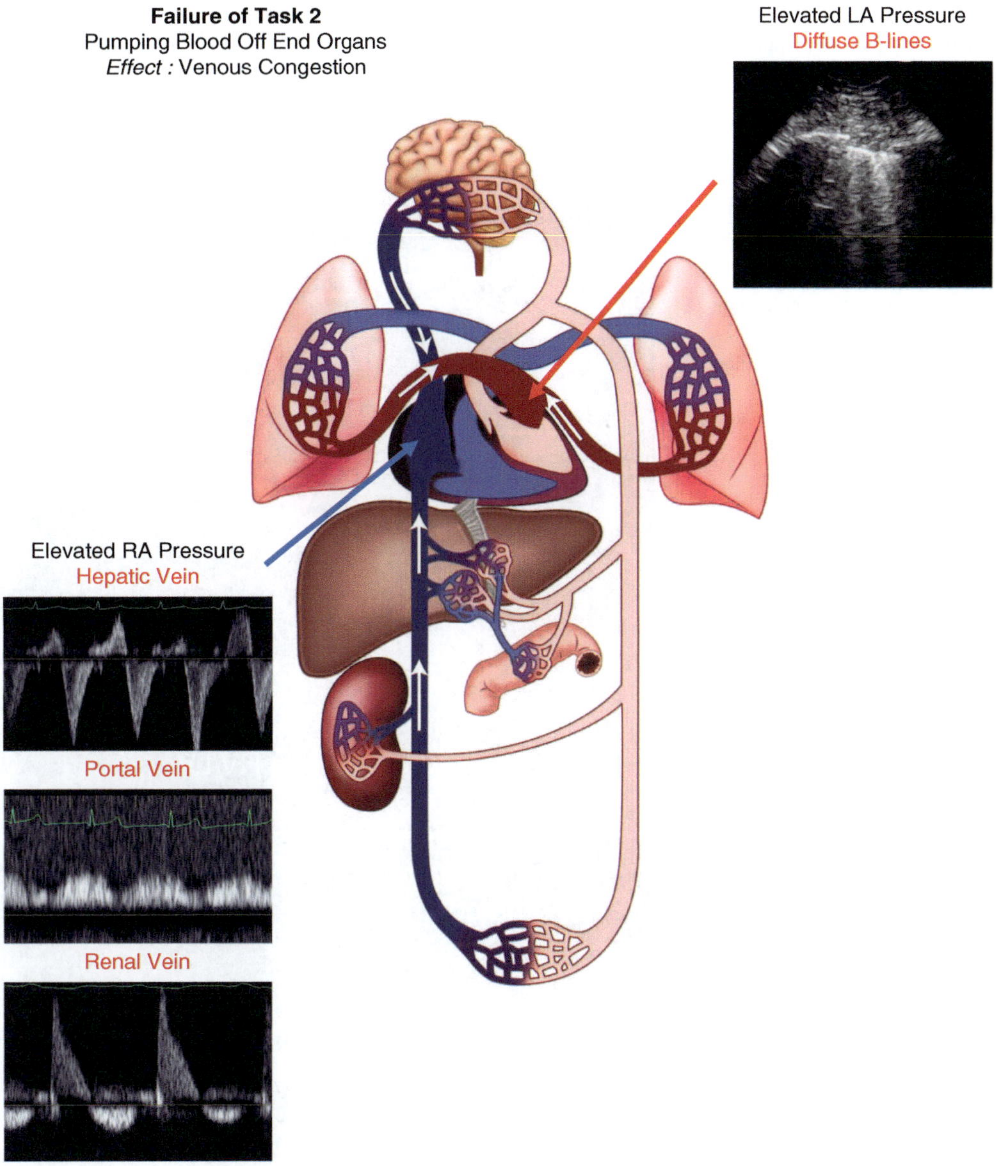

Fig. 3 Venous congestion, failure of Task 2. Venous congestion occurs when left or right atrial pressure is elevated. White arrows: blood flowing into the RA and LA; blue arrow: RA, red arrow; LA. Red type relevant ultrasound findings

    - *Pulsed wave Doppler (PWD) flow through the mitral valve*
    - *Tissue Doppler at the mitral annulus*
- Left ventricle (LV): Thicker walled, accustomed to higher pressure flow
  - Actively relaxes in diastole to receive blood from the LA
  - Contracts in systole to pump oxygenated blood into the aorta, through arteries and arterioles back into the end organ capillary beds
    1. *Ultrasound assessments*
       - *Size of the LV*
       - *LV ejection fraction*
       - *LV velocity time integral (LV VTI)*

Cardiac Cycle (Fig. 4)

- Ventricular Systole
  - The ventricles *both* contract.
  - When ventricular pressure exceeds central vascular pressure, the pulmonic and aortic valves open.
  - Blood is ejected into the pulmonary artery and aorta.
  - The atria fills in systole.
    - *Ultrasound assessments*
      - Elevations in right atrial pressure will cause decreased systolic venous flow assessed with PWD.
        - Hepatic, portal, and renal measurements
  - The RV and LV are getting smaller.
  - The LA and RA are getting bigger.
- Ventricular Diastole

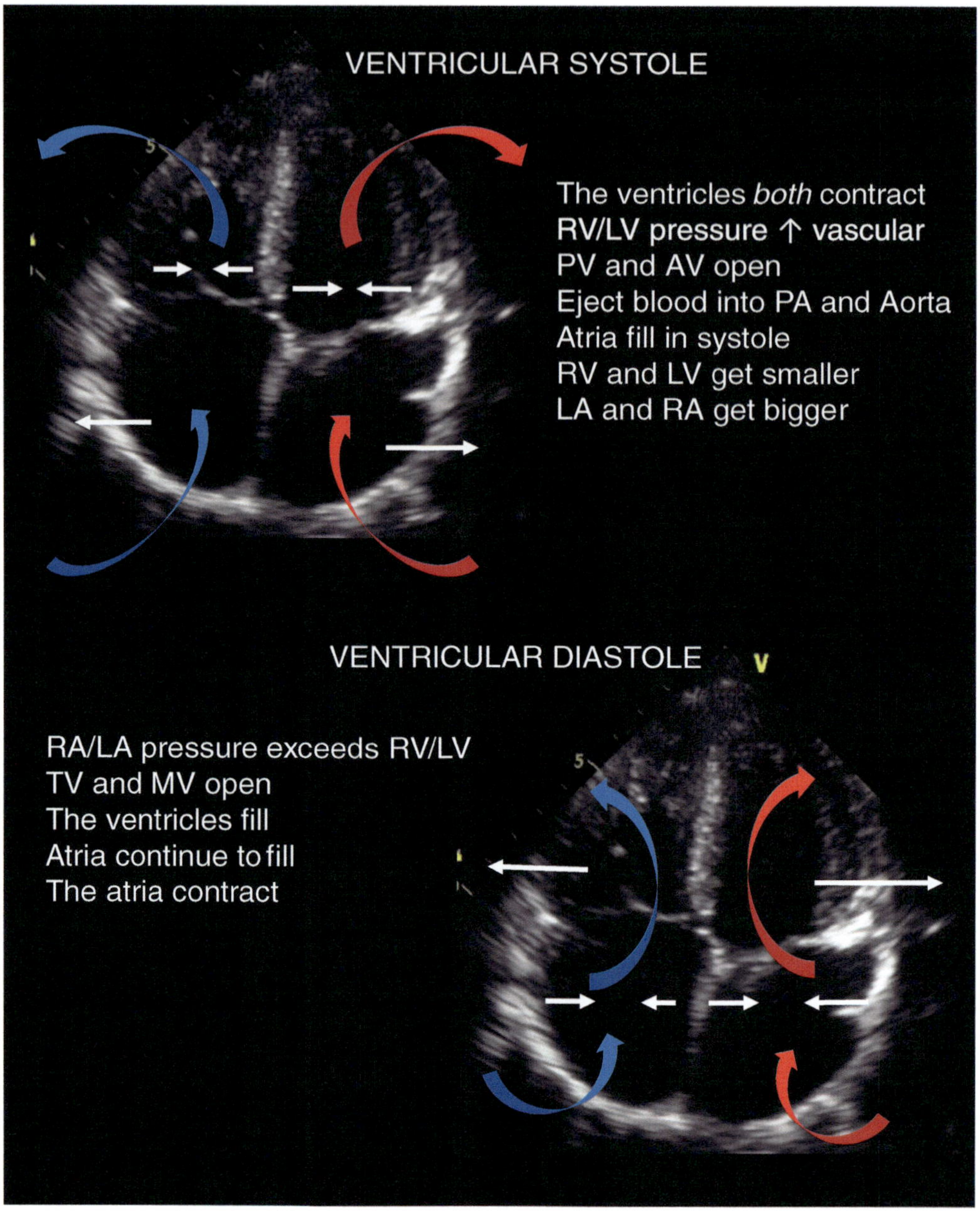

Fig. 4 The cardiac cycle: systole and diastole. Upper Panel: Ventricular systole. The ventricles both contract at the same time. The RV sends blood into the pulmonary artery. The LV ejects it into the aorta. The left and right atria fill throughout systole. White arrows: cardiac wall movement. Blue arrows: deoxygenated blood flow. Red arrows: oxygenated blood flow. Lower panel: Ventricular diastole. The ventricles rapidly descend, the tricuspid and mitral valves open, and blood rapidly fills the ventricles. The atria contract

  - Atrial pressure exceeds ventricular pressure.
  - The tricuspid and mitral valves open.
  - Both the RV and LV rapidly descend pulling blood in.
    - *Ultrasound assessments*
      - Pulsed wave Doppler through the MV
        - Early flow (E), atrial contraction flow (a)
      - Tissue Doppler
        - Early ventricular movement (E′)
  - Atrial filling continues in diastole until atrial contraction
- Electrocardiogram (ECG) (Fig. 5)
  - The actual contraction of the ventricles and atria occurs after the electrical signal.
  - The ECG is used to define systole and diastole. This helps with hepatic vein Doppler, measuring VTI and diagnosing tamponade. It can also be used to identify the E′, E, and a waves used diastolic function assessment.

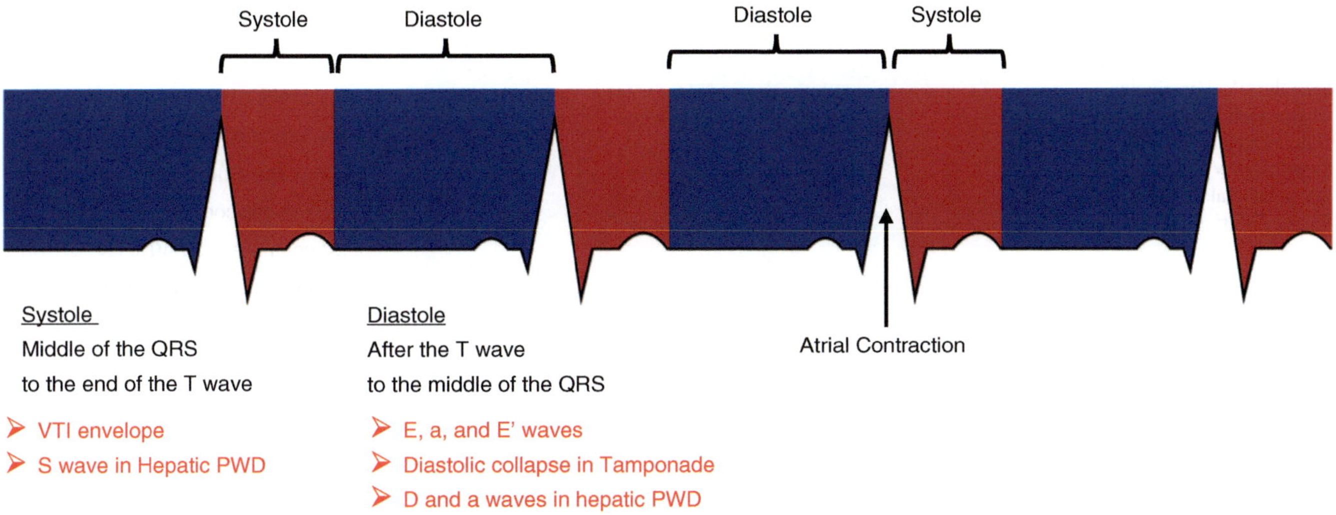

Fig. 5 EGC and the cardiac cycle. The electrical activity of the heart proceeds systole and diastole. Diastole occurs from the end of the T-wave to the middle of the QRS. Systole occurs from the middle of the QRS through the T-wave

- Systole
  - Middle of the QRS through the T-wave
- Diastole
  - End of the T-wave to the middle of the QRS
  - The atrial contraction occurs in the middle of the QRS.

Ventricular Interdependence and Cardiac Desynchrony

- The heart is a carefully folded structure in the limited space of the pericardium, located in the limited space of the thorax.
  - Ventricular interdependence results from several factors
    1. The LV and RV pump in parallel, while blood flows in series
       - RV filling determines LV end diastolic volume.
    2. The fixed space of the pericardium
       - There is limited space to expand.
       - Increased filling of one ventricle decreases filling of the other ventricle.
         - Enlarged RV from pressure-volume overload can inhibit LV filling in diastole.
         - Either from pulmonary embolus (PE) or elevated PA pressure from hypoxia
    3. The ventricles are interconnected by the septum and myofibrils (Fig. 6)
       - The LV is thick walled with the myofibrils spiraling into a helical alignment designed for forceful contraction against high systemic vascular resistance.
       - The RV is thinner walled and wrapped around the LV.
       - The LV primarily controls septal function.
    4. The ventricles contract at the same time (Fig. 7).
       - LV contraction contributes 20–40% of RV output.
         - RV free wall longitudinal movement accounts for the rest. This is assessed with TAPSE or tissue Doppler.
       - RV contraction contributes 5–10% of the LV output.
       - In cardiac desynchrony, the ventricles are not contracting together, so the synergistic effect is lost

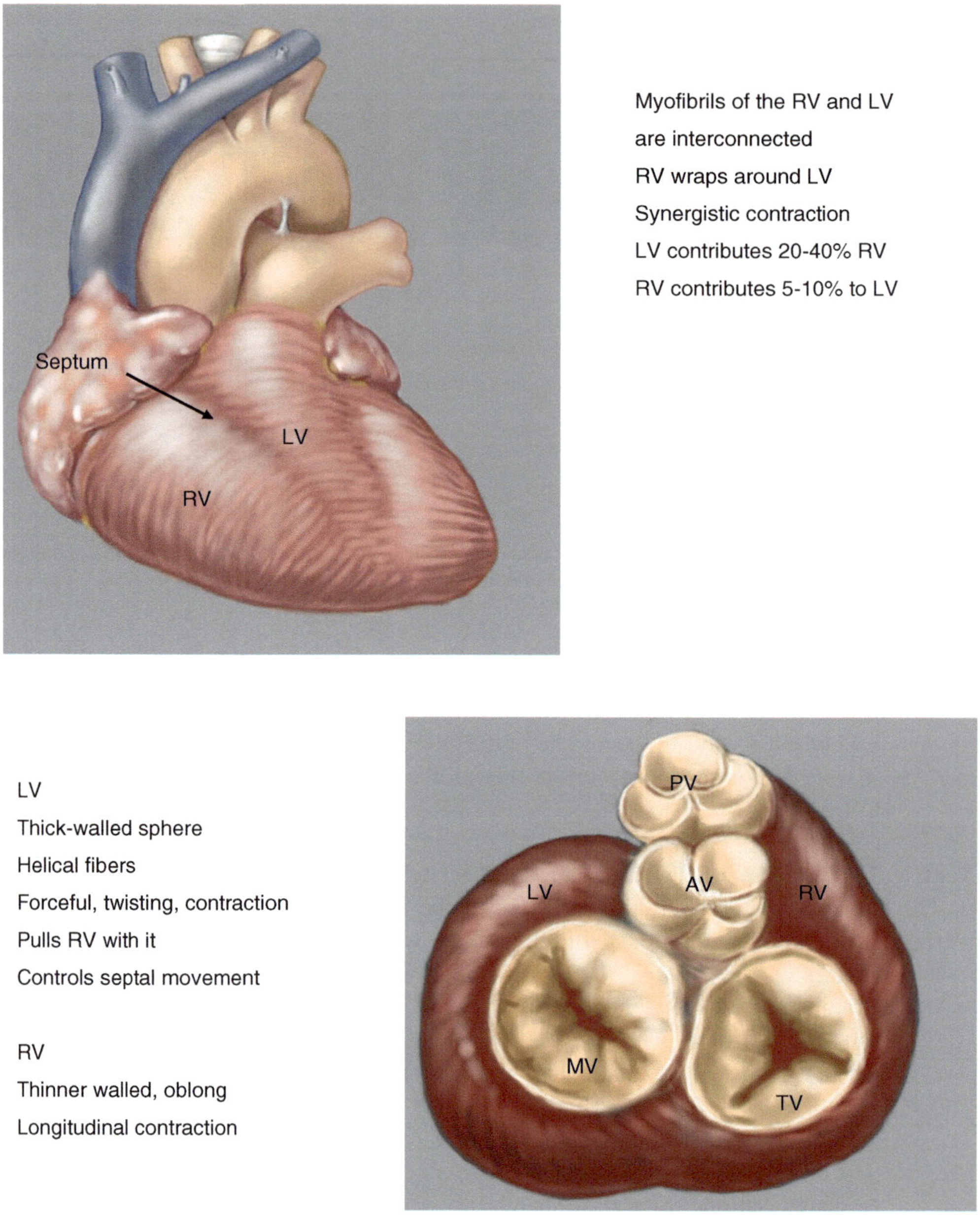

Fig. 6 LV and RV interdependence. The LV is larger and more muscular than the RV. Ventricular contraction is synergistic. RV right ventricle, LV left ventricle, PV pulmonic valve, AV aortic valve, MV mitral valve, TV tricuspid valve

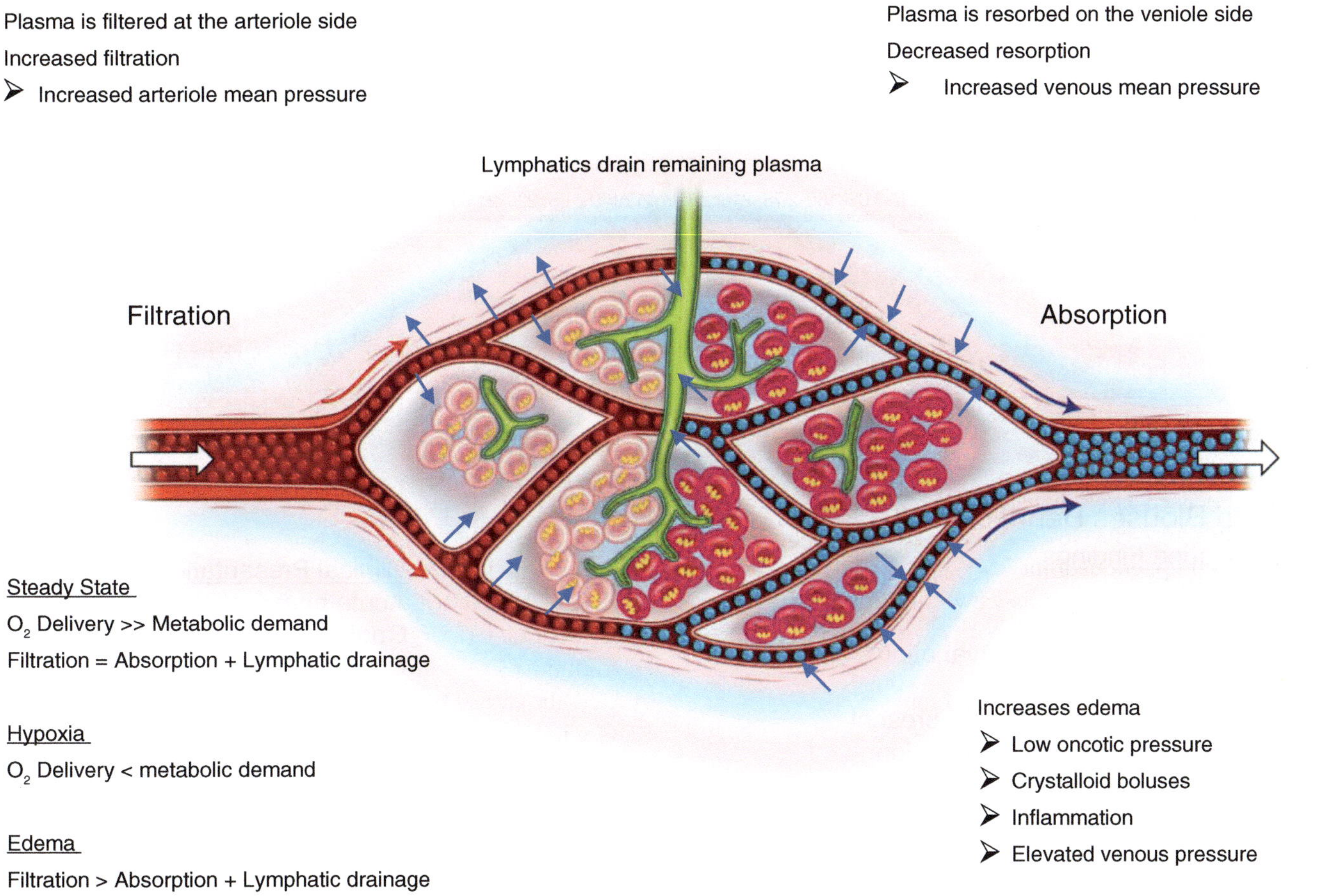

Fig. 7 Normal capillary perfusion. Blood passes from the arteriolar side of the capillary bed. As tissue is oxygenated, plasma filters out into the interstitium. It is resorbed at the venule side of the bed. Excess fluid is drained by lymphatics

3 The Capillary Bed

Plasma *filters* the vascular space into the interstitium on the arteriolar side and is *reasorbed* in the venule side of the capillary. Residual interstitial plasma is drained by the lymphatics. Venous congestion and inflammatory mediators can cause an increase in interstitial fluid which exceeds lymphatic drainage leading to organ edema and dysfunction. Conversely, shock states can increase end organ oxygen demand causing O_2 delivery (DO_2) dependent shock, worsened by hypovolemia.

- Normal flow (Fig. 8)
  - Blood and plasma flow easily across the capillary bed
  - At the capillary arteriole
    - Plasma is filtered out of the vascular space into the interstitium
  - At the venule side of the capillary
    - Plasma is resorbed back into the vascular space
  - Minimal tissue edema
    - Easily drained in the lymphatics
  - Adequate cellular oxygenation
- Hypoperfusion (Fig. 9 Upper Panel)
  - Task 1 failure contributes to cellular hypoxia
  - O_2 delivery dependent hypoperfusion
    - Increased oxygen demand
      - Inflammatory states
        - Sepsis
        - Trauma
      - Global or regional
    - Exacerbated by hypovolemia
    - Exacerbated by low perfusion pressure
      - Vasodilation, low systemic vascular resistance
    - Exacerbated by cardiac dysfunction
      - LV EF < 40%
      - Severe RV dysfunction with a small underfilled LV
  - Clinical effects
    - Ischemia
    - Organ injury and death
  - Clinical Presentation

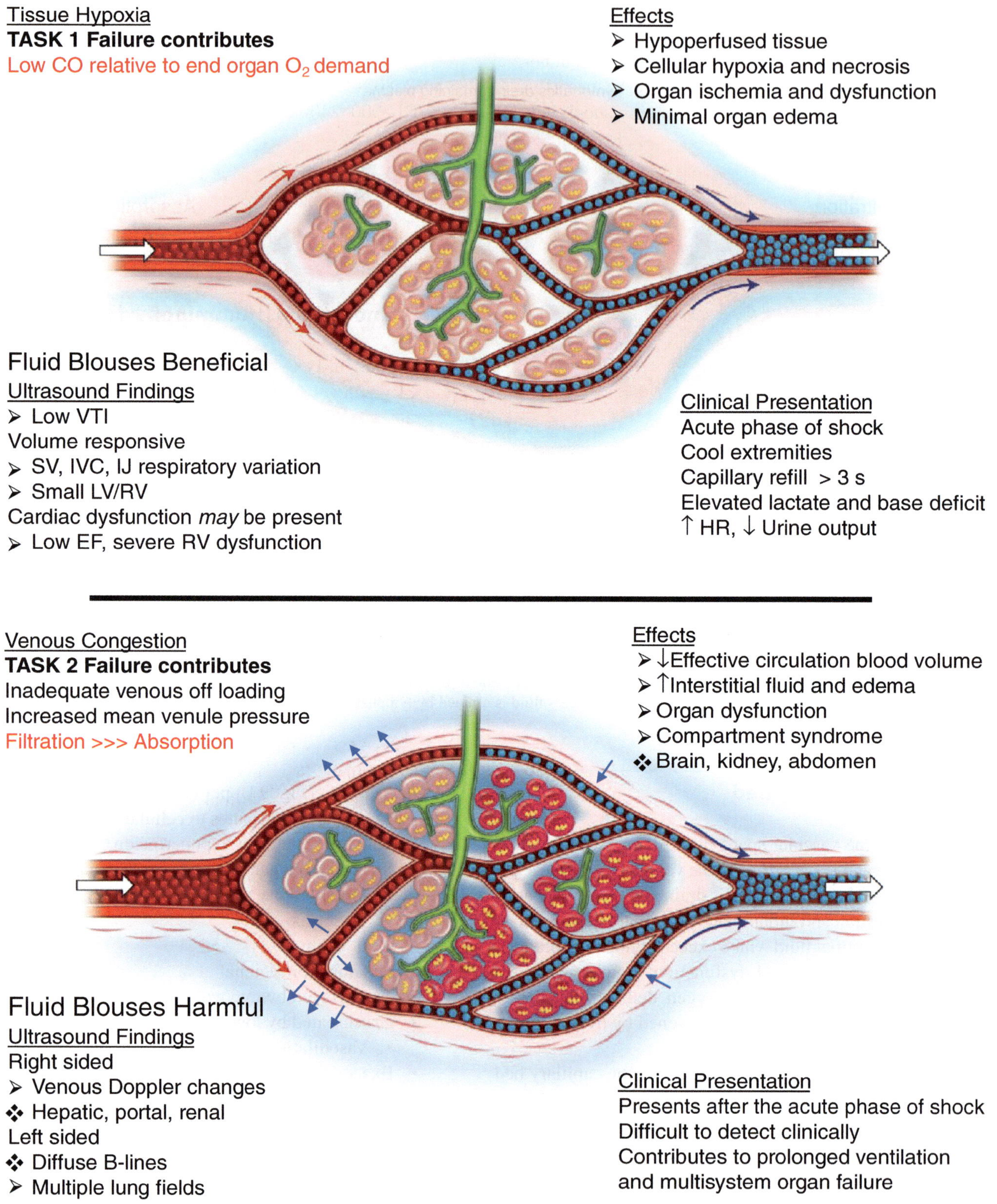

Fig. 8 Capillary hypoperfusion and venous congestion. Upper panel: Capillary hypoperfusion. Capillary perfusion occurs when oxygen delivery is less the end organ demand. It can be caused by a Type 1 failure of the circulation. Lower panel: Venous congestion. Venous congestion occurs when elevated mean venous pressure causes a decreased plasma absorption relative to filtration. It can be caused by elevated left or right atrial pressure

- Presentation and treatment are discussed in detail in Chap. 23.
- Hypoperfusion presents with findings of cellular hypoxia.
  - Increased heart rate, decreased urine output, delayed capillary refill, elevated lactate, and elevated base deficit
- *Ultrasound Findings*
  - Low VTI, small underfilled LV
  - Volume responsive
    - Stroke volume (SV), IVC, and internal jugular vein (IJ) respiratory variation
  - Cardiac dysfunction may be present.
    - *LV EF < 40%, severe RV dysfunction*
- Treatment
  - The most important treatment is identification and treatment of the cause of shock
  - Resuscitation is supportive
  - Fluid boluses are often indicated
  - Blood transfusion may be indicated
  - Systemic vasopressors if vasodilated
  - Inotropic support if moderate/severe cardiac dysfunction is present
- Venous congestion (Fig. 9, Lower Panel)
  - Failure of Task 2 contributes to venous congestion
  - High atrial pressure leads to elevated venous pressure
    - Increases mean capillary pressure on the venous side
    - Decreases *resorption* of plasma
      - Exceeds lymphatic drainage
      - Exacerbated with low oncotic pressures
        - Crystalloid fluid boluses
        - Low albumin
        - Inflammation
    - Cardiac dysfunction may be present, but often occurs with normal function
    - Increases tissue edema
    - Increases compartment pressure
      - Abdomen, kidney, central nervous system
    - Decreases effective circulating blood volume
    - Causes organ dysfunction
  - Clinical Presentation
    - The clinical presentation of venous congestion is more occult than hypoperfusion
    - Will present differently if the congestion is from elevated right atrial pressure or elevated left atrial pressure
    - Left-sided venous congestion
    - Right-sided venous congestion
  - *Ultrasound Findings*
    - Right-sided venous congestion
      - Changes in venous blood flow returning to the RA assessed with pulsed wave Doppler
        - *Hepatic*
          - Systolic flow < diastolic flow
          - Retrograde systolic flow
        - *Portal*
          - *Portal pulsatility > 30%*
        - *Renal*
          - *Biphasic or monophasic pulsatile flow*
    - Left-sided venous congestion
      - *Diffuse B-lines in multiple lung fields*
  - Treatment
    - Minimizing fluid boluses
    - Diuresis
    - Optimize cardiac function
- Non-DO_2-dependent cellular hypoxia
  - Refractory shock
  - Inflammatory mediators cause mitochondrial dysfunction unable to take up oxygen even with adequate perfusion
    - Elevated lactate
    - Elevated base deficit
    - Does not improve despite adequate O_2 delivery
  - Increasing oxygen delivery will not improve end organ hypoxia
  - Supportive management
    - Identify and treat the cause of shock
    - Support SV and CO while limiting venous congestion
    - Fluid boluses are not indicated and may be harmful

Effect of Mechanical Ventilation

Mechanical ventilation introduces a rapid increase in thoracic pressure which has significant cardiovascular effects. Blood flows along a gradient from higher pressure to lower pressure. Changes in thoracic pressure effect the pressure gradients into and out of the chest, while changes in *lung volume* can increase PA pressure and cause RV dysfunction.

- *Decreases work of breathing*
  - Relieves respiratory muscles decreasing whole body oxygen consumption
  - More oxygen available for other organ perfusion
  - Weaning/decreasing ventilatory support increases myocardial work and can worsen cardiac function
- *Increases intrathoracic pressure (ITP)* (Table 1)

Table 1 Hemodynamic changes with increased intrathoracic pressure

	RAP	RA Filling	RV function	PA pressure	LV Afterload	LV EF	Net effect SV/CO
↑ ITP	↑	↓↓	–	–	↓	↑	↓
↓ ITP	↓	↑	–	–	↑	↓	↑

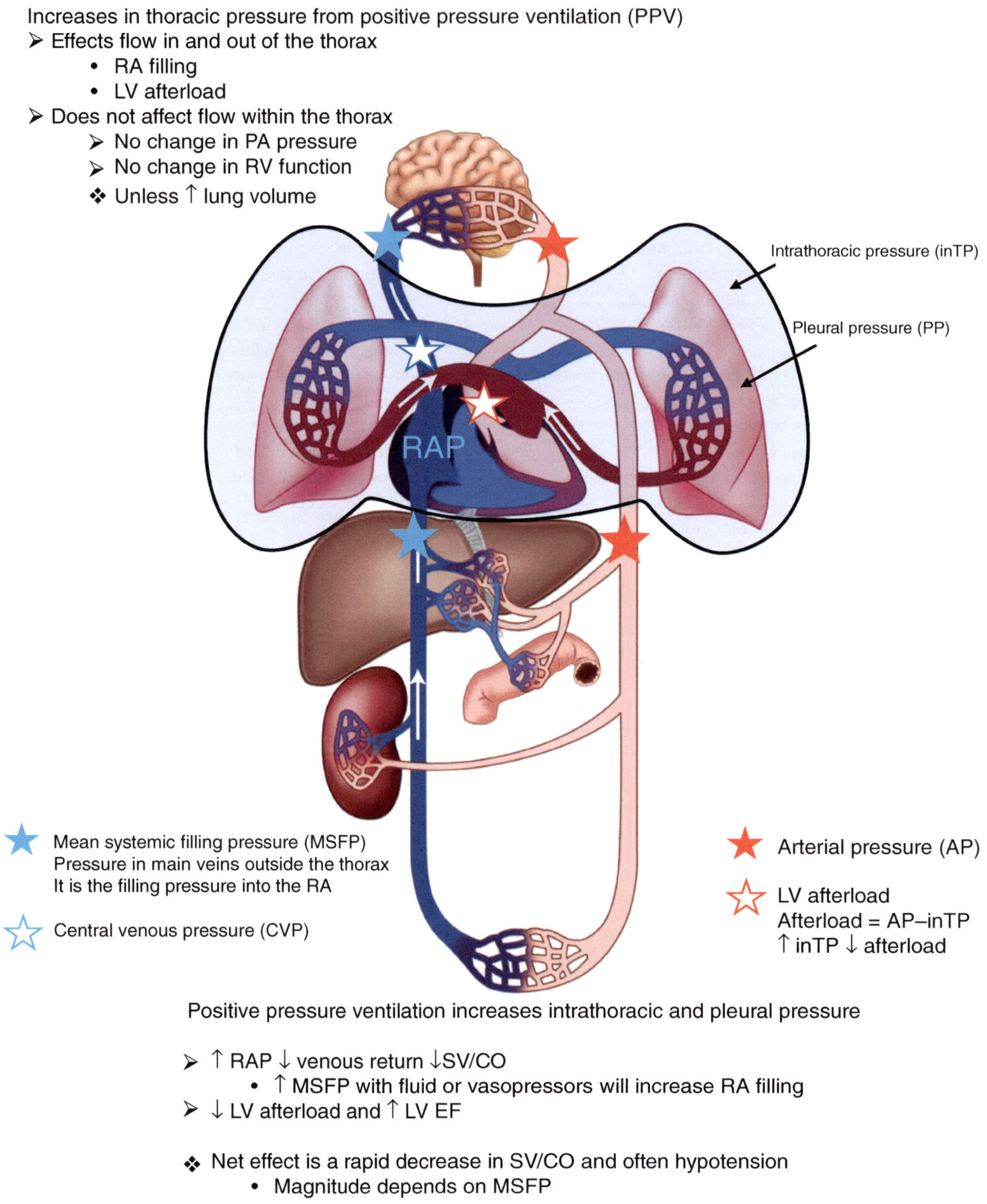

Fig. 9 Hemodynamic effects of mechanical ventilation. Positive pressure ventilation increases intrathoracic pressure, pleural pressure, and right atrial pressure. This intern effects blood flow into the RA and out of the LV

Table 2 Changes in the pulmonary artery pressure gradient (PG) with mechanical ventilation

	Hypoxia	Collapse	Recruitment	↑ Lung Volume
PA PG	↑	↑	↓	↑

1. Intrathoracic pressure changes effect blood flow *into* and *out of* the thorax
   - Effects RA filling and LV ejection
2. No effect on blood flow within the heart or thoracic cavity *unless* lung volume is increased
   - No effect on RV function
     - Both the RV and the pulmonary artery are exposed to the increased pressure, so there is no change in the pressure gradient
3. Increase in RAP causes a decrease in venous return
   - Magnitude of decrease is dependent on mean systemic filling pressure (MSFP) in the central veins outside the thorax
   - Normally, the venous system is low pressure, so the MSFP is low
     - Driving pressure for flow into the RA is only 4–8 mmHg.
     - Small changes in ITP from positive end expiratory pressure (PEEP) can cause profound decreases in venous filling.
   - Volume administration will elevate MSFP increasing filling pressure and counteracting the decrease in SV and cardiac output (CO).
   - But it will also cause venous congestion.
   - Pre-existing RV dysfunction can induce greater changes in RAP.
4. Decrease LV afterload and increase LV EF.
   - LV afterload is systemic vascular pressure minus ITP.
   - Increases in ITP will decrease LV afterload improving EF.
   - Weaning mechanical ventilation can increase afterload decreasing LV EF.
5. Mode of ventilation does not influence hemodynamic effects of ITP.
   - All modes increase the ITP.
   - While increased pressure is important, how that pressure is achieved (i.e., wave flow patterns) does not affect venous return.

- *Effect on Pulmonary Artery Systolic Pressure* (Table 2)
  - The RV is designed for low pressure flow. Acute elevations in the pressure gradient between the RV and the PA from hypoxia or alveolar overdistension can cause new RV dysfunction and profoundly worsen existing dysfunction.

Table 3 Changes in intrathoracic pressure with negative and positive pressure ventilation

	Inspiration	Expiration
NPV (natural airway)	↓ ITP	↑ITP
PPV (mechanical ventilation)	↑ITP	↓ITP
Abdominal Pressure	↑venous pressure ↑abdominal blood return	↓venous pressure ↓abdominal blood return

    1. The PA pressure relative to the RV pressure or the pressure gradient is the important metric.
       - Both the PA pressure and the RV pressure are increased with increases in ITP, but the gradient will remain the same.
       - While ITP itself will not change the gradient, its effect on hypoxia, lung recruitment, and alveolar over distention can cause significant changes.
  - The net effect of mechanical ventilation on PA pressure is variable.
    1. Improved oxygenation will *decrease* PA pressure by decreasing hypoxia induced vasoconstriction.
    2. Recruitment maneuvers which open collapsed lung will *decrease* PA pressure by stenting open arteries and improving vascular compliance.
    3. Increased lung volumes and alveolar over distention will *increase* PA pressure by decreasing the space available for blood flow.
    4. Ventilator strategies which open collapsed lung while reducing over distention will decrease the PA pressure gradient and facilitate RV off-loading even if high intrathoracic pressure is used.
       - Increasing PEEP and optimizing mean airway pressure can decrease the PA pressure gradient.
- Effect of breathing (Table 3)
  - Natural breathing is negative pressure ventilation (NPV), whereas positive pressure ventilation (PPV) is used by ventilators.
  - The mean stroke volume may not change, but the beat to beat variation can be impressive.
  - Inspiration
    1. NPV decreases ITP and RAP, increasing filling.
    2. PPV increases ITP and RAP, decreasing filling.
  - Expiration
    1. NPV increases ITP and RAP, decreasing filling.
    2. PPV decreases ITP and RAP, increasing filling.
  - Abdominal mean systemic venous pressure
    1. In inspiration, the diaphragm drops in both NPV and PPV increasing abdominal venous pressure which increases blood return.

- Respiratory variation as a marker of volume responsiveness
  1. Volume responsiveness
     - Likelihood stroke volume will increase with a fluid bolus.
     - Respiratory changes in SV, IVC, and the IJ predict volume responsiveness.
- Hypotension with induction and intubation
  - Induction agents cause vasodilation and decrease systemic vascular resistance (SVR).
  - As described above, increased ITP will decrease right ventricular filling and decrease CO.
  - Combination of decrease in CO and SVR can cause an acute decrease in MAP.
  - Unmask pre-existing conditions like aortic stenosis.
- Decreasing ventilatory support, weaning, and extubation
  - Decreasing ventilatory support will increase cardiac work and LV afterload which can precipitate LV failure and pulmonary edema.

Suggested Reading

Mahmood SS, Pinsky MR. Heart-lung interactions during mechanical ventilation: the basics. Ann Transl Med. 2018;6(18):349. https://doi.org/10.21037/atm.2018.04.29.

Spiegel R, Teeter W, Sullivan S, Tupchong K, Mohammed N, Sutherland M, Leibner E, Rola P, Galvagno SM Jr, Murthi SB. The use of venous Doppler to predict adverse kidney events in a general ICU cohort. Crit Care. 2020;24(1):615. https://doi.org/10.1186/s13054-020-03330-6. PMID: 33076961; PMCID: PMC7574322.

Vallabhajosyula S, Pruthi S, Shah S, Wiley BM, Mankad SV, Jentzer JC. Basic and advanced echocardiographic evaluation of myocardial dysfunction in sepsis and septic shock. Anaesth Intensive Care. 2018;46(1):13–24. https://doi.org/10.1177/0310057X1804600104.

Walley KR. Sepsis-induced myocardial dysfunction. Curr Opin Crit Care. 2018;24(4):292–9. https://doi.org/10.1097/MCC.0000000000000507.

Echo-Based Shock Physiology

Sarah B. Murthi

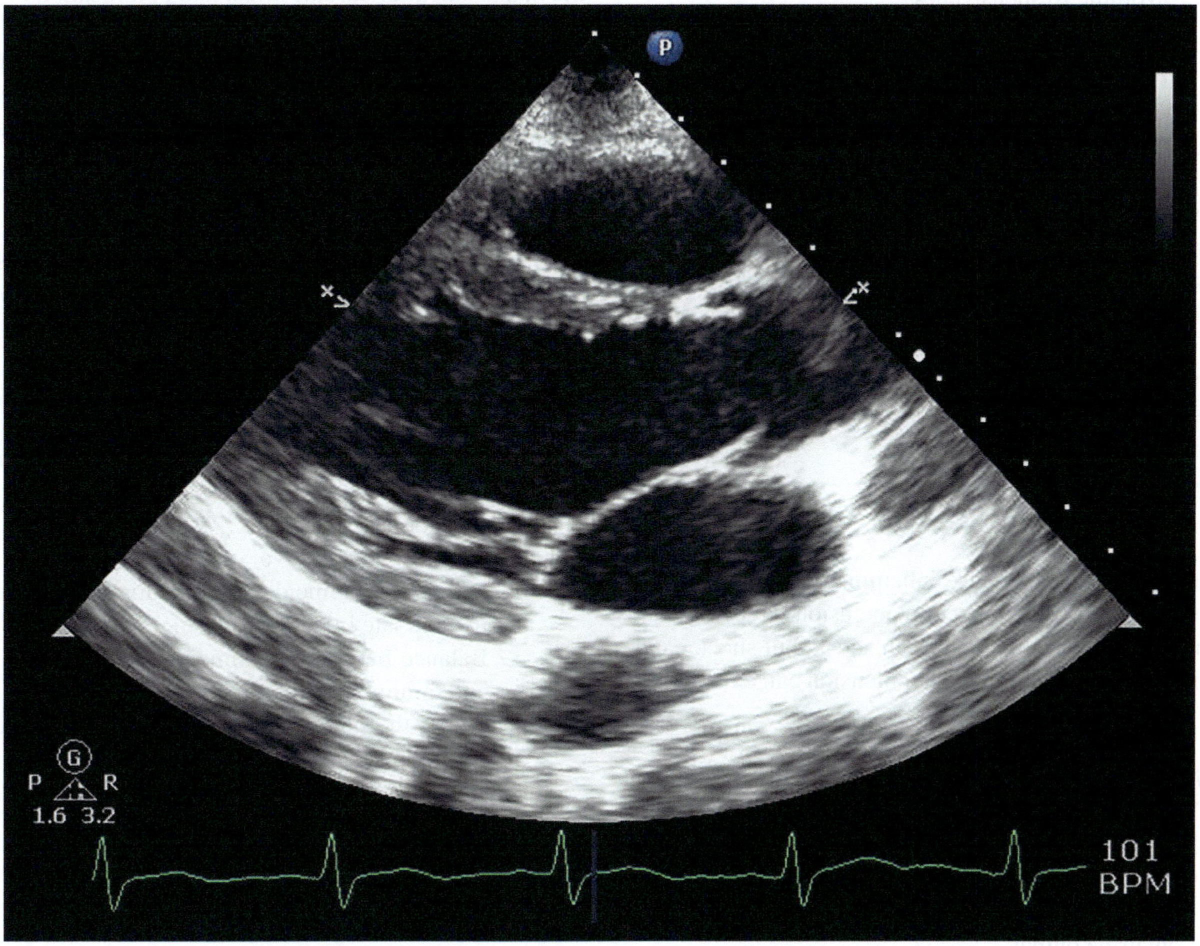

S. B. Murthi (✉)
Department of Surgery, Program in Trauma and Critical Care, R Adams Cowley Shock Trauma Center, University of Maryland School of Medicine, University of Maryland Medical Center, Baltimore, MD, USA
e-mail: smurthi@som.umaryland.edu

A. Salerno et al. (eds.), *Atlas of Critical Care Echocardiography*, https://doi.org/10.1007/978-3-030-74687-2_23

Abbreviations

CO	Cardiac Output
DO_2	Oxygen Dependent
Epi	Epinephrine
FAST	Focused Abdominal Sonogram for Trauma
ICU	Intensive Care Unit
MAP	Mean Arterial Blood Pressure
NE	Norepinephrine
OR	Operating Room
RUSH	Rapid UltraSound for Hypotension
SV	Stroke Volume
SVR	Systemic Vascular Resistance
Vaso	Vasopressin
VR	Volume Responsiveness

1 Introduction

Shock is a life-threatening condition from an inciting cause (i.e., infection, trauma) which results in organ hypoxia progressing to dysfunction and death if untreated. Ideal therapy is identification and treatment of the cause while optimizing perfusion to protect end organs. Optimizing perfusion, also called resuscitation, involves judicious use of fluids, inotropes, and vasopressors to mitigate venous congestion while encouraging oxygen delivery to the capillary beds of end organs.

2 Presentation of Shock

As shock progresses a dense inflammatory process is activated causing vasodilation and hypotension. Hypotension is commonly the presenting feature in shock, but shock can be present without it. Conversely hypotension can exist without organ hypoperfusion.

- **Clinical evidence of shock:** findings of cellular hypoxia
  - Elevated lactate
  - Elevated base deficit
  - Cold, clammy skin
  - Capillary refill <3 seconds
  - Low urine output
  - Tachycardia
  - Mental status changes
- **Hypotension**
  - Hypotension can be a presenting symptom, but it is not required for diagnosis:
    - Decreased capillary perfusion pressure further worsens cellular hypoxia.
  - Primarily a vasodilatory process:
    - Inflammatory mediators decrease systemic vascular resistance (SVR).
  - Low stroke volume (SV) and cardiac output (CO) can contribute to low mean arterial blood pressure (MAP):
    - Cardiac dysfunction
    - Hypovolemia, defined as a low SV
- **Not all shock has hypotension and not all hypotension causes shock.**

3 Optimizing Perfusion vs. Resuscitation

The terms resuscitation and resuscitate are used to describe the management of cardiac arrest and optimization of perfusion in shock. But these are two very different populations and treatment protocols. We recommend using the phrase "optimize perfusion" to describe the vital supportive management of shock. For clarity "resuscitation" can be reserved for cardiopulmonary resuscitation, and the specific treatments around cardiac arrest. Also thinking of optimizing perfusion as resuscitation results in considering it curative rather than supportive. This mind-set can cause inadequate source control and excessive fluid administration risking venous congestion and contributing to late organ dysfunction.

- Treatment of shock
  - Rapidly diagnose and treat the cause:
    - The single most important intervention in treatment of shock
  - Support organ perfusion:
    - Vital but not curative
    - Decreases the incidence of multisystem organ failure and late infection
    - Balance between maximizing cardiac output (CO) and minimizing venous congestion
    - Allow the end organs to recover without causing further damage
  - The goal is optimizing flow across capillary beds:
    - Cannot force cellular uptake of oxygen
    - Support flow *across* the capillary bed while treating the cause
      1. Balancing oxygen delivery (DO_2) and
      2. Venous return
    - Primary therapies
      1. Fluid
         - Crystalloid, colloid boluses
         - Transfusion with blood products
           - In shock related to acute blood loss
      2. Inotropic agents
         - Dobutamine and epinephrine (epi)
         - Milrinone

- In cardiogenic shock with normal or elevated mean arterial blood pressure (MAP)
  3. Systemic vasopressors
     - Norepinephrine (NE) and vasopressin (Vaso)
     - Phenylephrine, often referred to by its brand name Neo-Synephrine (NEO)
       - Pure vasoconstrictor, limited uses including hypotension with aortic stenosis
  - Often more than one intervention is indicated, for example, fluid and a vasopressor, because the stroke volume is low AND the patient is also vasodilated.
  - Other and future therapies, immunotherapies, and anti-inflammatory agents to balance the dense inflammatory cascades in shock are beyond the scope of this book:
    1. Corticosteroids, thiamine, and vitamin C among others
    2. Source of ongoing research
- The best support strategy is dictated by the phase of shock.

4 Phases of Shock (Fig. 1)

- **Prehospital**
  - Time between onset and presentation.
  - Length of time determines the depth of shock.
  - Some emergency medical services (EMS) can initiate treatment.
    - *Ultrasound: FAST and RUSH can help triage.*
- **Acute: Diagnosis and treatment of the cause**
  - Time: 0–6 hrs. Location: Emergency department/operating room.
  - Time frame longer in surgical patients.
  - Diagnosis of cause is the primary focus:
    - *Ultrasound: FAST and RUSH*
  - More likely to be in O_2 delivery (DO_2)-dependent shock:
    - More likely to be volume responsive (VR), or respond to a fluid bolus with an increase in stroke volume (SV)
  - Less like to have venous congestion and fluid intolerance.

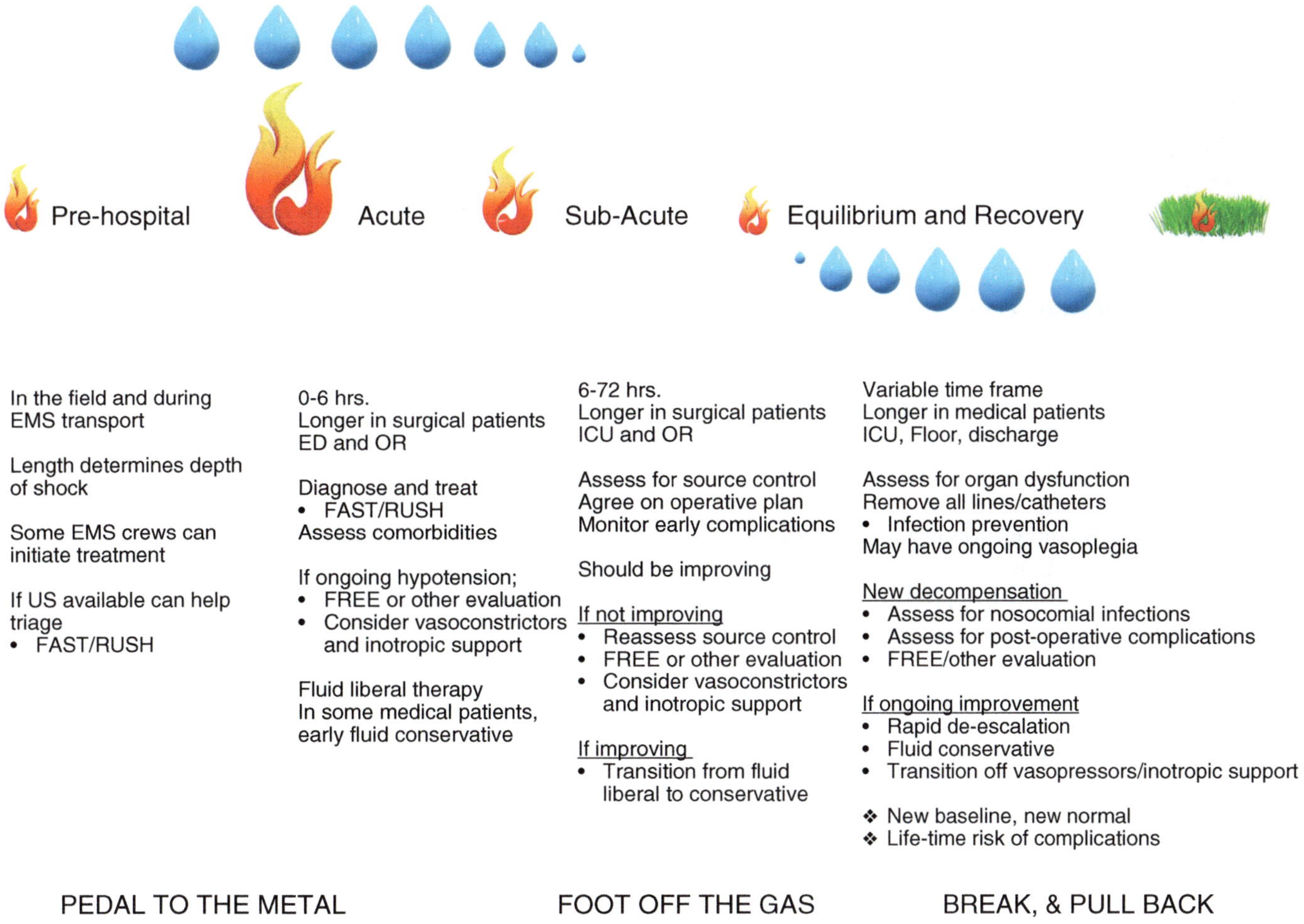

Fig. 1 Phases of shock. Depicted are the four phases of shock from before the hospital through to long-term recovery

  - If long prehospital course:
    - More likely hypovolemic leading to low SV
  - If suspected comorbidities or ongoing unexplained hypotension:
    - *Ultrasound: FREE or other cardiac evaluation*
      - Assess need for vasoconstrictors and/or inotropic agents.
  - **Perfusion strategy: Full go, pedal to the metal**
    - Diagnose and treat source.
    - Push SV and CO.
    - Fluid-liberal strategy.
    - In some medical patients, transition early to fluid conservative.
- **Subacute: Optimize while allowing organ recovery**
  - Time: 6–72 hrs. Location: Intensive care unit (ICU)
  - Timeframe variable; longer in surgical, shorter in medical patients:
    - Can be several days if multiple operations are required for source control
  - The primary cause has been identified and treatment has started:
    - Source may not be completely addressed.
      - Surgical patients
        - Possibility of planned reoperations for source control
        - Risk of bleeding and other early postoperative complications
  - May still have elements of DO_2-dependent shock.
  - Vasoplegia and cardiac dysfunction may be contributing:
    - *Ultrasound: FREE or other cardiac evaluation*
      - Assess need for vasoconstrictors and/or inotropic agents.
  - **Perfusion strategy: Foot off the gas**
    - Ensure source completely treated.
    - Maintain SV and CO.
    - Fine-tune support to limit venous congestion.
    - Dial back on fluid administration.
  - As soon as evidence of end-organ hypoperfusion trends down:
    - Tailor fluid administration to mitigate edema and venous congestion.
    - Begin transitioning to a fluid-conservative strategy.
- **Equilibration and recovery: De-escalation return to new normal**
  - Time: 24 hrs–10 days Location: ICU to discharge; lifetime risks
  - Timeframe variable, can be in the ICU for weeks to months
  - Course related to pre-existing conditions and depth of shock
  - Organ dysfunction manifests
  - May require vasopressors for ongoing vasoplegia
  - High risk of nosocomial infection, organ dysfunction, and postoperative complications (in surgical patients)
  - Fluid-conservative strategy
  - **Perfusion strategy: Gently break, start pulling back**
    - Monitor for new sources
      - Nosocomial infections
    - Assess for organ injury:
      - That is, acute renal injury
    - Risk of postoperative complications
    - Fluid-conservative strategy

5 Medical vs. Surgical Shock

Shock can be categorized by cause: septic, hemorrhagic, or traumatic. But it may also be useful to think of it as medical or surgical (Fig. 2). Surgical shock places the patient at high risk of needing an intervention which complicates acute and subacute perfusion management (Table 1).

- **Surgical shock: High risk of needing an invasive procedure to treat the cause of shock**
  - Healthier patients, more complex initial course.
  - Acute and subacute phases can last for days to weeks.
  - Perfusion management needs to be adjusted around each operation.
  - Risk of hemorrhage, more likely to require transfusions.
  - Risk of reoperation exists throughout the course:
    - Consider whenever unexplained deterioration.
- **Medical shock: Low risk of needing an intervention**
  - Sicker patients, more straightforward initial management.
  - Pre-existing lung disease complicated by pneumonia is very common.
    - Less tolerant of elevations in left atrial pressure
      1. Pulmonary edema resulting in worsening respiratory status can be fatal.
    - May benefit from fluid conservative strategy even in the acute phase
  - Worsening of pre-existing diseases resulting in prolonged stays.
- **Septic shock**
  - Both surgical and medical sources of infection.
  - Research; considered as a single group:
    - Many more medical patients in large, randomized trials
    - Less known about ideal perfusion management in surgical patients
  - Surgical patients require an operation, often multiple operations for source control:
    - More complex fluid management
- **Surgical septic and traumatic shock are both forms of surgical shock**

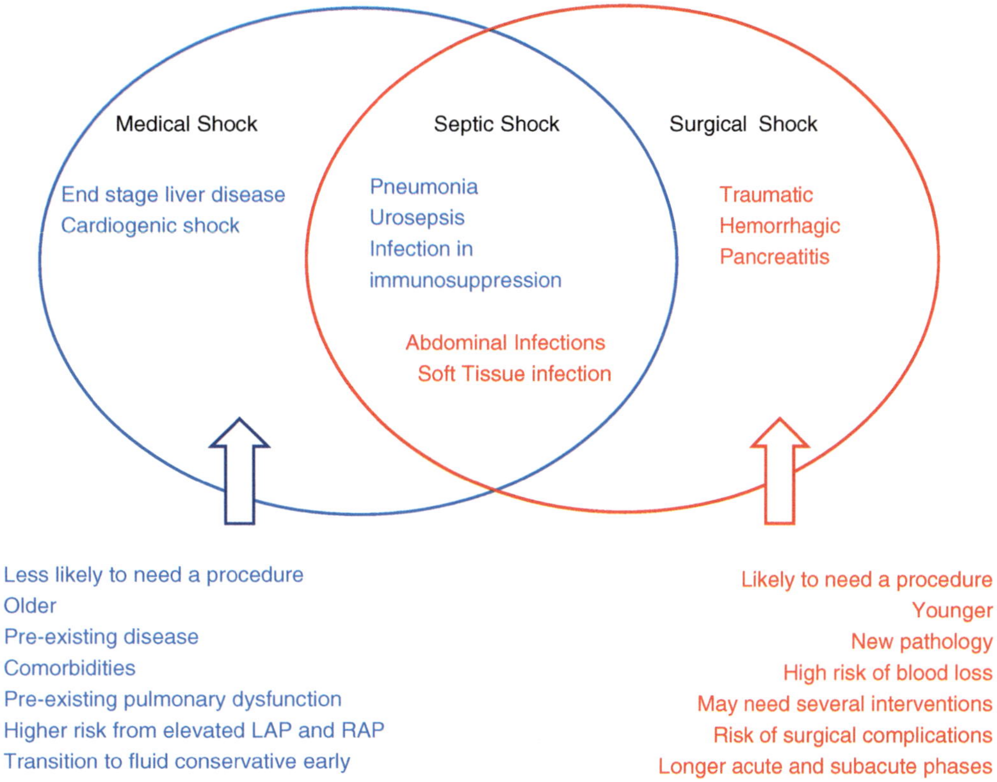

Fig. 2 Medical and surgical shock. *Blue circle and text*, Medical shock. *Red circle and text*, Surgical shock

Table 1 Medical versus surgical shock

	Examples	Patient population	Course
Medical shock	Pneumonia Urosepsis End-stage liver disease Cardiogenic	Older Comorbidities Often pre-existing lung dysfunction	Worsening of a pre-existing condition Prolonged stay
Surgical shock	Abdominal infection Soft tissue infection Trauma Hemorrhage Pancreatitis	Younger Less comorbidities	Longer in the acute and subacute phases May need multiple operations Risk of surgical complications

- Different initial operative and medical management
- Similar perfusion optimization in all phases:
  - High risk of operative intervention to address the source of shock.
  - Taylor management around frequent operations.
  - Monitor for adequate source control.
  - Monitor for surgical complications.
  - Good care requires communication between the ICU, surgical, and operating room teams.
  - Good care also requires close working relationships with interventional radiology and other consulting procedure-based specialties.

6 Therapies to Optimize Perfusion in Shock

There are four essential elements in perfusion optimization:

1. Source control
2. Volume administration
   - DO_2 shock + VR.
   - *Ultrasound: measure VR and stroke volume. Assess for venous congestion.*
3. Systemic vasoconstrictors (Fig. 3)
   - Low systemic vascular resistance (SVR)
   - *Ultrasound: estimate SVR*
4. Inotropic agents (Fig. 3)
   - DO_2 shock + cardiac dysfunction.
   - *Ultrasound: detect and differentiate types of dysfunction.*

Current guidelines for sepsis and other shock states recommend a stepwise approach. For example, give 2 liters of fluid and then start a vasoconstrictor; maximize vasoconstrictors, and then start an inotropic agent. While this is reasonable with only a catheter to help manage the patient, hemodynamic echo allows us to be smarter.

- Volume responsive *and* vasodilated:
  - Give fluids *and* start a vasopressor.

	Action		Site	HR	Contractility	SVR	Other Efects
Norepinephrine Vasoconstrictor Mild inotrope	α1 β1 β2	++++ ++ +	Heart Vasculature	↑	↑	↑↑↑	Digital necrosis ↑ Coronary flow Prolonged; myonecrosis
Epinephrine Inotrope Vasoconstrictor	α1 β1 β2	++++ ++++ +	Heart Vasculature	↑↑↑	↑↑↑ Predominant effect at low doses < 4.0 mcg/min or < 0.06 mcg/kg/min	↑ Predominant effect at higher doses	↑↑ Arrythmias ↑ Coronary flow Prolonged; myonecrosis ↑ lactate (liver production) ↑ Hyperglycemia ↓ Splanchnic perfusion
Dobutamine Inotrope	α1 β1 β2	+ ++++ ++	Heart Vasculature	↑↑↑	↑↑↑	↓	↑↑ Arrythmias ↓ Pulmonary vascular resistance ↑ Myocardial O_2 consumption
Phenylephrine Vasoconstrictor	α1 β1 β2	++++ No No	Vasculature	↓	↓	↑↑↑	↑↑ Pulmonary vascular resistance
Milrinone Inotrope	Inhibits Phosphodiesterase ↑ cAMP ↑ cellular calcium		Myocyte Vasculature	None	↑↑↑	↓↓↓	↓ RAP ↓ Pulmonary vascular resistance Coronary vasodilator Bronchial dilation
Vasopressin Vasoconstrictor	V_1 V_2		Vasculature	None	No effect	↑↑↑	↓ Pulmonary vascular resistance ↓ Renal vasoconstriction ↑ Renal fluid resorption
Angiotensin II Vasoconstrictor	Ang II RAS pathway	Ang II	Vasculature Adrenal glands	None	No effect	↑↑↑	Aldosterone release ↑ Renal fluid resorption Venoconstriction Increases NE sensitivity

Fig. 3 Systemic vasopressors and inotropic agents in shock

- Cardiac dysfunction *and* vasodilated:
  - Start a vasoconstrictor *and* inotropic support.

Source Control The most important intervention for perfusion is source control.

- Essential element in perfusion optimization
- If the patient is not improving as expected in the subacute phase:
  - Re-evaluate; is the source completely addressed?
  - Do not assume a failure of resuscitation.
- New decompensation in the recovery phase
  - New infection? Postoperative complication?

Fluid Bolus Fluid boluses can increase SV and CO but will result in tissue edema. Boluses are primarily used to increase perfusion in DO_2 organ hypoxia in the acute and subacute phases.

- Positive effects
  - Unique property: Increases SV and mean arterial blood pressure (MAP), while increasing myocardial perfusion (via an increase SV and central venous pressure).
  - Rapid administration does not require central line.
  - Excellent in the acute phase to push SV and CO while identifying and treating the cause of shock.
- Negative effects
  - Increase in MAP is transient:
    - Buys time, does not treat hypotension from vasodilation
    - Leads to repeated boluses causing edema
  - Tissue edema:
    - Decreases oncotic pressure while increasing mean capillary pressure
    - Increases atrial pressure may lead to venous congestion:
      - Increases capillary filtration while decreasing resorption
        - Can overwhelm lymphatic drainage
      - Increased left atrial pressure (LAP)
        - Pulmonary edema and respiratory dysfunction
        - *Ultrasound findings; diffuse B-lines*
      - Increased right atrial pressure (RAP)
        - Hepatomegaly, nephrosarca, and bowel edema
        - *Ultrasound findings: hepatic, portal, and renal venous Doppler waveform changes*

- Primary indication for a fluid bolus
  - Evidence of organ hypoperfusion
    - Tachycardia, decreased urine output, and delayed capillary refill
    - Elevated lactate and/or base deficit
  - *Not* hypotension after the acute phases
    - Fluid will only transiently increase MAP.
    - Need to examine patient and assess for systemic vasodilation.
    - Vasoplegia is better treated with a vasoconstrictor.

Systemic Vasoconstrictors Vasodilation from inflammatory mediators causing hypotension is common in all shock. Systemic vasoconstrictors can increase the MAP improving perfusion to capillary beds.

- Positive effects
  - Increase in vascular tone, increase in MAP, and improved perfusion
- Negative effects
  - Vasoconstriction causing ischemia and hypoperfusion
- Primary indication
  - Hypotension with low systemic vascular resistance
- Common agents
  - *Norepinephrine (NE)*
    - Most common initial agent in vasodilatory shock
    - Predominant α1 effect; some β1
      - Increase in MAP via increase in SVR
      - Some increase in contractility and HR
    - Less tachyarrhythmias, and less coronary hypoperfusion compared to epinephrine
    - 0.01–3.3 mcg/kg/min
  - *Vasopressin (Vaso)*
    - Often added at higher doses of NE
    - Decreases NE requirement
    - Less cerebral, coronary, pulmonary, and renal vasoconstriction
      - Stimulates endothelial nitric oxide release
    - Increases fluid resorption in the kidney
    - Vasopressor: 0.03–0.1 units/minute
    - Vasoplegia in septic shock 0.04 units/minute
      - No survival benefit at higher doses
  - *Angiotensin II*
    - Works in the renin-angiotensin-aldosterone (RAS) pathway
      - Direct vasoconstriction
      - Synergy with catecholamines (NE and Epi)
      - Release of antidiuretic hormone and aldosterone
      - Volume expansion (kidney sodium and water resorption)
    - Effective as a salvage agent in patients with refractory vasodilatory shock
    - 5–40 ng/kg/min

Inotropic Agents

- *Epinephrine (Epi)*
  - Effects α1 and β1 equally but:
  - β1 predominant at lower doses
    - < 4.0 mcg/min, or < 0.06 mcg/kg/min if weight-based dosing
    - Increase in HR, SV, and CO
  - α1 effects predominant at higher doses
  - Use Epi at inotropic doses for cardiac dysfunction and titrate NE to counteract vasodilation:
    - NE has fewer negative effects and is a safer vasoconstrictor.
  - Only inotrope which is also a vasoconstrictor
    - Ideal in patients with depressed function and a low SVR
    - Common finding in septic shock
  - Other effects
    - Elevation lactate from increased liver production, not from hypoperfusion, but it complicates trending the value
    - Tachyarrhythmias and hyperglycemia
- *Dobutamine*
  - Primarily β1 with some β2.
  - Increase in HR, SV, and CO.
  - Decrease in SVR and decrease in pulmonary vascular resistance.
  - Effect on MAP is variable.
  - Arrhythmogenic and increases myocardial O_2 demand.
  - Reasonable to use dobutamine to increase CO and NE to treat vasodilation.
  - 2–20 mcg/kg/min.
- *Milrinone*
  - Direct cellular action on the myocyte and vasculature.
  - Increase in contractility with no increase in HR.
  - Potent vasodilator, decreases pulmonary vascular resistance.
  - Decreases MAP, will likely need to add a vasoconstrictor (NE or vasopressin).
  - Ideal for right heart failure with elevated pulmonary artery pressure, and a normal or high MAP.
  - Used in catecholamine-resistant heart failure with shock
  - Long half-life and profound vasodilatory effect make it hard to use milrinone in non-cardiogenic shock.
  - Dosing based on creatinine clearance.
- *Inotropic support in septic shock with hypotension*
  - Current guidelines are to add inotropic support after vasoconstrictors have been maximized.
  - But vasodilation and cardiac dysfunction often coexist:
    - Adding inotropic support in patients with dysfunction earlier may be beneficial.
  - Also, if LV and RV systolic function are excellent, or even normal, there is little rationale for adding

inotropic support because the patient is requiring high doses of vasoconstrictors to mitigate severe vasodilation:
    - Instead continuing to escalate NE may be the best option.
    - Also, other measures to address refractory vasodilation may be indicated:
        - Stress dose steroids, or adding angiotensin II, for example
  - We recommend assessing cardiac function and output in all patients with shock and/or hypotension:
    - Judicious use of fluid boluses to protect SV and CO:
        - Assess for volume responsiveness and venous congestion in the subacute and recovery phases.
    - Vasoconstrictors to mitigate vasodilation.
    - Add inotropic support if end-organ hypoperfusion and cardiac dysfunction are present.
  - If vasodilation and dysfunction are present, NE/dobutamine and NE/Epi (inotropic doses) are reasonable:
    - No data outcome difference between the choices of inotropic support.
    - Epinephrine is also a vasoconstrictor so it will help treat vasodilation.
    - Dobutamine allows independent titration of inotropic and vasoconstrictor support.
- Ongoing or new hypotension after the acute phase
  - Do not reflexively give fluid.
    - Effect on blood pressure may be from elevation in central venous pressure and not an increase in stroke volume:
        - Blood pressure may increase *without* improving capillary perfusion.
        - May worsen perfusion if venous congestion is present.
        - Effect on blood pressure will be transient leading to excessive fluid administration.
  - Examine the patient and review the clinical history and labs:
    - If evidence of end-organ hypoperfusion is present, consider fluid bolus and possibly starting/increasing a systemic vasopressor.
    - If no evidence of end-organ hypoperfusion, consider starting/increasing a systemic vasoconstrictor.
    - Consider FREE or assessment of cardiac function and cardiac output.
    - Determine the cause of hypotension.

7 Hypotension vs. Shock

Shock can exist without hypotension and hypotension can be present without shock. Confusing hypotension and shock results in late diagnosis of shock and incorrect treatment of vasoplegia with fluid. In the *acute phase,* all effort is in diagnosing and treating the cause of shock. Using fluid to increase SV and CO and central venous pressure to increase the MAP is reasonable. But with ongoing hypotension or new hypotension already in the hospital, using fluid to prop up blood pressure leads to organ edema and dysfunction.

Suggested Reading

Busse LW, McCurdy MT, Ali O, Hall A, Chen H, Ostermann M. The effect of angiotensin II on blood pressure in patients with circulatory shock: a structured review of the literature. Crit Care. 2017;21(1):324. Published 2017 Dec 28. https://doi.org/10.1186/s13054-017-1896-6.

Den Ouden DT, Meinders AE. Vasopressin: physiology and clinical use in patients with vasodilatory shock: a review. Neth J Med. 2005;63:4–13.

Overgaard CB, Dzavík V. Inotropes and vasopressors: review of physiology and clinical use in cardiovascular disease. Circulation. 2008;118(10):1047–56. https://doi.org/10.1161/CIRCULATIONAHA.107.728840. PMID: 18765387

Pollard S, Edwin SB, Alaniz C. Vasopressor and inotropic management of patients with septic shock. P T. 2015;40(7):438–50.

The Focused Rapid Echocardiographic Evaluation (FREE)

Sarah B. Murthi

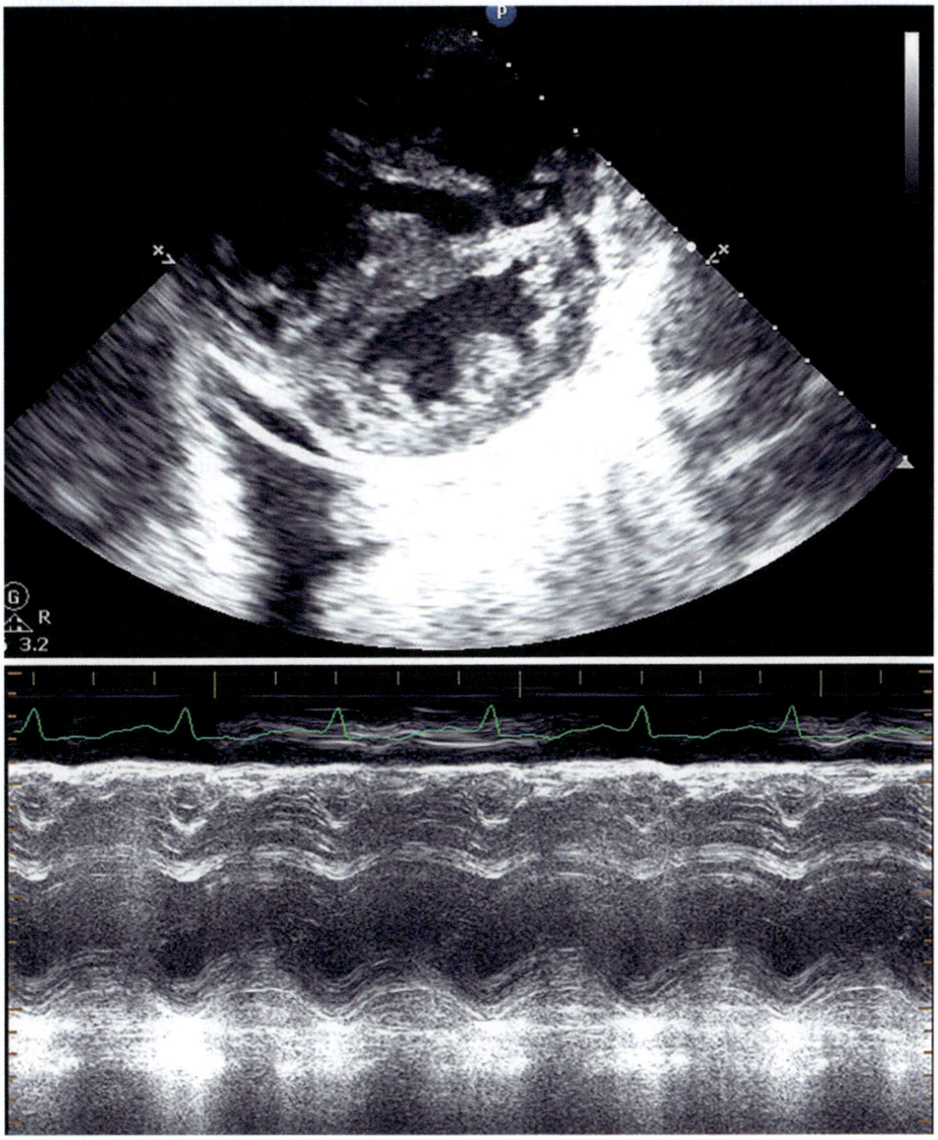

S. B. Murthi (✉)
Department of Surgery, Program in Trauma and Critical Care,
R Adams Cowley Shock Trauma Center, University of Maryland
School of Medicine, University of Maryland Medical Center,
Baltimore, MD, USA
e-mail: smurthi@som.umaryland.edu

A. Salerno et al. (eds.), *Atlas of Critical Care Echocardiography*, https://doi.org/10.1007/978-3-030-74687-2_24

Abbreviations

CI	Cardiac Index
CO	Cardiac Output
ECG	Electrocardiogram
ED	Emergency Department
EF	Ejection Fraction
FREE	Focused Rapid Echocardiographic Evaluation
HR	Heart Rate
ICU	Intensive Care Unit
IVC	Inferior Vena Cava
LV	Left Ventricle
LVOT D	Left Ventricular Outflow Tract Diameter
LVOT	Left Ventricular Outflow Tract
POCUS	Point-of-Care UltraSound
RA	Right Atrium
RV	Right Ventricle
SVI	Stroke Volume Index
SVR	Systemic Vascular Resistance
TAPSE	TransAnnular Plane Systolic Excursion
VTI	Velocity Time Integral

1 Introduction

The Focused Rapid Echocardiographic Evaluation (FREE) is a comprehensive exam used to guide fluid, systemic vasopressors, and inotropic use in complex shock and respiratory failure. It is more relevant in the intensive care unit (ICU) than it is in the emergency department (ED). When a patient initially presents to the ED with undifferentiated shock, all care must be dedicated to diagnosing and treating the cause. Protocols like the RUSH and the FAST are essential. Further a more fluid-liberal strategy is usually indicated. But after initial management, many patients still exhibit evidence of ongoing hypoperfusion which could be caused by cardiac dysfunction, vasoplegia, and hypovolemia either alone or in combination. Also, in the ICU a more fluid-conservative strategy may lead to better outcomes. The FREE can be performed either by the treating physician or a consult service with expertise in both echocardiography and point-of-care ultrasound (POCUS).

2 Uses

- Ongoing complex shock
- Severe respiratory failure with hypotension
- End-organ hypoperfusion
- Organ dysfunction
- Extend use of vasopressors
- Patients with shock who are not responding to standard therapy

3 FREE Protocol

The FREE has four different parts: (1) pre-imaging assessment, including determination of the fluid strategy, (2) ultrasound exam, (3) analysis, and (4) treatment recommendations.

4 Pre-imaging Assessment

Prior to doing the echo, review the clinical course and examine the patient. Even if you are imaging your own patient, take a few minutes to understand what phase of shock the patient is in; see Chap. 23. Are you more concerned about end-organ hypoperfusion, or is respiratory failure the primary issue? Has the cause of shock been identified and treated? Are measures of cellular hypoperfusion worsening or improving?

Clinical Data

- Age, sex, height, and weight:
  - Needed to calculate cardiac index (CI) and stroke volume index (SVI)
  - Can be used to estimate the left ventricular outflow tract diameter (LVOT D)
- Heart rate (HR), rhythm, systolic blood pressure, and diastolic blood pressure:
  - Needed to calculate the cardiac output (CO) and systemic vascular resistance (SVR)
- Assess capillary refill:
  - Helps understand if the patient is in delivery-dependent shock
- Note vasoactives, type, and dose.
- Note inotropes, type, and dose.
- Note if receiving renal replacement therapy.
- Record ventilator settings:
  - Relates to best fluid strategy.
  - Also, the ventilator can affect the inferior vena cava (IVC) findings.

Fluid Strategy The fluid strategy is based on the patient's clinical course and status, rather than the echo findings. The strategy is used with the hemodynamic dynamic profiles to generate treatment recommendations.

Fluid Liberal

- The primary concern is end-organ hypoperfusion.
- Early in shock:
  - Acute and subacute phases
- Concern for cellular hypoperfusion:
  - Capillary refill >3 seconds
  - Lactate increasing
  - Base deficit increasing

- Risk of needing surgery to treat cause of shock.
- Severe respiratory failure is not a major issue.

Fluid Conservative

- The primary concern is venous congestion.
- Severe respiratory failure is a primary issue.
- Equilibrium and recovery phases of shock.
- No evidence of cellular hypoperfusion:
  - Capillary refill <3 seconds
  - Lactate normal or improving
  - Base deficit normal or improving
- Minimal risk of needing surgery.

5 Ultrasound Imaging in the FREE (Fig. 1)

The following windows and measurements are described in detail in their corresponding chapters. Below is a list that summarizes the current FREE protocol. While imaging the patient, continue to assess and examine her. Is her skin warm? Is the ventilator alarming? Blood pressure or heart rate variability?

All Imaging

- Phased array probe.
- Cardiac presets:
  - Except lung imaging which is done in abdominal presets
- ECG leads attached.
- Save a clip of every window:
  - 5 seconds or 5 beats
- Save every measurement.

Parasternal Long Axis

- Assess LV EF.
- Assess RV function.
- Measure the LVOT D.
- Color flow over the mitral valve.
- Color flow over the aortic valve.
- Assess for aortic stenosis.

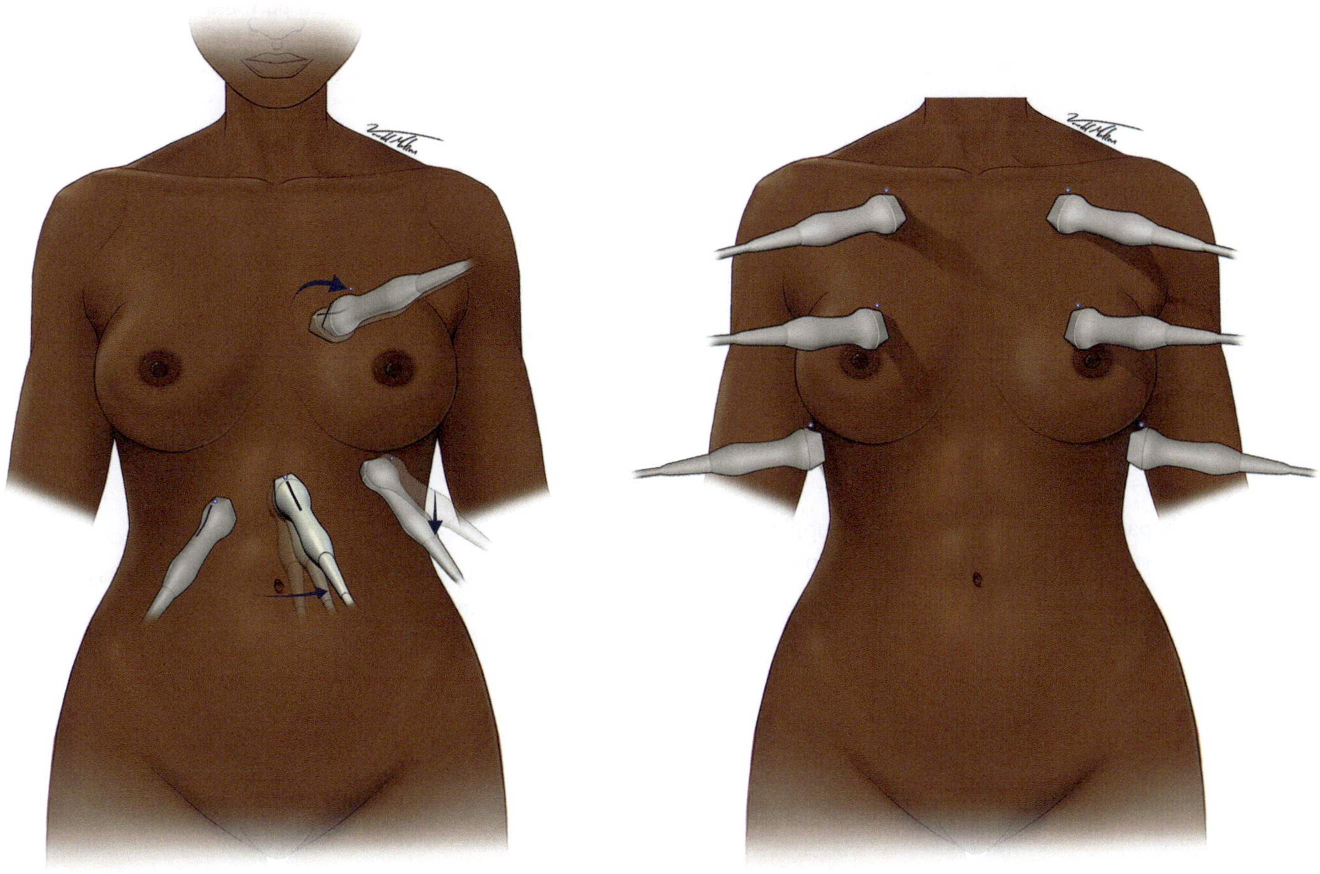

Fig. 1 The FREE windows. *Left panel*: Cardiac FREE windows. Upper transducer; parasternal long axis and parasternal short axis. Below the breast; apical 4 and apical 5. Middle transducer; subxiphoid and inferior vena cava. Left lower; portal and hepatic veins. *Right panel*: Lung windows. Right and left upper, middle, lower anterior lung fields

Parasternal Short Axis

- Assess at the level of the papillary muscles:
  - *Optional*: obtain the aortic, body, and apical window.
- Assess LV EF.
- Assess RV function; look for septal flattening.

Apical 4

- Assess RV function.
- Assess LV EF.
- Color flow Doppler through the mitral valve.
- Color flow Doppler through the tricuspid valve.
- Measure transannular plane systolic excursion (TAPSE).
- *Optional*: pulmonary artery systolic pressure assessment:
  - Consider if RV dysfunction, especially if LV, is underfilled.
  - Continuous wave Doppler of the tricuspid jet.
- *Optional*: diastolic function assessment:
  - Pulsed wave Doppler through the mitral valve
  - Tissue Doppler through the lateral mitral annulus

Apical 5

- Measure the LV velocity time integral (VTI) with pulsed wave Doppler.
- *Optional*: measure the aortic valve VTI with continuous wave Doppler:
  - Consider if concern for aortic stenosis.

Subxiphoid

- Assess LV EF.
- Assess RV function.
- Assess for pericardial fluid; if present assess for tamponade physiology.

Liver

- Assess the IVC for respiratory variation.
- Assess the hepatic vein with pulsed wave Doppler.
- Assess the portal vein with pulsed wave Doppler.

Lung

- Switch to abdominal presets.
- Adjust depth to >10 cm to evaluate for B lines.
- Image the apex and middle and lower anterior chest on the left thorax.
- Image the apex and middle and lower anterior chest on the right thorax.

6 Measurements and Analysis

The threshold values used are rounded and intuitive rather than precise, for example, a SVI of 35 ml rather than the normal value of 34 ml. Ultrasound is not exact enough for high precision. We feel that rounded cut points are simpler and a better way of understanding quantitative ultrasound metrics. See Chap. 27 for more details.

Cardiac Function

- Stroke volume
- Cardiac output/cardiac index
- LV EF
- Global assessment of RV function
- TAPSE
- *Optional*: LV diastolic function

Volume Status

- Volume responsiveness
  - LV VTI
  - Respiratory stroke volume variation
  - IVC
    - Less reliable in surgical patients
    - Less reliable with prolonged ventilation
      - Especially if mean airway pressure is high
- Venous congestion
  - Right side
    - Hepatic venous waveform
    - Portal venous waveform
  - Left side
    - B lines

Vascular Resistance

- Systemic vascular resistance
- *Optional*: Pulmonary artery systolic pressure

Anatomic Findings

Anatomic findings (partial list of possible findings). Assess for pathology that could affect hemodynamics; it is not a detailed anatomic survey:

- Pericardial fluid
  - Assess for tamponade physiology.
- Moderate to severe aortic stenosis
- Moderate to severe mitral valve regurgitation
- Clot in the RA or RV

7 Hemodynamic Profiles and Treatment Recommendations

As part of the analysis for the FREE, the clinical data and the echo data are combined to create a hemodynamic profile. Based on the fluid strategy and the hemodynamic profile, reproducible recommendations are made. Profiles and treatment strategies are discussed in detail in the following chapters.

Normal

- Also known as a happy heart
  - *Normal function, normal volume status, and normal systemic vascular resistance*
- Treatment recommendations if hypoperfusion is present
  - No indication for inotropic support
  - No indication for adding/increasing systemic vasopressors
- Fluid liberal
  - If no indication of venous congestion:
    - Consider fluid bolus.
  - If venous congestion is present:
    - Maintain fluid status or careful removal of fluid.
      - Clinical context determines if fluid strategy is to maintain or remove fluid.
- Fluid conservative
  - Consider careful removal of fluid.

Vasodilated

- Also known as vasodilated/high output
  - Normal function, *vasodilated*, any stroke volume
    - Often high output
    - Often high EF
    - Usually HR > 100
- Treatment recommendations if concern for hypoperfusion:
  - Vasopressors are indicated if MAP < 65 mmHg.
  - No indication for inotropic support.
- Fluid liberal
  - If volume responsive and no e/o venous congestion:
    - Fluid bolus
  - If venous congestion is present:
    - Maintain fluid status or careful removal of fluid:
      - Clinical context determines if fluid strategy is to maintain or remove fluid.
- Fluid conservative
  - If SV low (<35 ml):
    - Maintain fluid status.
  - If SV normal or high >35 ml:
    - Consider careful removal of fluid.

Hummingbird

- Also known as a teeny, tiny underfilled heart
  - High HR, low stroke volume, and normal or high systemic vascular resistance
- Treatment recommendations
  - No indication for inotropic support
  - No indication for vasoconstrictors
- Fluid liberal or fluid conservative
  - Fluid bolus
    - HR is high and SV is low; the myocardium is at risk.

Dysfunctional

- Also known as a sad heart
  - Cardiac function may be contributing to shock or respiratory failure.
  - LV EF < 55%, moderate or severe RV dysfunction, and bradycardia.
- Treatment recommendations if concern for hypoperfusion:
  - Varies depending on type of pathology.
  - Inotropic may be indicated.
  - Vasopressors are indicated if SVR < 800:
    - Epinephrine is likely the best inotropic agent.
  - Depending on the pathology found, other recommendations may be appropriate.
- Fluid liberal
  - +Volume responsive or indeterminant and no venous congestion
    - Fluid bolus
  - −Volume responsive or e/o venous congestion
    - Maintain fluid status or careful removal of fluid.
- Fluid conservative
  - Careful removal of fluid

Mixed Profiles

- If dysfunction is present, place in Dysfunctional Profile as primary
  - Also Vasodilated
  - Also Hummingbird
- If vasodilated with normal function, place in Vasodilated Profile:
  - Also, Hummingbird
    - Fluid and vasopressors are indicated.

8 Operationalizing the FREE

- Billable exam
  - Satisfies criteria for a complete transthoracic echocardiogram
    - Technical and professional fees
  - Need a method of saving reports and images and linking to the electronic medical record
- Consider setting up a service or program
  - At least able to provide imaging/support during rounds
  - Teaching and education
  - Administrative issues
    - Quality assurance
    - Billing

9 Tips and Pointers

The FREE requires expertise in both critical care and echocardiography to perform and interpret. The hemodynamic profiles become intuitive and can lead to rapid decision-making with partial data. The profiles allow reproducible decision-making without having all the data.

10 Special Considerations

This exam is intended to be used after the acute management of shock, not during initial evaluation. How to provide high-quality quantitative echo at the bedside in the ICU will vary from institution to intuition.

Suggested Reading

Glaser JJ, Cardarelli C, Galvagno S Jr, Scalea TM, Murthi SB. Bridging the gap: hybrid cardiac echo in the critically ill. J Trauma Acute Care Surg. 2016;81(5 Suppl 2 Proceedings of the 2015 Military Health System Research Symposium):S157–61. https://doi.org/10.1097/TA.0000000000001020. PMID: 27768664

Murthi SB, Frankel HL, Narayan M, Lissauer M, Furgusen M, Fatima SH, et al. Making the financial case for a surgeon-directed critical care ultrasound program. J Trauma Acute Care Surg. 2014;76(2):340–44; discussion 344-6. https://doi.org/10.1097/TA.0000000000000115. PMID: 24458042.

Murthi SB, Markandaya M, Fang R, Hong CM, Galvagno SM, Lissuaer M, et al. Focused comprehensive, quantitative, functionally based echocardiographic evaluation in the critical care unit is feasible and impacts care. Mil Med. 2015;180(3 Suppl):74–9. https://doi.org/10.7205/MILMED-D-14-00374. PMID: 25747636

Olivieri PP, Patel R, Kolb S, Fatima S, Galvagno SM, Haase DJ, et al. Echo is a good, not perfect, measure of cardiac output in critically ill surgical patients. J Trauma Acute Care Surg. 2019;87(2):379–85. https://doi.org/10.1097/TA.0000000000002304. PMID: 31349350

Fluid Strategies in the FREE

Brooke Anderson and Sarah B. Murthi

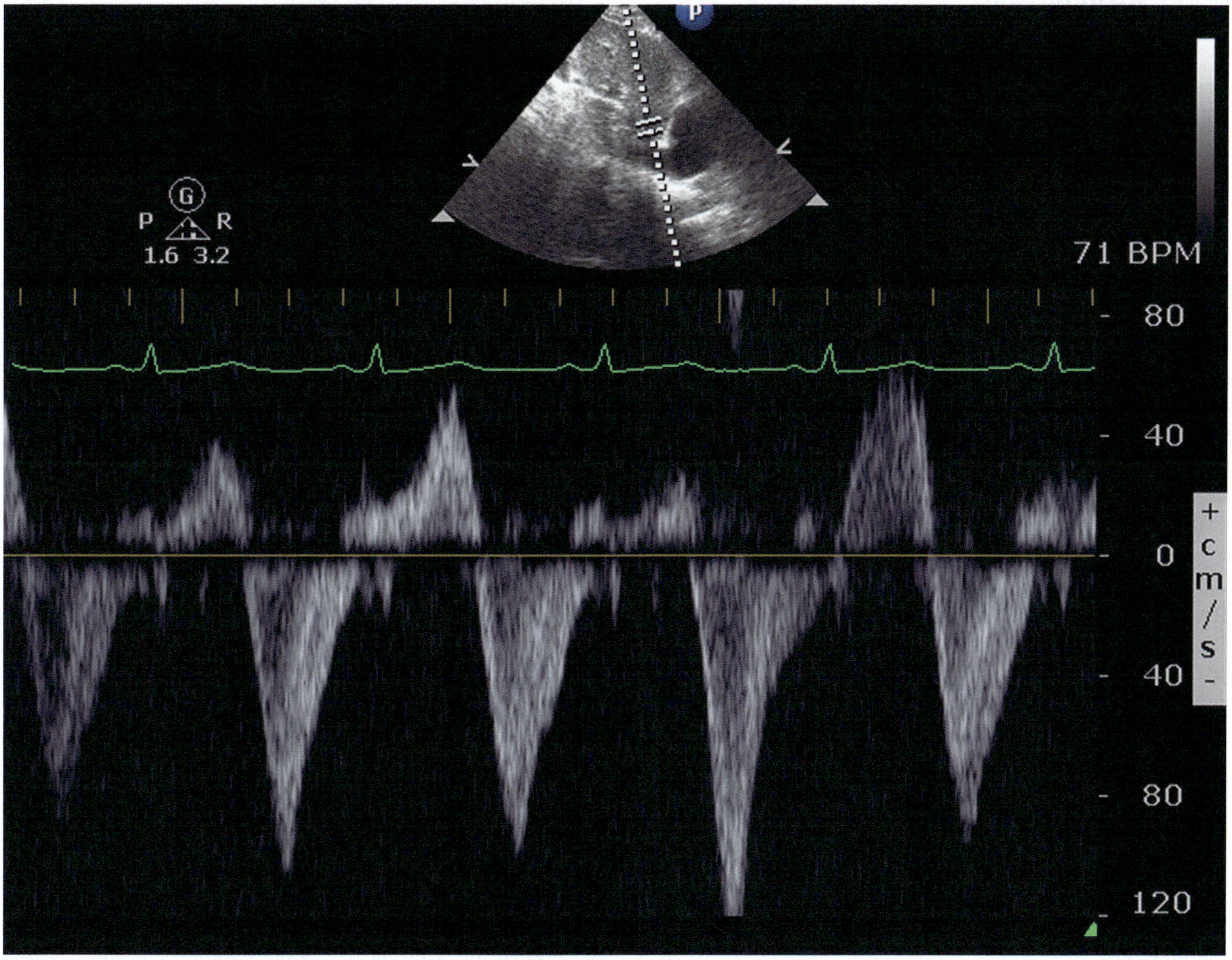

B. Anderson
R. Adams Cowley Shock Trauma Center, University of Maryland, Baltimore, MD, USA

S. B. Murthi (✉)
Department of Surgery, Program in Trauma and Critical Care, R Adams Cowley Shock Trauma Center, University of Maryland School of Medicine, University of Maryland Medical Center, Baltimore, MD, USA
e-mail: smurthi@som.umaryland.edu

A. Salerno et al. (eds.), *Atlas of Critical Care Echocardiography*, https://doi.org/10.1007/978-3-030-74687-2_25

Abbreviations

CO	Cardiac output
CVP	Central venous pressure
DO_2	Oxygen delivery
FREE	Focused Rapid Echocardiographic Evaluation
HR	Heart rate
RAP	Right atrial pressure
SV	Stroke volume
SVR	Systemic vascular resistance
VR	Volume responsiveness

1 Introduction

The Focused Rapid Echocardiographic Evaluation (FREE) is both an ultrasound exam and a style of resuscitation. It allows using fluid, vasoconstrictors, and inotropes together, personalized to the patient. It aims to optimize flow across the capillary beds by considering both arterial delivery and venous return. Treatment recommendations for fluid can change based on the strategy. Fluid-liberal strategies make sense early in shock, if there is clear evidence of end-organ hypoperfusion, and if severe respiratory failure is not a primary issue. Conversely fluid-conservative therapies are reasonable after the primary cause of shock has been addressed, and when severe respiratory failure is present. This chapter describes the resuscitation philosophy behind the FREE and how to select the correct fluid strategy. The following chapters discuss how to incorporate the strategy and echo to generate treatment recommendations.

2 Effects of a Fluid Bolus

A fluid bolus is not a physiologic intervention. It is not filling up something empty. Like every medical therapy, it has risks and benefits and should only be administered when the benefits outweigh the risks. The benefit is an increase in stroke volume, and the risk is organ edema leading to dysfunction.

Volume Responsiveness (VR) The likelihood a fluid bolus will increase cardiac stroke volume (SV) and thus cardiac output (CO).

Effect of a Fluid Bolus A fluid bolus will *always* increase the mean arterial blood pressure (MAP) at least transiently because it causes an increase in right atrial pressure (RAP) and central venous pressure (CVP).

- MAP = ((SV × HR) x SVR) + CVP
  - SV × HR = CO
- Increase in CVP
  - Leads to venous congestion if RAP is already elevated
- Increase in SV
  - Only in + VR patients
  - Increase in CO; assuming HR remains the same
- Increase in MAP
  - Because of an increase in CVP and CO (only in VR patients)
  - If the primary reason the MAP increases is because of the CVP:
    - It is not improving organ perfusion and may be harming it by causing venous congestion
      - *Even though the MAP increases*
- **Positives**
  - Improves organ perfusion. If the patient is volume responsive it will increase the SV, CO and oxygen delivery
- **Negatives**
  - Increases organ edema
    - Decreases intravascular oncotic pressure
    - Increase in atrial pressure causing venous congestion
- **A fluid bolus is likely to be beneficial**
  - If oxygen delivery (DO_2)-dependent shock is present
  - And the patient is volume responsive
  - With no venous congestion:
    - Left atrial and right atrial pressure is normal
- **A fluid bolus is likely to be harmful**
  - The patient is not volume responsive
  - Or venous congestion is present:
    - Left and/or right atrial pressure is elevated
- **Removing fluid is likely to be beneficial**
  - If venous congestion is present
  - If edema is present
  - After the acute phase of shock
- **Removing fluid is likely to be harmful**
  - If DO_2-dependent shock is present
  - And the patient is volume responsive

3 Fluid Liberal vs Fluid Conservative (Figs. 1 and 2)

There is no easy answer to who benefits from a fluid bolus, but part of the solution lies in the patient. Are you – as the treating physician – most concerned with end-organ hypoperfusion *or* the risks of venous congestion? For the FREE the fluid strategy is used with the hemodynamic profile to generate treatment recommendations as discussed in the following chapters.

Fluid Liberal The primary concern is end-organ hypoperfusion:

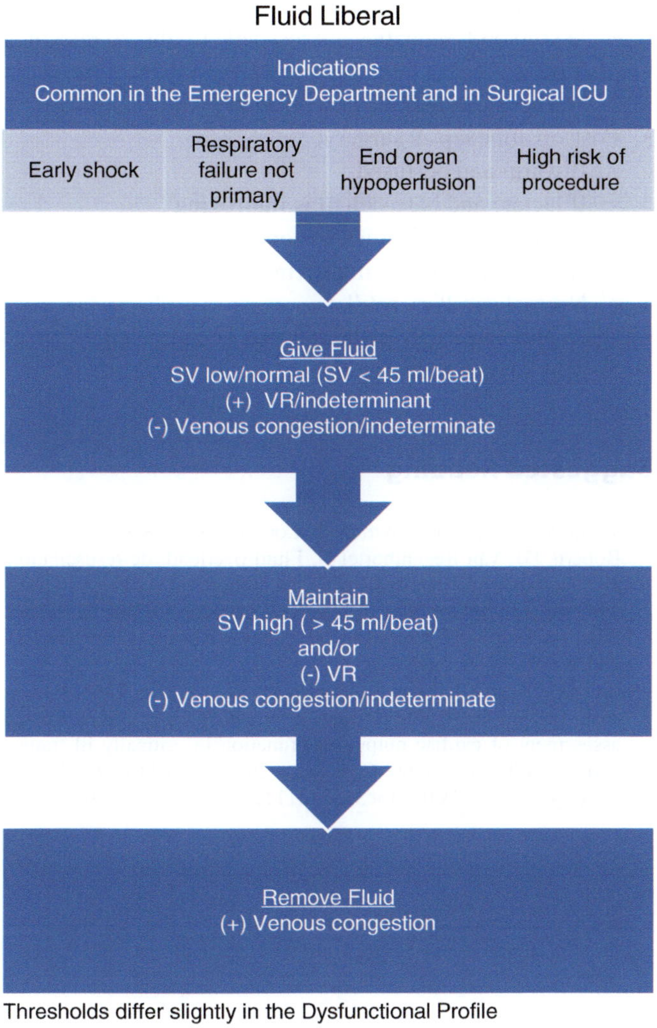

Fig. 1 Fluid liberal. Indications and treatment recommendations for a fluid-liberal strategy. If using the FREE, the thresholds are slightly different in the Dysfunctional Profile; see Chap. 23

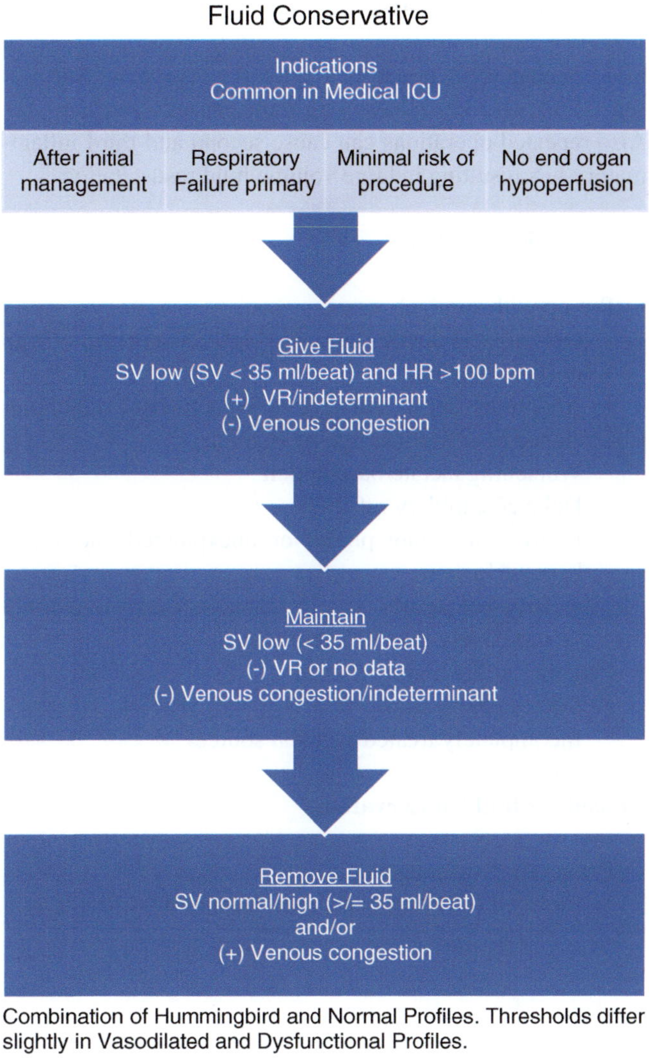

Fig. 2 Fluid conservative. Indications and treatment recommendations for a fluid-conservative strategy. If using the FREE, the thresholds are slightly different in the Vasodilated and Dysfunctional Profiles (*see* Chap. 22)

- Early in shock as the primary cause is being diagnosed and treated
- Evidence of end-organ hypoperfusion:
  - Worsening lactate/base deficit
  - Delayed capillary refill
- Risk of needing surgery
- Severe respiratory failure is not present

Fluid Conservative The primary concern is venous congestion:

- After initial shock management
- Respiratory failure is a primary issue
- Minimal risk of needing surgery
- Concern for bowel congestion/edema

There is more evidence to suggest that fluid boluses are harmful than there is suggesting benefit.

As soon as the patient appears to be perfusing well, and measures of tissue hypoxia (lactate/base deficit) are improving, consider transitioning to a fluid-conservative strategy.

Do not use repeated fluid boluses to prop up the MAP:

- *The effect is transient, leading to repeated fluid boluses*
- *If the reason for increase in MAP is an increase in CVP, it will not improve perfusion*
- *It will lead to edema and organ dysfunction*
- *Assess SVR and consider starting a vasoconstrictor*

In the FREE the fluid strategy is used with other findings to create treatment suggestions based on the hemodynamic profile described in detail in Chap. 26.

4 Surgical Patients

Fluid management in surgical patients is complex. Surgical sepsis and pancreatitis have long acute phases (*see* Chap. 22). Also repeated operations can cause second and third inflammatory hits resulting in large volume fluid resuscitation.

Consider Fluid Liberal

- Pre-op with surgical sepsis:
  - Optimize SV and CO prior to high-risk operation in an unstable patient
  - Abdominal sepsis and necrotizing soft tissue infections
- Evidence of end-organ hypoperfusion:
  - Worsening lactate/base deficit
  - Delayed capillary refill
  - If after the acute phase, or unexplained end organ hypoperfusion:
    - Re-evaluate for surgical source control. Do not reflexively give fluid boluses.
- Ongoing inflammatory source:
  - Severe pancreatitis
  - Incompletely treated surgical source

Consider Fluid Conservative

- Pre-op for liver transplant:
  - Elevated RAP can make transplant more difficult
- Post-op from lung surgery:
  - Disrupted lymphatics are less able to absorb intestinal fluid
    - Elevated LAP may be injurious
- Post-op after sepsis surgery:
  - If warm and perfused
  - If lactate and base deficit is improving
- No evidence of end-organ hypoperfusion:
  - Lactate/base deficit improving
  - Normal capillary refill
- Open abdomen after pathology has been treated:
  - May improve closure rates

Suggested Reading

Malbrain ML, Marik PE, Witters I, Cordemans C, Kirkpatrick AW, Roberts DJ, Van Regenmortel N. Fluid overload, de-resuscitation, and outcomes in critically ill or injured patients: a systematic review with suggestions for clinical practice. Anaesthesiol Intensive Ther. 2014;46(5):361–80. https://doi.org/10.5603/AIT.2014.0060. PMID: 25432556

Murthi SB, Hess JR, Hess A, Stansbury LG, Scalea TM. Focused rapid echocardiographic evaluation versus vascular catheter-based assessment of cardiac output and function in critically ill trauma patients. J Trauma Acute Care Surg. 2012;72(5):1158–64. https://doi.org/10.1097/TA.0b013e31824d1112. PMID: 22673240

Hemodynamic Profiles in the FREE

Sarah B. Murthi

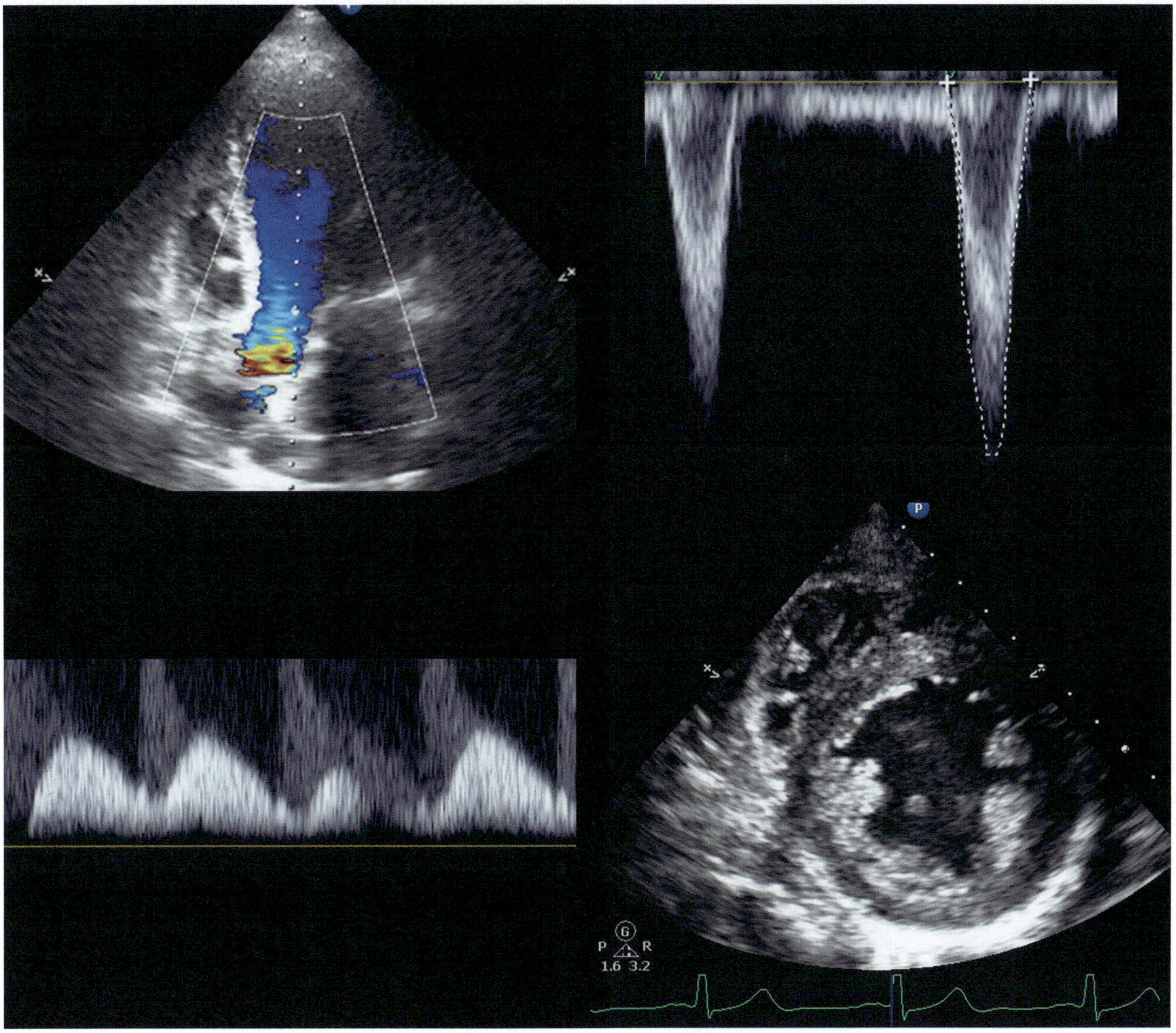

S. B. Murthi (✉)
Department of Surgery, Program in Trauma and Critical Care,
R Adams Cowley Shock Trauma Center, University of Maryland
School of Medicine, University of Maryland Medical Center,
Baltimore, MD, USA
e-mail: smurthi@som.umaryland.edu

A. Salerno et al. (eds.), *Atlas of Critical Care Echocardiography*, https://doi.org/10.1007/978-3-030-74687-2_26

Abbreviations

CI	Cardiac Index
CO	Cardiac Output
D	Diastole
FREE	Focused Rapid Echocardiographic Evaluation
HR	Heart Rate
IVC	Inferior Vena Cava
LV	Left Ventricle
MAP	Mean Arterial Blood Pressure
Ml	Milliliter
PASP	Pulmonary Artery Systolic Pressure
RV	Right Ventricle
S	Systole
SV	Stoke Volume
SVI	Stroke Volume Index
SVR	Systemic Vascular Resistance
SVRI	Systemic Vascular Resistance Index
SVVr	Respiratory Stroke Volume Variation
TAPSE	Transannular Plane Systolic Excursion
VR	Volume Responsiveness
VTI	Velocity Time Integral

1 Introduction

After performing thousands of critical care echocardiograms, we began placing them into categories to allow more consistent treatment recommendations. The categories became hemodynamic profiles which consider clinical information including heart rate (HR), and mean arterial blood pressure (MAP), combined with ultrasound findings. The profile is then used with the fluid strategy to create recommendations about inotropic support, systemic vasopressors, and fluid management.

2 Hemodynamic Profiles

There are four types: normal ×3, vasodilated, underfilled, and dysfunctional (Fig. 1). If end-organ hypoperfusion is present, then recommendations about the use of vasopressors and inotropic support are made to optimize organ blood flow. Fluid management recommendations are made based on the strategy: fluid liberal or fluid conservative (*see* Chap. 25). Generally, a fluid-liberal strategy is indicated if end-organ hypoperfusion is present.

The decisions about end-organ hypoperfusion and fluid strategy are made by the healthcare provider taking care of the patient. If the same provider is doing the imaging and interpretation, then we recommend taking a few minutes before the ultrasound to review the history and labs and do a quick physical to answer these two questions: (1) "Am I concerned about end-organ hypoperfusion?" (2) "What is the best fluid strategy in *this* patient at *this* time?" We have a critical care ultrasound service that does FREEs during rounding hours. A member of the ultrasound team reviews the chart, briefly examines the patient, and discusses the case with the primary team before and after the exam.

- Evidence of end-organ hypoperfusion
  - HR > 100
  - MAP < 65 mmHg and/or use of vasopressors
  - Capillary refill time >3 seconds
  - Cold/clammy extremities
  - Elevated/increasing lactate and/or base deficit
  - Decreased urine output
- Fluid strategy
  - Fluid liberal
    - Early in shock.
    - If end-organ hypoperfusion is present.
    - Plan for high-risk surgery.
    - Respiratory failure is not the primary issue.
  - Fluid conservative
    - After the cause of shock has been identified and treated.
    - Respiratory failure is a primary issue.
    - No indication of end-organ hypoperfusion.
    - Base deficit and lactate down trending.

Fig. 1 Hemodynamic profiles. The four echo-based hemodynamic profiles are described

Normal x 3

Primary finding

Normal cardiac function

Normal SVR

Normal preload

Cardiac function (Normal)

- LV EF >55% , CI > 2.5 L/min
- Normal RV function

SVR (Normal)

- 800-1200 dynes -sec/cm^5

Preload (Normal)

- SVI > 35 ml/m^2/beat, VTI > 20 cm

Underfilled (Hummingbird)

Primary finding

Normal cardiac function

Normal/high SVR

Low preload

Cardiac function (Normal)

- LV EF >55%, often > 70%
- Normal RV function

SVR (Normal/High)

- > 800 dynes - sec/cm^5
- Often > 1200

Preload (Low)

- SVI < 35 mL/m^2/beat, VTI < 20 cm
- Small underfilled LV/RV

Vasodilated

Primary finding

Low SVR, often high CO

Cardiac function (Normal/High)

- LV EF >55%, often > 70%
- Normal RV function
- CI > 2.5 L/min /m^2

SVR (low)

- < 800 dynes - sec/cm^5

Preload (low, normal or high)

- SVI < 35 mL/m^2/beat, VTI <20 cm
    - **Vasodilated and Hummingbird**

Dysfunctional (Sad Heart)

Primary finding

Cardiac dysfunction

Cardiac function

- LV EF < 55%
- RV dysfunction
- Significant anatomic pathology

SVR (low, normal or high)

- If low <800 dynes - sec/cm^5
    - **Dysfunctional and Vasodilated**

Preload (low, normal or high)

- Low SVI/VTI could be due do cardiac dysfunction

3 Assessing the Profiles

Partial data is the norm in critical care echocardiography. The idea is to use what data you have available to profile the patient. There is no true difference between a stroke volume index (SVI) of 33 and 35 ml/m^2/beat, even though 34 is the cutoff between low and normal. Really, low normal is the best way to think of that entire range of stroke volumes. The assessments should be made using human judgment based on the preponderance of the information available, tailored to the individual patient.

The most problematic assessment is volume responsiveness. Most patients fall into the indeterminate or mixed category. We still find it useful in some patients, so it is included in the assessments. Volume responsiveness is a source of active research, and hopefully a more definitive method of assessment will emerge soon. We are currently investigating using positional changes in the IJ as another measure of volume responsiveness.

To define the Vasodilated Profile, the systemic vascular resistance (SVR) must be assessed, so the left ventricular (LV) velocity time integral (VTI) must be measured to allow estimation of the stroke volume (SV) and SV index (SVI). The SV × HR and the SVI × HR can then be used to calculate the cardiac index (CO) and cardiac index (CI), respectively. The CO is needed to estimate the SVR (see Table 1). So, if the VTI cannot be measured, vasodilation cannot be assessed. Normal, hummingbird, and dysfunctional can be called using global assessments.

Table 1 Reference values

	Equations	Normal Values
LV EF	Visual estimation	50-70 %
RV TAPSE	M mode	> 17 mm
LV VTI	PW Doppler	18-25 cm
Stroke Volume	3.14 (LVOTD/2)^2 X LV VTI	70-140 mL/beat
Stoke Volume Index	SV/BSA	35-45 mL/m^2/beat
Cardiac Output	(SV X HR)/1000	4-7 L/min
Cardiac Index	CO/BSA	2.5-4.0 L/min/m^2
SVR	((MAP-RAP)/CO) X 80 *Estimate RAP	800-1200 dynes -sec/cm^5
SVR Index	((MAP-RAP)/CI) X 80 *Estimate RAP	2000-2400 dynes -sec/cm^5/m^2
PASP	4 x (TR jet Vmax)^2 + RAP * Estimate RAP	< 30 mmHg normal
SVVr	$((VTI_{max} - VTI_{min})/VTI_{min}) \times 100$	<10 % less likely 10-15 indeterminant >15% more likely volume responsive
IVC variation	$((IVC_{max} - IVC_{min})/IVC_{min}) \times 100$	<20% less likely 20-50% indeterminant >50% more likely volume responsive
B lines	2D, Thoracic windows	Diffuse, multiple lung fields (>3 B-lines, in > 3 lung fields) likely left sided venous congestion
Hepatic Venous PW	PW Doppler, Liver window	S > D, normal S < D, likely right sided venous congestion S above the baseline, likely severe venous congestion
Portal Venous PW	PW Doppler, Liver window Visual call or $((PV_{max} - PV_{min})/PV_{max}) \times 100$	Pulsatility index > 30%; likely right sided venous congestion To-fro around the baseline, likely severe venous congestion

*Estimate RAP at 5, 10, 15 mmHg. We most often use 10 for simplicity

The most common assessments used in the FREE and the normal values are listed. *Blue metrics* are measures of cardiac function. *Green values* are assessments of vascular resistance. *Yellow measures* assess volume responsiveness, and *pink* are measures of venous congestion

We have recently started assessing measures of venous congestion. We find it useful in determining if fluid boluses are likely to be harmful and when diuresis may be beneficial. For a more detailed description of assessing elevated left atrial pressure using B-lines, see Chap. 16, and for an explanation of assessing elevated right atrial pressure, see Chap. 17. The findings of right and left sided venous congestion are independent of each other meaning B line can be present and the right sided venous flow patterns can be normal or abnormal. We use an indication of venous congestion or fluid intolerance to indicate that fluid boluses may be harmful, and that diuresis may be indicated.

4 Normal × 3 (Happy Heart)

The normal × 3, or happy heart, has normal function, normal preload, and normal systemic vascular resistance (Figs. 1 and 2). A surprising number of patients with shock fall into this category.

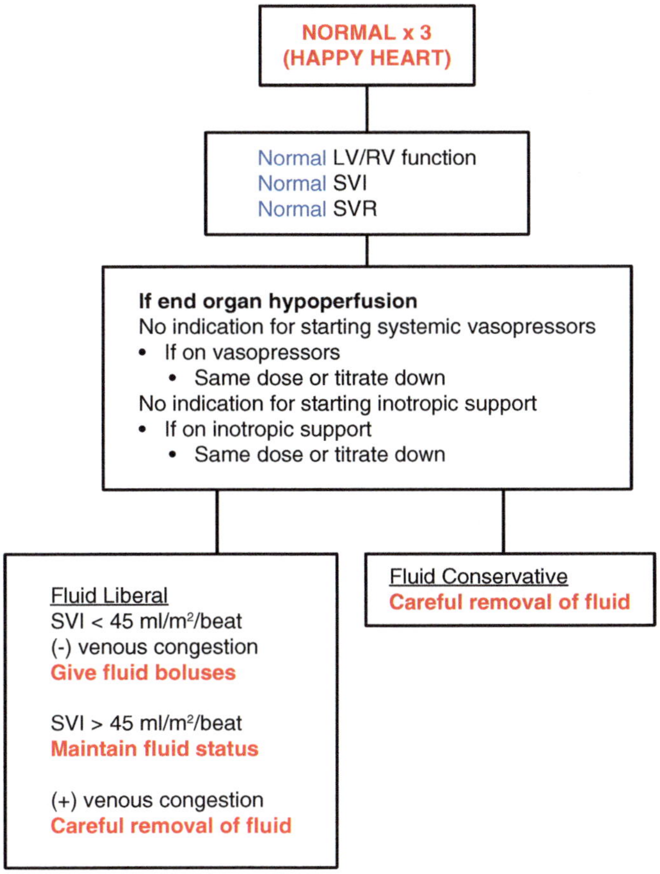

Fig. 2 Treatment recommendations for the Normal Profile (happy heart)

Vital signs

- HR 75–100 (usually)
- MAP > 65 mmHg

Cardiac Function (Normal)

- CI > 2.5 L/min /m^2
- (and) LV ejection fraction (EF) > 55%
- (and) Right ventricular (RV) function normal
  - Global assessment
  - Transannular plane systolic excursion (TAPSE) > 17 mm

Systemic Vascular Resistance and Systemic Vascular Resistive Index (Normal)

- SVR 800–1200 dynes -sec/cm^5
- SVRI 2000–2400 dynes -sec/cm^5/m^2

Preload (Normal)
Normal or high SV

- SVI > 35 mL/m^2/beat and/or VTI >20 cm

5 Underfilled (Hummingbird)

The hummingbird or underfilled heart is characterized by normal LV and RV function, a low stroke volume, and high heart rate. Usually the MAP is normal or high and the systemic vascular resistance is high. This puts the myocardium itself at risk of ischemia, so fluid boluses are recommended in both the fluid-liberal and fluid-conservative strategies (Fig. 3).

Vital Signs

- HR > 100 bpm
- MAP > 65 mmHg

Cardiac Function (Normal)

- LV EF > 55%, usually >70%
- (and) RV function normal
  - Global assessment normal
  - TAPSE >17 mm

Systemic Vascular Resistance (Normal or High)
Normal or high

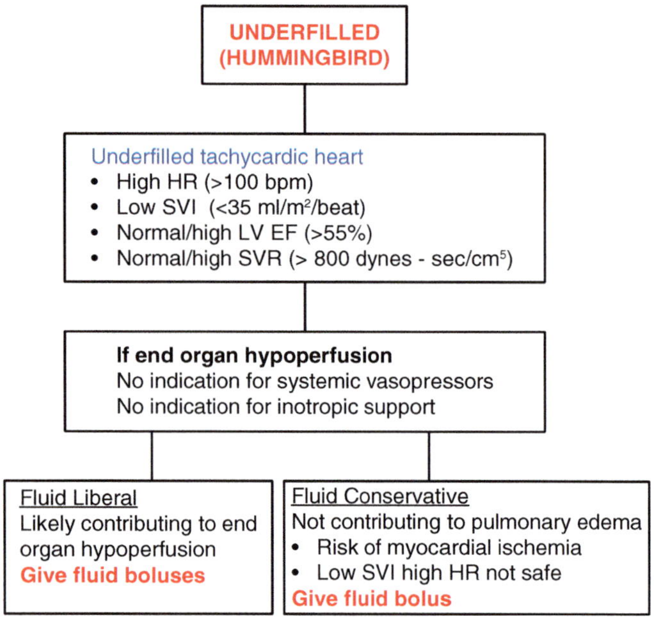

Fig. 3 Treatment recommendations for the underfilled profile (hummingbird)

SVR

- >800 dynes -sec/cm^5
- Often high (>1200)

SVRI

- >2000 dynes -sec/cm^5/m^2
- Often high (>2400)

Preload (Low SV, (–) Venous Congestion)

Stroke volume is low:

- SVI <35 mL/m^2/beat
- VTI <20 cm
- No evidence of venous congestion
  - Minimal B-lines
  - Hepatic S > D
  - <30% portal pulsatility

6 Vasodilated

Any heart with a low systemic vascular resistance and normal LV and RV function is placed in the vasodilated category. Usually the cardiac output is high, and the cardiac function is excellent. We often see vasodilated, high output hearts in sepsis and other inflammatory states including severe trauma. Because the SVR is low, systemic vasopressors may be indicated (Fig. 4). If the stroke volume is also low, then the patient is considered to have a mixed Vasodilated-Hummingbird Profile, and fluid in addition to vasopressors is indicated in both the liberal and conservative fluid strategies.

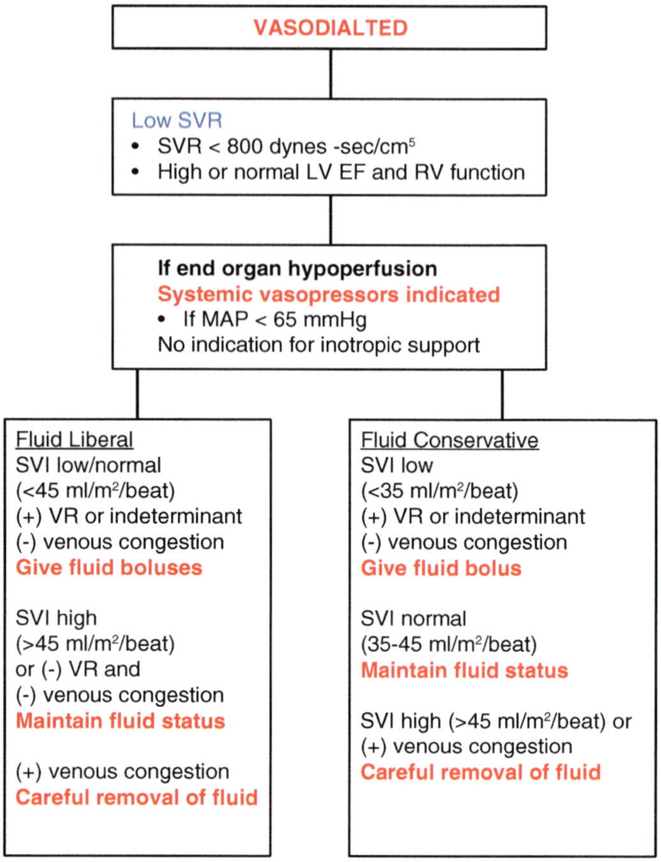

Fig. 4 Treatment recommendations for the Vasodilated Profile

Vital Signs

- HR >100 (usually)
- MAP <65 mmHg (usually)

Cardiac Function (Normal, Excellent)

- Cardiac index >2.5 L/min/m^2
  - Often >4.0
- (and) LV EF > 55%
  - Often >75%
- (and) global RV assessment
  - Normal
  - RV TAPSE >17 mm

Systemic Vascular Resistance (Low)

- SVR < 800 dynes -sec/cm^5
- SVRI < 2000 dynes -sec/cm^5/m^2

Preload

- Can be any SV or VTI
- Low SV < 35 ml/m²/beat or VTI <20 cm
    - Mixed vasodilated/hummingbird; vasodilated and underfilled

7 Dysfunctional (Sad Heart)

Cardiac dysfunction which could be contributing to end-organ hypoperfusion is present in the dysfunctional or sad heart. Classically this is a moderate to severe LV or RV dysfunction, and inotropic support is the primary recommendation. If the SVR is low, then systemic vasopressors may also be indicated. The treatment recommendations will vary depending on the type of dysfunction identified (Fig. 5).

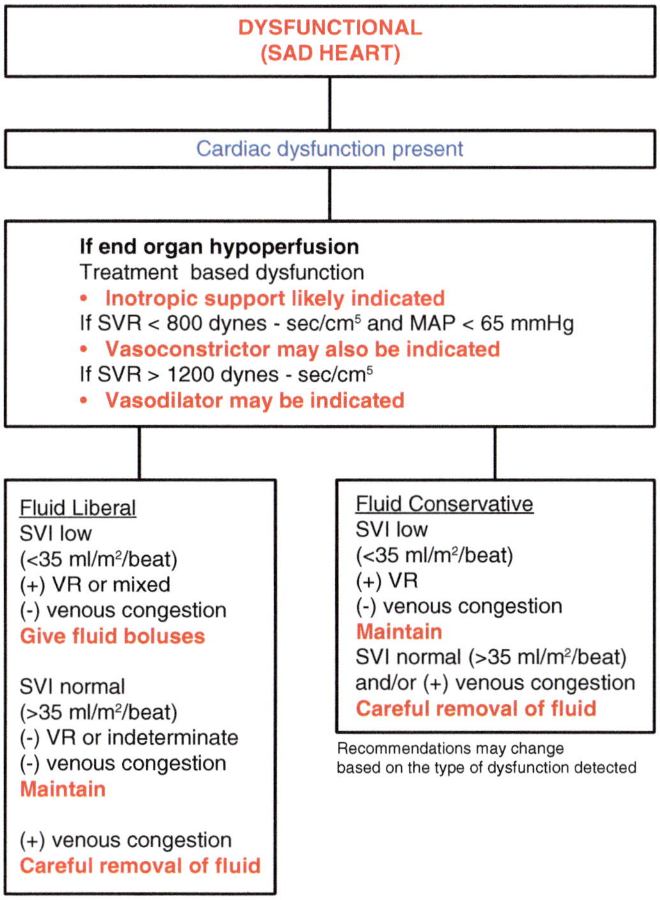

Fig. 5 Treatment recommendations for the Dysfunctional Profile (sad heart)

Vital sign criteria (any)

Cardiac function (dysfunction is present)

- LV EF <55%
- Usually ≤40%, often <30%
- RV dysfunction
    - Usually moderate or severe
    - TAPSE <17 mm
- HR < 65 BPM and cardiac index <2.5 L/min/m²
    - Bradycardic with a low output
- Anatomic pathology that could affect cardiac output
    - Moderate/severe aortic stenosis
    - Moderate/large pericardial effusion

Systemic vascular resistance (any)

- If SVR <800 dynes -sec/cm⁵
    - Mixed dysfunctional/vasodilated

Preload

- Can be any SV or VTI

Treatment recommendations

- More than any other category, the treatment recommendations really depend on the specific findings causing dysfunction. Below are the most common recommendations we make for low LV EF and moderate to severe RV dysfunction.

End-organ hypoperfusion

- *Inotropic support may be indicated:*
    - LV EF <55%
    - RV dysfunction
        - If PASP elevated and/or LV appears underfilled:
            - Consider measures to reduce pulmonary artery systolic pressure (PASP).
            - Pulmonary vasodilator.
    - Consider starting dobutamine or epinephrine.
- If SVR low <800 (mixed dysfunctional/vasodilated):
    - *Vasoconstrictors may also be indicated.*
    - Epinephrine may be ideal inotropic agent because it is also a vasoconstrictor.
    - Also, the combination of dobutamine and norepinephrine is reasonable.
- If SVR high >1200 dynes -sec/cm⁵/m²:
    - Vasodilators to reduce afterload may be indicated.
- Address anatomic findings:
    - Specific to the finding, see Chap. 18.

8 Mixed Profiles

The beauty of hemodynamic echocardiography is that it allows understanding when more than one factor is contributing to shock.

- Any dysfunction, or anatomic pathology which could affect cardiac output:
  - Place in the dysfunctional category.
  - If also vasodilated:
    - Dysfunctional/vasodilated
      - Inotropic support and vasoconstrictors are indicated.
- If vasodilated with normal function:
  - Place in the vasodilated category.
  - If also low Stroke Volume:
    - Vasodilated/hummingbird
      - Fluid and vasoconstrictors are indicated.
- Normal and Hummingbird Profiles
  - Have normal function
  - And normal SVR

Suggested Readings

Murthi SB, Markandaya M, Fang R, Hong CM, Galvagno SM, Lissuaer M, Stansbury LG, Scalea TM. Focused comprehensive, quantitative, functionally based echocardiographic evaluation in the critical care unit is feasible and impacts care. Mil Med. 2015;180(3 Suppl):74–9. https://doi.org/10.7205/MILMED-D-14-00374.

Olivieri PP, Patel R, Kolb S, Fatima S, Galvagno SM, Haase DJ, Ramani GV, Ludmir J, Alkhatib H, Herr D, Bruno DA, Scalea TM, Murthi SB. Echo is a good, not perfect, measure of cardiac output in critically ill surgical patients. J Trauma Acute Care Surg. 2019;87(2):379–85. https://doi.org/10.1097/TA.0000000000002304.

Spiegel R, Teeter W, Sullivan S, Tupchong K, Mohammed N, Sutherland M, Leibner E, Rola P, Galvagno SM Jr, Murthi SB. The use of venous Doppler to predict adverse kidney events in a general ICU cohort. Crit Care. 2020;24(1):615. https://doi.org/10.1186/s13054-020-03330-6. PMID: 33076961; PMCID: PMC7574322

The Focused Rapid Echocardiographic Evaluation (FREE): Clinical Examples

Sarah B. Murthi

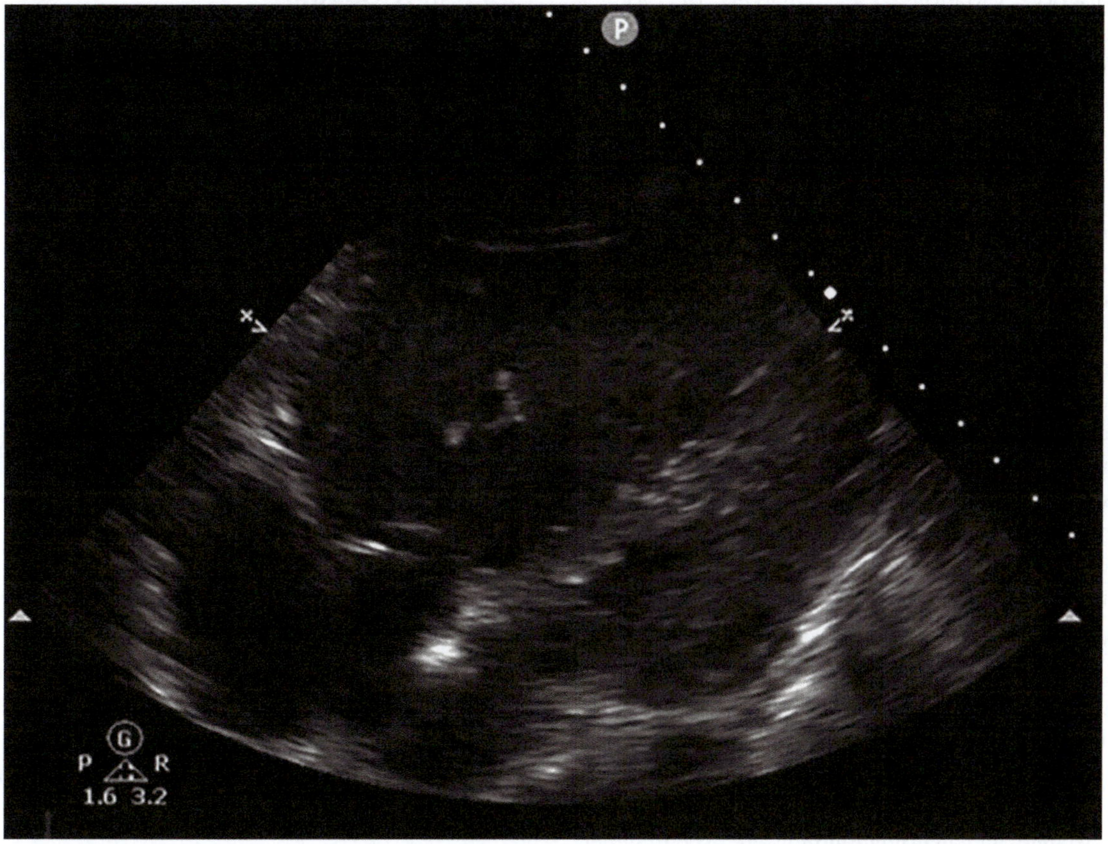

Supplementary Information The online version of this chapter (https://doi.org/10.1007/978-3-030-74687-2_27) contains supplementary material, which is available to authorized users.

S. B. Murthi (✉)
Department of Surgery, Program in Trauma and Critical Care, R Adams Cowley Shock Trauma Center, University of Maryland School of Medicine, University of Maryland Medical Center, Baltimore, MD, USA
e-mail: smurthi@som.umaryland.edu

A. Salerno et al. (eds.), *Atlas of Critical Care Echocardiography*, https://doi.org/10.1007/978-3-030-74687-2_27

Abbreviations

BP	Blood pressure
BSA	Body surface area
CI	Cardiac index
CRRT	Continuous renal replacement therapy
FREE	Focused rapid echocardiographic evaluation
HR	Heart rate
Ht	Height
ICU	Intensive care unit
IVC	Inferior vena cava
LVOT D	Left ventricular outflow tract diameter
MAP	Mean arterial blood pressure
PAC	Pulmonary artery catheter
PASP	Pulmonary artery systolic pressure
PEEP	Positive end expiratory pressure
POCUS	Point-of-care ultrasound
SVI	Stroke volume index
SVR	Systemic vascular resistance
SVV	Stroke volume variation
TAPSE	Transannular plane systolic excursion
UTA	Unable to assess
VR	Volume responsiveness
VTI	Velocity time integral
Wt	Weight

1 Introduction

Using the focused rapid echocardiographic evaluation (FREE) is easier than explaining it. Below are examples of guiding complex resuscitation tailored to patient need with ultrasound. The scenarios are adapted from clinical cases using FREEs to direct management. Even though measurements contained in the FREE evolve the structure remains the same; patient assessment, selection of a fluid strategy, ultrasound evaluation of cardiac function, volume status, vascular resistance, and anatomic findings are used to generate recommendations about the use of fluid, vasopressors, and inotropic support.

All of the calculations listed below are described in their respective chapters. We created and use a free phone application called resuscitation ultrasound (resUS) to preform them on a routine basis. Ultrasound systems are designed for cardiology and radiology applications, so doing this type of exam is cumbersome but not intellectually hard. Almost all systems have a programmable calculation package, so you can create a protocol and automate some of the calculations to tailor ultrasound exams to intensive care unit (ICU) needs.

Critically ill patients, especially those who have had surgery, are notoriously difficult to image with transthoracic echo. In most patients some of the windows and metrics cannot be obtained based on patient anatomy. The FREE is comprehensive so that enough data can be obtained in most patients to allow informed decisions.

We have found the FREE can answer the clinical question >90% of the time and changes care about 50% of the time it is performed. Also, the protocol allows excellent interobserver variability in treatment recommendations. Using a comprehensive, multi-window exam, critical information needed to make carefully reasoned exams can be obtained in most patients.

2 Quantitative Measurements in the FREE

The FREE uses quantitative echo. Table 1 lists some of the most used metrics and the break points for low, intermediate, and high. We feel the use of rounded numbers and large categories is easier and encourages thinking about measurement in point-of-care ultrasound (POCUS) as it is; semiquantitative rather than precise.

Qualifications About Quantification

- Echo can generate precise numbers which exceed its sensitivity:
  - The sensitivity is based on reproducibility between observers.
- Large ranges with intuitive cut points are ideal when categorizing groups of patients:
  - Allows for interobserver variability.
  - In reality the precise cut points are imprecise:

Table 1 Reference values for the FREE

	Low	Intermediate	High
VTI (cm)	<20 Low	20–25 Normal	>25 High
SVI (ml/m^2)	<35 Low	25–45 Normal	>45 High
CI (L/min/m^2)	< 2.5 Low	2.5–4.5 Normal	>4.5 High
TAPSE (mm)	<17 Dysfunctional	–	–
SVR (dynes -sec/cm^5)	<800 Vasodilated	800–1200 Normal	>1200 Vasoconstricted
SVV (%)	<10 Unlikely VR	10–15 Indeterminant	>15 Likely VR
IVC (%)	<15 Unlikely VR	15–25 Indeterminant	>20 Likely VR

VTI velocity time integral, *SVI* stroke volume index, *CI* cardiac index, *TAPSE* transannular plane systolic excursion, *SVR* systemic vascular resistance, *SVV* stroke volume variation, *IVC* inferior vena cava, *VR* volume responsive

    - There is no reproducible difference between a calculated SVR of 810 and 790 even though they fall on either side of the threshold between normal and low:
      - Both are better understood as low normal.
  - There will be indeterminate values especially in metrics like volume responsiveness.
- Trending more precise changes in the same patient overtime is reasonable:
  - Trending changes in VTI with the addition of inotropic support, for example
  - Especially if the same person is obtaining the metric
- Thresholds for dysfunction like TAPSE and E-point septal separation are drawn from large population studies using the 95% confidence interval and lower threshold for fifth percentile. So, they only detect severe dysfunction:
  - While a TAPSE <17 mm detects severe dysfunction, a TAPSE >17 mm does not mean normal RV function.
- Use more than one metric and check all measurements against careful visual inspection:
  - Does the TAPSE make sense with how RV function as it appears in all of the windows obtained?
- Know where the errors lie in the metrics being used, so they can be used more accurately.

The calculations used below are described in their respective chapters. When an estimation of right atrial pressure or central venous pressure is needed, we use 10 mmHg. A free phone application called Resuscitation Ultrasound that we created is used to perform the calculations.

3 Case 1: Trauma Patient with Decreased Urine Output

The patient is a 73-year-old male with end-stage liver disease who fell from standing. His injuries include a subdural hematoma and nasal fractures. He is admitted to the ICU for frequent neurologic assessments. He has a urine output of <30 cc for the last 2 hours and he is cool to the touch. His capillary refill is 3 seconds. His hemoglobin is stable. A FREE is performed.

Indication for the FREE

- Decreased urine output

Vital signs

- HR 97 bpm
- BP 119/55 mmHg
- MAP 76 mmHg

Ht 181 cm, Wt 62 kg, and BSA 1.8 m^2
Vasoconstrictors/inotropic support: None
Ventilator: Not intubated, on 4L nasal cannula

Fluid Strategy

- Fluid liberal
  - Recent trauma with evidence of end-organ hypoperfusion (decreased urine output)
  - Minimal respiratory dysfunction

FREE Findings (Fig. 1)

- Cardiac function
  - LV: EF 55–70%
  - RV: Normal by visual assessment and TAPSE
  - Hemodynamics
    - VTI, low (17 cm); LV outflow tract diameter (LVOT D), 1.80 cm
    - SVI, low (24 ml/m^2); CI, low (2.3 L/min/m^2); and SVR, high (1265 dynes -sec/cm^5)
- Volume assessments
  Volume responsiveness
  - SV: Low
  - SVV: Likely VR (16%)
  - IVC: Likely VR (100% collapse)

Venous congestion
  - Hepatic flow normal
  - Portal flow normal
  - Minimal B-lines
- Systemic vascular resistance
  - SVR: high
  - Pulmonary artery systolic pressure (PASP): Not assessed; RV function and size normal
- Anatomic findings
  - Mild mitral regurgitation

Profile Hummingbird

- Normal LV and RV systolic function
- Low stroke volume, high heart rate, and high systemic vascular resistance

Treatment Suggestions

- Consider fluid bolus.
- No indication for systemic vasoconstrictors.
- No indication for inotropic support.

Clinical Course
After the FREE the patient is bolused with 500 cc of crystalloid three times over 8 hours resulting in an increase in urine output. His neurologic exam is improving, and he is not intubated.

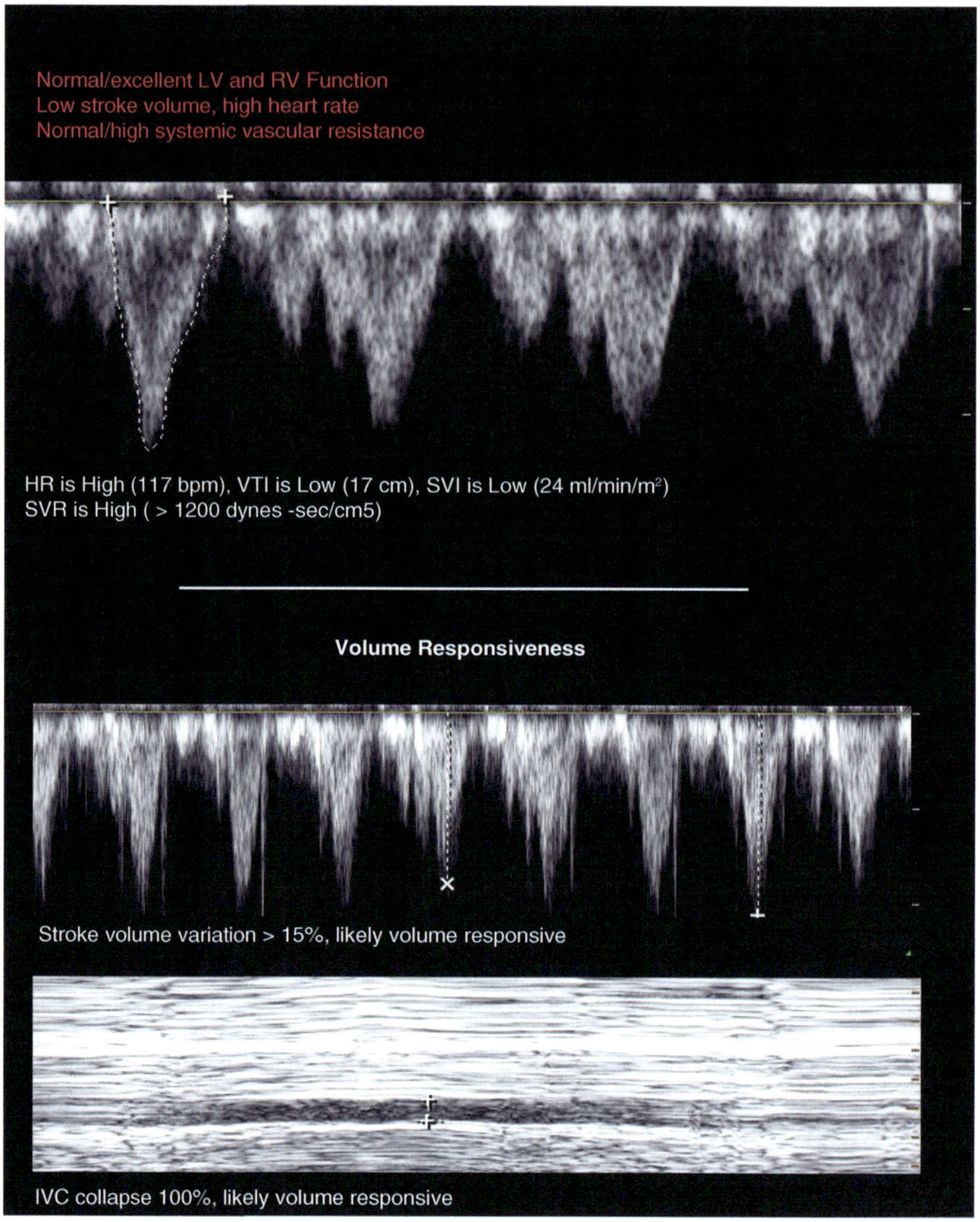

Fig. 1 Case 1: Hummingbird/underfilled. This patient is in the Hummingbird Profile because left and right ventricular function are normal (not shown), the HR is high, the SVI is low, and SVR is high. He also appears volume responsive (lower 2 panels). See text for details on medical management

Teaching Point

In the Hummingbird Profile, the echo itself suggests fluid is beneficial because the heart rate is high, and the stroke volume is low putting the myocardium itself at risk. Fluid is suggested in both the liberal and conservative strategies. By definition cardiac function is normal, and the systemic vascular resistance is normal/high, so inotropic support and vasoconstrictors are not indicated.

4 Case 2: Overdose with Respiratory Failure and Hypotension

R.O. is a 39-year-old female admitted to the ICU after acetaminophen overdose. She is intubated for airway protection on admission. During the procedure she aspirates. Four hours later she has developed hypotension and increasing ventilatory requirements. A FREE is performed.

Indications for the FREE

- Ongoing hypotension and respiratory failure

Vital signs

- HR 117 bpm
- BP 101/60 mmHg
- MAP 74 mmHg

Ht 170 cm, Wt 68 kg, and BSA 1.79 m^2

Vasoconstrictors/inotropic support: Norepinephrine 0.08 mcg/kg/min

Ventilator: Pressure control rate of 20, positive end expiratory pressure (PEEP) 14 cmH_2O, RR 18, and FiO_2 40%

Fluid Strategy

- Fluid liberal
  - Arguments could be made to use either strategy. In this case the critical care team selected a fluid-liberal strategy to encourage hepatic and renal blood flow.

FREE Findings (Fig. 2)

- Cardiac function
  - LV: EF >70%
  - RV: Normal by visual assessment and TAPSE
  - Hemodynamics
    - VTI, 23.8 cm; LVOT D, 1.85 cm
    - SVI, normal (36 ml/m^2); CI, normal (4.2 L/min/m^2); and SVR, low (680 dynes -sec/cm^5)
- Volume assessments

Volume responsiveness

- SVV: Unlikely VR
- IVC: Unlikely VR (2.42 cm, no collapse)

Venous congestion (Fig. 3)

- Hepatic vein flow: Abnormal (retrograde systolic flow)
- Portal vein flow: Abnormal (pulsatile)
- Diffuse B-lines

- Systemic vascular resistance
  - SVR: Low
  - PASP: Not assessed; RV function and size normal
- Anatomic findings
  - Normal valvular function; no pericardial effusion

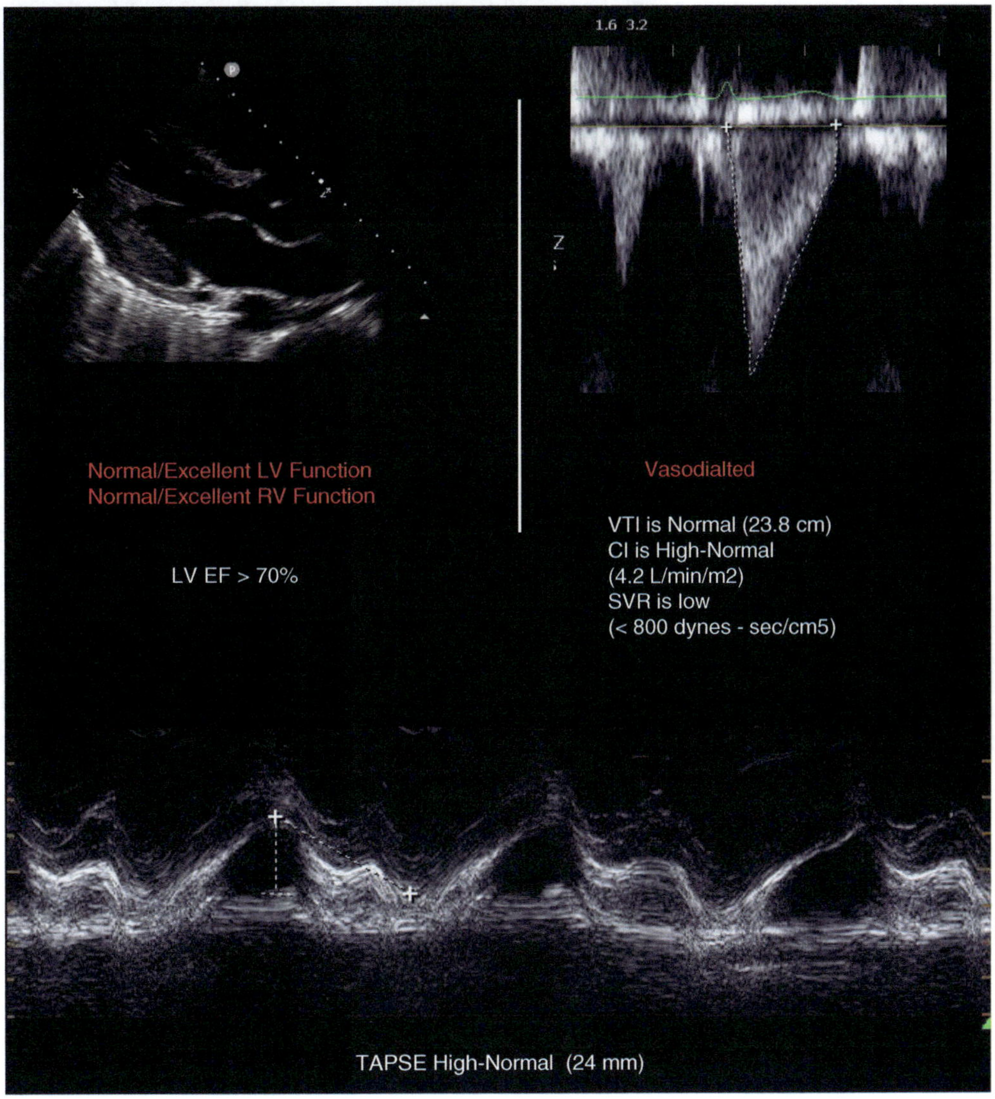

Fig. 2 Case 2: Vasodilated. This patient is placed in the Vasodilated Profile because he is vasodilated with normal/excellent LV and RV function. See text for details on medical management

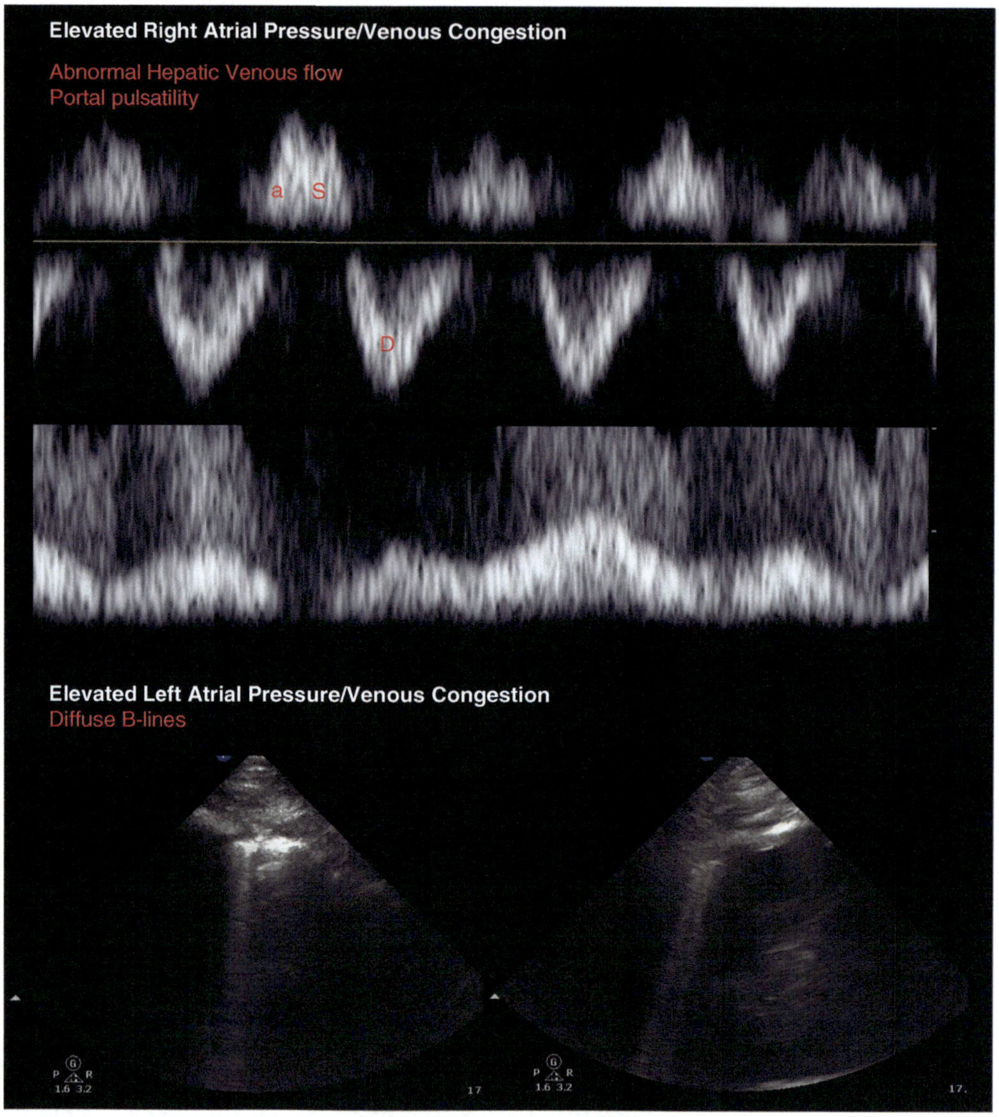

Fig. 3 Case 2: Severe venous congestion Upper panel: Abnormal hepatic venous flow. Middle panel: Portal pulsatility. Lower panel: Diffuse B-lines. In addition to being vasodilated, the patient in Case 2 also had evidence of severe right-sided venous congestion and severe left-sided venous congestion. Note that right sided and left sided congestion can appear either independently or at the same time

Profile Vasodilated

- Normal LV and RV function
- Low systemic vascular resistance
- Indications of left- and right-sided venous congestion

Treatment Suggestions

- Consider careful removal of fluid:
  - Even though a fluid-liberal strategy is selected, diuresis is recommended because there is evidence of left- and right-sided venous congestion.
- Continue vasoconstrictors; titrate to maintain a MAP of 65 mmHg:
  - Diuresis will likely lower the right atrial pressure, and the MAP may further decrease requiring an increase in norepinephrine.
- No indication for inotropic support.

Clinical Course After the FREE the patient is given Lasix and norepinephrine is continued. Over the next 24 hours, R.O.'s fluid balance is 1 liter negative, while her norepinephrine requirements and ventilatory needs have decreased.

Teaching Points In the Vasodilated Profile, the fluid recommendations can be to give fluid, maintain fluid status, and diuresis depending on the fluid strategy and volume assessments.

- The FREE allows consideration of fluid and vasopressors separately even though both can affect the blood pressure.
- In this case the patient has indications of both elevated left- and right-sided venous congestion. This is not always the case, sometimes there are diffuse B-lines present, and right-sided flows are normal and vice versa.

- The hypotension is from vasodilation rather than low cardiac output, and there is evidence of right- and left-sided venous congestion. So continuing vasopressors while removing fluid is the best way to optimize tissue perfusion.

5 Case 3: Postoperative from a Major Ventral Hernia Repair with Hypotension

The patient is a 64-year-old female who underwent an 8-hour enterocutaneous fistula takedown and ventral hernia repair. Four hours postoperatively he has ongoing hypotension with a vasopressor requirement despite 4 liters of crystalloid. Her urine output is marginal; her skin is warm and perfused. A FREE is performed.

Indication for the FREE

- Hypotension requiring vasopressors

Vital signs

- HR 67 bpm
- BP 117/44 mmHg
- MAP 68 mmHg

Ht 164 cm, Wt 55 kg, and BSA 1.6 m^2

Vasoconstrictors/inotropic support: Norepinephrine 0.15 mcg/kg/min

Ventilator: Synchronous intermittent mechanical ventilation, PEEP 10 cmH_2O, and FiO2 40%

Fluid Strategy

- There is a conflict among the team.
- The surgeons are concerned that the current fluid-liberal strategy will cause abdominal compartment syndrome; the critical care team is concerned limiting fluid boluses will harm organ perfusion:
    - The FREE is often performed to settle a debate about the best resuscitation plan.

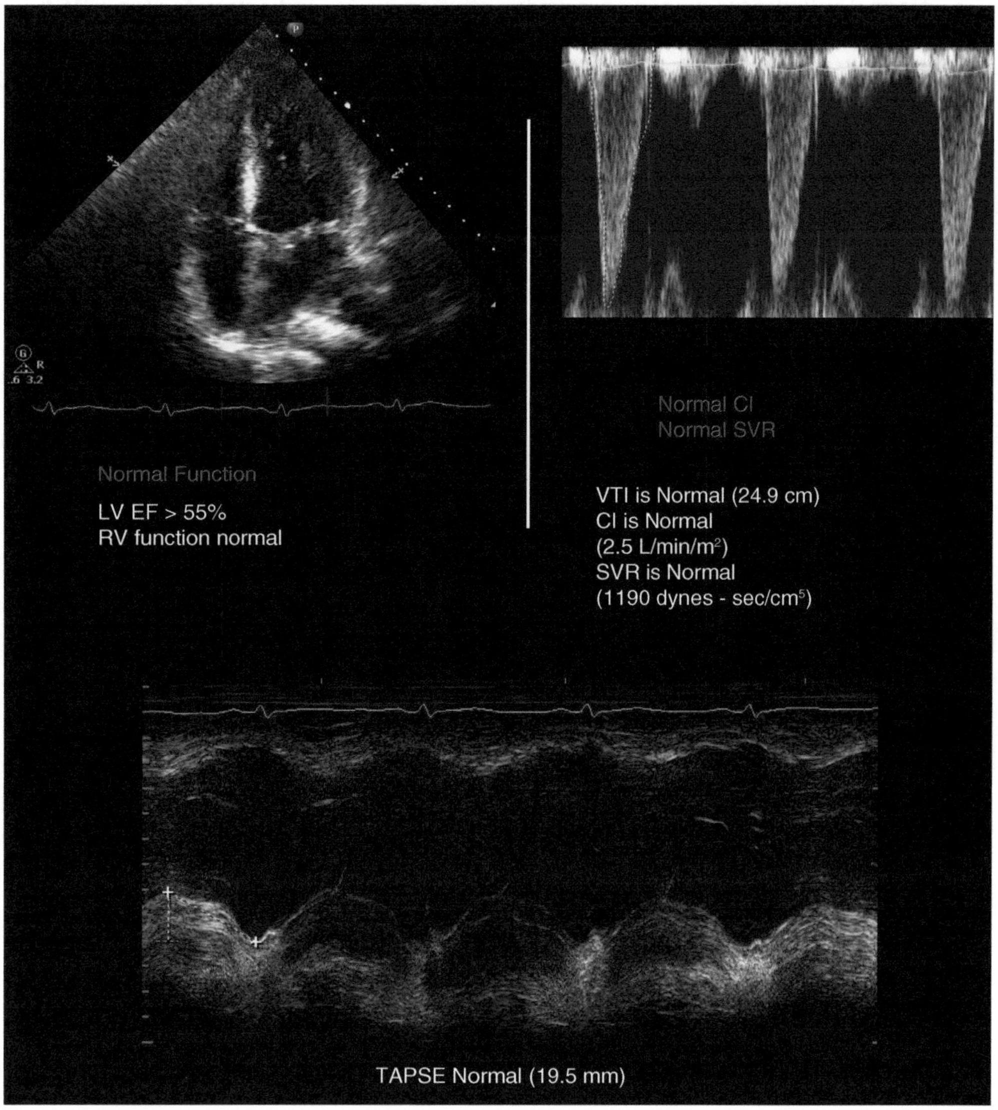

Fig. 4 Case 3: Normal x 3. This patient is in the Normal Profile because she has normal cardiac function, normal cardiac output, and normal systemic vascular resistance

FREE Findings (Fig. 4)

- Cardiac function
  - LV: EF 55–70%
  - RV: Normal by visual assessment and TAPSE
  - Hemodynamics
    - VTI, 24.9 cm; LVOT D, 1.73 cm
    - SVI, normal (37 ml/m^2); CI, normal (2.5 L/min/m^2); and SVR, normal (1190 dynes -sec/cm^5)
- Volume assessments

  Volume responsiveness
  - SVV: Unlikely VR (5%)
  - IVC: Unlikely VR (1.93 cm, no collapse)

  Venous congestion
  - Hepatic vein flow: Normal (systolic > diastolic)
  - Portal vein flow: Normal (not pulsatile)
  - Minimal B-lines
- Systemic vascular resistance
  - SVR: Normal (while on systemic vasopressors)
  - PASP: Not assessed; RV function and size normal
- Anatomic findings
  - Normal valvular function; no pericardial effusion

Profile Normal × 3

- Normal LV and RV function
- Normal systemic vascular resistance
  - On norepinephrine.
  - This is noted and referenced in the treatment recommendations. The profile itself is based on vital signs and echo findings.
- Minimal indications of venous congestion, or elevated atrial pressure

Treatment Suggestions

- Fluid liberal
  - Maintain fluid status:
    - Stroke volume is normal and does not appear volume responsive.
- Fluid conservative
  - Consider careful removal of fluid.
- No indication for increasing systemic vasopressors
- No indication for adding or increasing inotropic support

Clinical Course

The team decides to maintain fluid status and monitor the patient closely. No further boluses were given. Over the next 24 hours, her urine output improves, and she is extubated. After extubation her norepinephrine requirement decreases, allowing us to titrate it off.

Teaching Points We do not consider the use of inotropic support or vasopressors at the time of the FREE in profiling the patient. It is based on vital signs and the echo, so this patient has a Normal Profile while on systemic vasopressors. We do record the vasoactives at the time of the FREE and reference them in the treatment recommendations.

6 Case 4: Hospital-Acquired Pneumonia and Hypotension

SB is a 78-year-old female who was admitted after a motor vehicle crash. Her injuries include multiple rib fractures causing respiratory compromise. An epidural catheter is placed for pain control, and she is monitored for respiratory failure. Two days after admission, she is transferred to the ICU for hypoxic respiratory failure. She is intubated, diagnosed with pneumonia, and started on antibiotics. Now she has increasing ventilatory requirements and requires norepinephrine. She is warm and perfused. Her urine output is normal but trending down. A FREE is performed.

Indication for the FREE

- Respiratory failure and hypotension

Vital signs

- HR 115 bpm
- BP 100/40 mmHg
- MAP 60 mmHg

Ht 165 cm, Wt 55 kg, and BSA 1.60 m^2

Vasoconstrictors/inotropic support: Norepinephrine 0.18 mcg/kg/min

Ventilator: Pressure control $FiO_2$60% and PEEP 12 cmH_2O

Fluid Strategy

- Debate among the team
  - The team is concerned about respiratory failure and end-organ hypoperfusion.

FREE Findings (Fig. 5)

- Cardiac function
  - LV: EF < 30% (Video 1)
  - RV: Normal by visual assessment and TAPSE
  - Hemodynamics
    - VTI, 13.5cm; LVOT D, 1.83 cm
    - SVI, low (22 ml/m^2); CI, normal (2.6 L/min/m^2); and SVR, normal (980 dynes -sec/cm^5)
- Volume assessments

  Volume responsiveness
  - SVV: Likely volume responsive (15%)

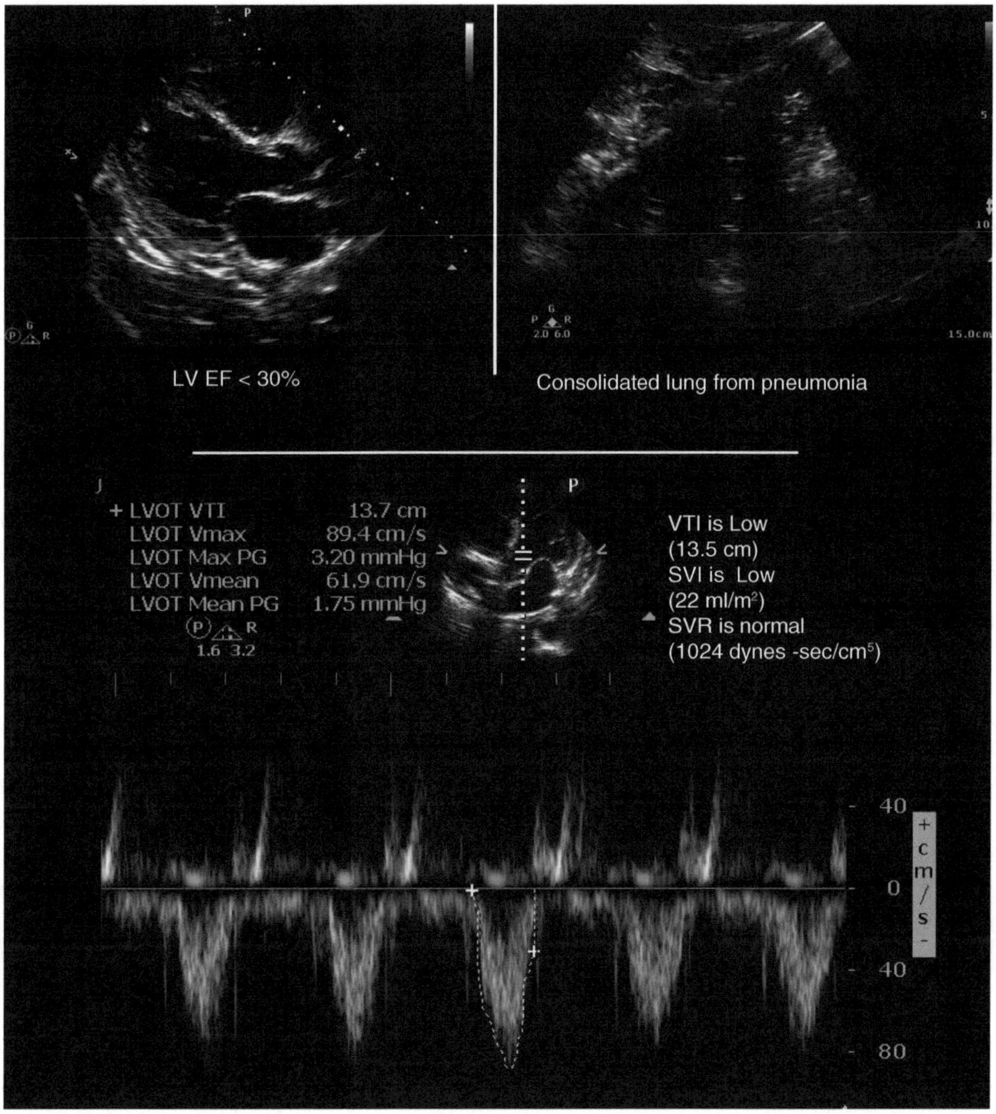

Fig. 5 Case 4: SB is in the Dysfunctional Profile because she has severe LV systolic dysfunction with an EF < 30%. Note the consolidated lung from pneumonia seen in the upper right panel

- ◦ IVC: Less likely volume responsive (2.3 cm, no collapse)

Venous congestion

- ◦ Hepatic vein flow: Normal (S > D)
- ◦ Portal vein flow: Normal (not pulsatile)
- ◦ B-lines minimal; consolidated lung seen in the right lower lung field
- Systemic vascular resistance
  - SVR: Normal
  - PASP: Unable to assess
- Anatomic findings
  - Normal valvular function; no pericardial effusion

Profile Dysfunctional

- LV EF < 30% and low stroke volume
- Normal systemic vascular resistance
  - On systemic vasopressors
- Volume assessment mixed
  - Stroke volume variation suggests volume responsive.
  - IVC suggests less likely volume responsive:
    - Rib fractures and high PEEP make this metric less reliable.
    - We are considering removing IVC assessments from the FREE and are evaluating positional internal jugular vein changes instead.
  - No evidence of left or right venous congestion.

Treatment Suggestions

- Fluid liberal:
  - Careful fluid bolus
- Fluid conservative:
  - Maintain fluid status

- Consider adding inotropic support to improve left ventricular function.
- No indication to increase systemic vasoconstrictors.

Clinical Course Inotropic epinephrine (0.05 mcg/kg/min) is started. Intermittent 250–500 cc boluses are given over the next 6 hrs. Repeat imaging shows an improvement in EF and an increase in VTI; B-lines remain minimal. Her urine output increases, and her norepinephrine requirement decreases.
Teaching Points Prior to the FREE, the plan had been to increase the NE and add vasopressin but as a result of the FREE, inotropic support is started instead:

- Low EF is the most common reason for the Dysfunctional Profile.
- Echo allows tailoring inotropic support and fluid to the patient.

7 Case 5: COVID-19 Requiring ECMO with Hypotension and Worsening Hypoxia

RD is a 48-year-old male who was admitted 10 days ago with progressive respiratory failure from COVID-19. Two days ago, he was placed on extracorporeal membrane oxygenation (ECMO) and is on continuous renal replacement therapy (CRRT). Over the last 24 hours, he has become progressively hypotensive and hypoxic. His capillary refill >3 seconds.

Indication for the FREE

- Respiratory failure and hypotension

Vital signs

- HR 105 bpm
- BP 100/45 mmHg
- MAP 63 mmHg

Ht 181 cm, Wt 70 kg, and BSA 1.9 m^2
Vasoconstrictors/inotropic support: Norepinephrine 0.08mcg/kg/min
Ventilator: Pressure control FiO_2 60%, PEEP 12 cmH_2O, and ECMO ongoing

Fluid Strategy

- Fluid conservative
  - Although he is hypotensive with some indication of end-organ hypoperfusion, his primary issue is respiratory failure.

FREE Findings (Fig. 6 and 7)

- Cardiac function
  - LV: EF < 70%
  - RV: Severely dysfunctional by visual assessment (Video 2)
    - TAPSE: 16.4 mm
  - Hemodynamics
    - VTI: Unable to assess (UTA)
    - SVI, CI, and SVR: UTA
- Volume assessments
  Volume responsiveness
  - SVV: UTA
  - IVC: UTA (ECMO cannula in place)

Venous congestion
  - Hepatic vein flow: Abnormal (retrograde systolic flow)
  - Portal vein flow: Abnormal (pulsatile)
  - B-lines diffuse. Thickened pleura; subpleural collections
- Systemic vascular resistance
  - SVR: UTA
  - PASP: Elevated (estimated >60 mmHg)
    - Septal flattening with a D-shaped LV
- Anatomic findings
  - Large clot seen in the RV, freely mobile

Profile Dysfunctional (Fig. 6)

- Severely depressed RV function
- Pulmonary artery hypertension
- Small LV with an EF > 70%
- Septal flattening/D-shaped LV
- Clot in RV, high risk of pulmonary embolus (PE)
- Unable to calculate SVI, CI, or SVR
- Right-sided venous congestion
- Unable to assess left atrial pressure
- Diffuse B-lines consistent with severe COVID (Fig. 7)

Treatment Suggestions

- Consider careful removal of fluid. There is evidence of elevated right atrial pressure and right ventricular pressure volume overload.
- Consider adding inotropic support to improve RV function.
- Consider measures to decrease pulmonary artery pressure:
  - Both pulmonary vasoconstriction from hypoxia and pulmonary embolus could be leading to RV failure with high pulmonary artery systolic pressure.
- Unable to comment on use of systemic vasopressors. Vascular resistance could not be calculated.

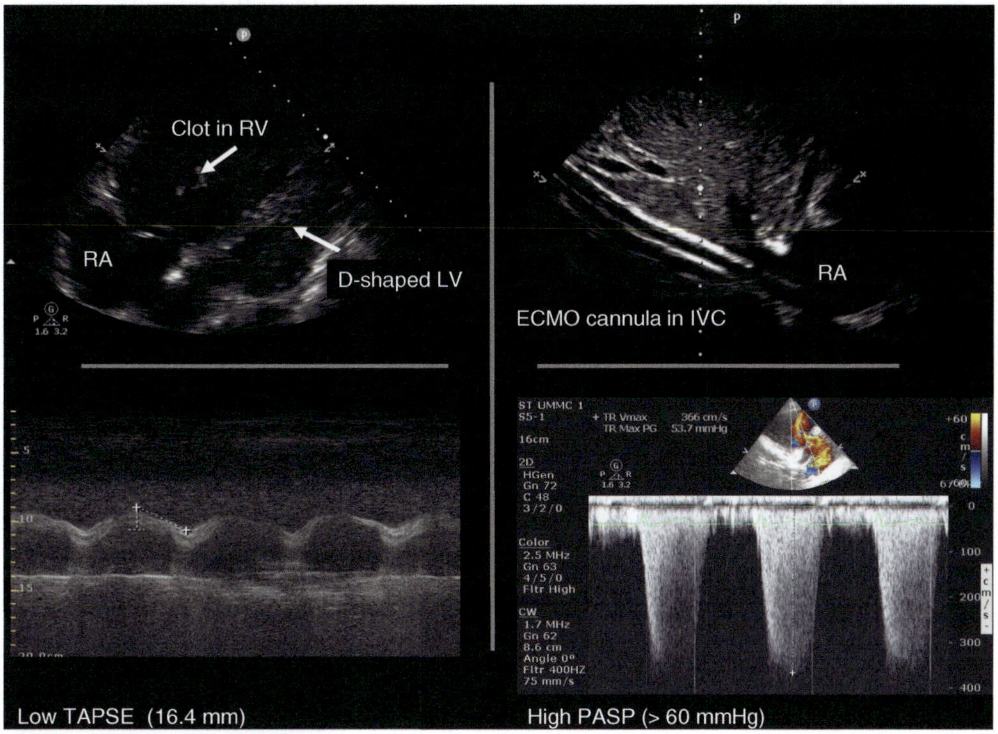

Fig. 6 Case 5: RD is in the Dysfunctional Profile because of severe RV failure. There is also clot in the RV seen in panel 1

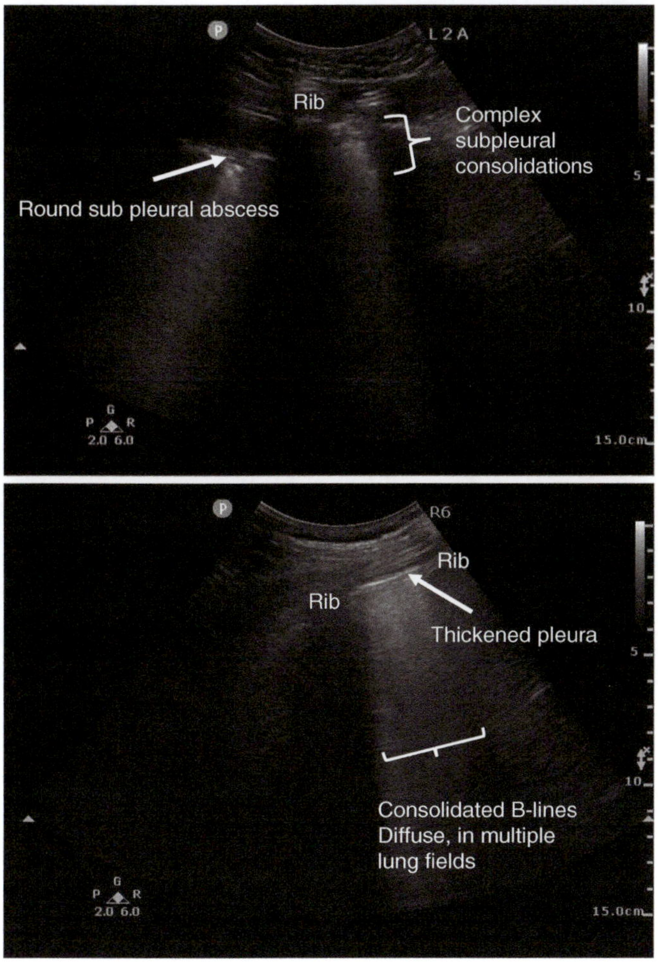

Fig. 7 Case 5: Lung findings in severe COVID-19

Additional Suggestions

- Consider placement of a pulmonary artery catheter (PAC).
- Consider full systemic anticoagulation. RV clot is seen, high risk of pulmonary embolus.

Clinical Course Inotropic epinephrine is started at 0.05 mcg/kg/min, as is epoprostenol (Flolan) to reduce pulmonary arterial pressure. Fluid is slowly removed via CRRT. RD is already on a heparin infusion, but the PTT goal is increased. After discussion of the risks and benefits, the decision is made to not place a PAC. The gravity of the situation is discussed with the family, and the goals of care are addressed. He initially improves, but 2 days later, he rapidly declines and dies.

Teaching Points The Dysfunctional Profile contains several types of dysfunction:

- Anything which impacts cardiac function including low EF, RV dysfunction, moderate/severe aortic stenosis, pericardial effusion with tamponde, and even bradycardia causing a low cardiac output is a reason for placement in the Dysfunctional Profile.
- The treatment suggestions vary depending on the dysfunction.
- Often some metrics cannot be collected; in this case the VTI so the SVI, CO, and SVR cannot be estimated. Even with partial data, the structure of the FREE allows coordinated decision-making.

Suggested Reading

Murthi SB, Markandaya M, Fang R, Hong CM, Galvagno SM, Lissuaer M, et al. Focused comprehensive, quantitative, functionally based echocardiographic evaluation in the critical care unit is feasible and impacts care. Mil Med. 2015;180(3 Suppl):74–9. https://doi.org/10.7205/MILMED-D-14-00374. PMID: 25747636

Murthi SB, Hess JR, Hess A, Stansbury LG, Scalea TM. Focused rapid echocardiographic evaluation versus vascular cather-based assessment of cardiac output and function in critically ill trauma patients. J Trauma Acute Care Surg. 2012;72(5):1158–64. https://doi.org/10.1097/TA.0b013e31824d1112. PMID: 22673240. PMID: 27768664

Glaser JJ, Cardarelli C, Galvagno S Jr, Scalea TM, Murthi SB. Bridging the gap: hybrid cardiac echo in the critically ill. J Trauma Acute Care Surg. 2016;81(5 Suppl 2 Proceedings of the 2015 Military Health System Research Symposium):S157–61. https://doi.org/10.1097/TA.0000000000001020.

Olivieri PP, Patel R, Kolb S, Fatima S, Galvagno SM, Haase DJ, et al. Echo is a good, not perfect, measure of cardiac output in critically ill surgical patients. J Trauma Acute Care Surg. 2019;87(2):379–85. https://doi.org/10.1097/TA.0000000000002304. PMID: 31349350

Spiegel R, Teeter W, Sullivan S, Tupchong K, Mohammed N, Sutherland M, et al. The use of venous Doppler to predict adverse kidney events in a general ICU cohort. Crit Care. 2020;24(1):615. https://doi.org/10.1186/s13054-020-03330-6. PMID: 33076961; PMCID: PMC7574322

Index

A. Salerno et al. (eds.), *Atlas of Critical Care Echocardiography*, https://doi.org/10.1007/978-3-030-74687-2

R

S

GPSR Compliance

The European Union's (EU) General Product Safety Regulation (GPSR) is a set of rules that requires consumer products to be safe and our obligations to ensure this.

If you have any concerns about our products, you can contact us on ProductSafety@springernature.com

In case Publisher is established outside the EU, the EU authorized representative is:

Springer Nature Customer Service Center GmbH
Europaplatz 3
69115 Heidelberg, Germany

Batch number: 10731528

Printed by Printforce, the Netherlands